ADVANCES IN
Surgery

Editor-in-Chief
John L. Cameron, MD

ELSEVIER

PHILADELPHIA LONDON TORONTO MONTREAL SYDNEY TOKYO

VOLUMES 1 THROUGH 52 (OUT OF PRINT)

VOLUME 55

1. Optimal Surgical Treatment for Type 2 Diabetes: Sleeve Gastrectomy or Gastric Bypass? *by Amanda Mueller, Sarah Palilla, and Jonathan Carter*

2. Advances in the Diagnosis and Management of Appendicitis in Children, *by Katherine He and Shawn J. Rangel*

3. Malignant Bowel Obstruction, *by Nadege T. Fackche and Fabian M. Johnston*

4. Nonoperative Treatment of Diverticulitis, *by Matthew Symer and Heather L. Yeo*

5. The Current Management of Visceral Artery Aneurysms, *by Bara Zuhaili and James H. Black III*

6. Mesenteric Ischemia: When and How to Revascularize, *by Kristofor A. Olson and Pedro G. Teixeira*

7. Watch-and-wait Management for Rectal Cancer After Clinical Complete Response to Neoadjuvant Therapy, *by Jonathan B. Yuval and Julio Garcia-Aguilar*

8. Paraesophageal Hernia: Current Management, *by Laura Mazer and Dana A. Telem*

9. Surgery During a Pandemic: Guidelines, *by Cole S. Brown and Andrew M. Cameron*

10. The Role of Node Dissection for Thyroid Cancer, *by Reese W. Randle and Susan C. Pitt*

11. Multimodal Pain Control in Surgery 2020, *by Hannah Decker, Christopher L. Wu, and Elizabeth Wick*

12. What is the Current Role of Hyperthermic Intraperitoneal Chemotherapy in Colorectal Cancer? *by Catherine H. Davis and H. Richard Alexander Jr*

13. Machine Perfusion in Liver Transplantation, *by Malcolm MacConmara and Parsia A. Vagefi*
14. What Is the Proper Technique for Primary Laparotomy Closure? *by Charlotte Horne and Eric Pauli*
15. Can Pancreatic Organoids Help in the Treatment of Pancreatic Cancer? *by Toni T. Seppä lä and Richard A. Burkhart*
16. Necrosectomy in the Management of Necrotizing Pancreatitis, *by Amy Y. Li, John R. Bergquist, and Brendan C. Visser*
17. Vascular Reconstructions for Traumatic Injuries, *by Ali Khalifeh and Todd E. Rasmussen*
18. Evolution of Point-Of-Care Ultrasound in Surgical Management, *by William A. Teeter and Thomas Scalea*
19. Breast Implant–Associated Anaplastic Large Cell Lymphoma, *by Melissa Camp*

VOLUME 54

1. Controversies in the Management of Diverticulitis *by Thomas Curran and Mary R. Kwaan*
2. Venous Thromboembolism Prevention and Treatment in Cancer Surgery *by Lawrence B. Brown, Michael B. Streiff, and Elliott R. Haut*
3. The Value of Surgical Coaching Beyond Training ? *by Jason C. Pradarelli, Yue-Yung Hu, Justin B. Dimick, and Caprice C. Greenberg*
4. Neoadjuvant Therapy: When Should It Be Used for Pancreatic Cancer?, *by Kristin N. Kelly, Francisco I. Macedo, and Nipun B. Merchant*
5. Islet Tumors: Resect or Follow?, *by Tiffany J. Sinclair and George A. Poultsides*
6. The Role of Artificial Intelligence in Surgery *by Daniel A. Hashimoto, Thomas M. Ward, and Ozanan R. Meireles*
7. What Is the Current Status of Lung Transplantation? *by Daniel A. Walker, Fatima G. Wilder, and Errol L. Bush*
8. Contemporary Management of Mitral Valve Disease, *by Brian D. Cohen, Michael A. Napolitano, J. James Edelman, Keegan V. Thourani, and Vinod H. Thourani*
9. Surgery Resident Wellness Programs: The Current State of the Field and Recommendations for Creation and Implementation *by Rebecca L. Williams-Karnesky, Alissa Greenbaum, and Jasmeet S. Paul*

10. Evidence-Based Management of Gallstone Pancreatitis, *by Lillian S. Kao and Jayne S. McCauley*

11. Management of Melanoma Patients with Positive Nodes, *by Rachel M. Lee, Keith A. Delman, and Michael C. Lowe*

12. Video Assessment of Surgeons and Surgery, *by Elif Bilgic, Sofia Valanci-Aroesty, and Gerald M. Fried*

13. Fascial Closure: New Surgery Paradigms *by Gregory A. Dumanian and Simon Moradian*

14. Enteral Feeding: Percutaneous Endoscopic Gastrostomies, Tubes, and Formulas, *by Colin G. DeLong and Eric M. Pauli*

15. Increasing Importance of Ethics in Surgical Decision Making *by Anghela Z. Paredes, Christopher T. Aquina, Luke V. Selby, Stephanie DiFilippo, and Timothy M. Pawlik*

16. Per Oral Pyloromyotomy for Gastroparesis, *by John H. Rodriguez and Jeffrey Ponsky*

17. What Is the Role of Neoadjuvant Radiation Therapy for Retroperitoneal Sarcoma? *by Sophia K. McKinley, Thomas F. DeLaney, and John T. Mullen*

18. New Models of Surgical Training, *by Christopher C. Stahl and Rebecca M. Minter*

VOLUME 53

1. Laparoscopic Hernia Repair *by Javier Otero, Andrew T. Huber, and B. Todd Heniford*

2. Ductal Carcinoma In Situ of the Breast: Controversies and Current Management *by Andrea V. Barrio and Kimberly J. Van Zee*

3. What Is the Role for Carotid Stenting Versus Endarterectomy? *by Kyla M. Bennett and John E. Scarborough*

4. Managing Complications of Bariatric Surgery, *by Richard M. Peterson and John D. Scott*

5. Trends in Palliative Surgical Care, *by Allison R. Wilcox and Sandra L. Wong*

6. Management of Difficult Dialysis Access Issues for Dialysis Patients *by Matthew J. Dougherty, Douglas A. Troutman, and Krystal C. Maloni*

7. Has Personalized Medicine for Pancreatic Cancer Arrived? *by Ashley Krepline and Susan Tsai*

8. Is Hyperthyroidism Diagnosed and Treated Appropriately in the United States?, *by Ammar Asban, Sophie Dream, and Brenessa Lindeman*

9. How Do We Prevent Burnout in Surgery? *by Gerard M. Doherty*

10. Elimination of Bile Duct Injury in Cholecystectomy, *by Maria S. Altieri and L. Michael Brunt*

11. Surgical Emergencies in the Pregnant Patient, *by Don J. Selzer and Dimitrios Stefanidis*

12. Transoral Endoscopic Thyroidectomy Vestibular Approach, *by Neeta J. Erinjeri and Robert Udelsman*

13. Firearm Violence in America: Is There a Solution? *by Rachel L. Choron, Sarabeth Spitzer, and Joseph V. Sakran*

14. Musculoskeletal Disorders in Minimally Invasive Surgery, *by H. Reza Zahiri, Alex Addo, and Adrian E. Park*

15. What's New in Trauma Resuscitation? *by Elizabeth Dauer and Amy Goldberg*

16. Anticoagulants and Surgery: So Many Agents, So Many Taking Them, *by Ronak B. Patel and Apostolos K. Tassiopoulos*

17. Status of 5-Year Survivors of the Whipple Procedure for Pancreatic Adenocarcinoma *by Winta T. Mehtsun, Daniel A. Hashimoto, and Cristina R. Ferrone*

18. Indications for Neoadjuvant Systemic Therapy for Breast Cancer, *by Kristalyn K. Gallagher and David W. Ollila*

19. Watchful Waiting for Inguinal Hernia, *by Alexander D. Schroeder, Dustin J. Tubre, and Robert J. Fitzgibbons Jr*

20. The Opioid Crisis: The Surgeon's Role, *by Ross F. Goldberg*

Editor: John Vassallo
Developmental Editor: Arlene Campos

Editorial Office:
Elsevier
1600 John F. Kennedy Blvd,
Suite 1800
Philadelphia, PA 19103-2899

International Standard Serial Number: 0065-3411
International Standard Book Number: 978-0-323-98739-4

ADVANCES IN
Surgery

CONTRIBUTORS

AIDIN BAGHBANI-OSKOUEI, MD, McGovern Medical School, The University of Texas Health Science Center at Houston, Houston, Texas, USA

KRISTEN M. BEYER, MBA, Northwell Health Cancer Institute, Lake Success, New York, USA

L. MICHAEL BRUNT, MD, Pruett Professor of Surgery, Chief, Section of Minimally Invasive Surgery, Department of Surgery, Washington University School of Medicine, St Louis, Missouri, USA

JAMES P. BYRNE, MD, PhD, FRCSC, Assistant Professor of Surgery, Division of Acute Care Surgery, Department of Surgery, Johns Hopkins Hospital, Baltimore, Maryland, USA

JENNWOOD CHEN, MD, Assistant Professor, Department of Surgery, University of Utah, Assistant Professor, Department of Surgery, Veterans Affairs, Salt Lake City, Utah, USA

MICHOL A. COOPER, MD, PhD, Assistant Professor of Vascular Surgery and Endovascular Therapy, University of Florida College of Medicine, Division of Vascular Surgery and Endovascular Therapy, Gainesville, Florida, USA

LYUDMYLA DEMYAN, MD, Department of Surgery, Northwell Health Cancer Institute, Lake Success, New York, USA

MARINA DIAS-NETO, MD, MSc, PhD, McGovern Medical School, The University of Texas Health Science Center at Houston, Houston, Texas, USA

ADRIAN DIAZ, MD, MPH, Department of Surgery, The Ohio State University Wexner Medical Center and James Comprehensive Cancer Center, Columbus, Ohio, USA; Center for Healthcare Outcomes and Policy, University of Michigan, Ann Arbor, Michigan, USA

KEVIN EMERICK, MD, Department of Otolaryngology, Massachusetts Eye and Ear Infirmary, Massachusetts, USA

ROBERT D. FANELLI, MD, MHA, FACS, FASGE, Vice Chair, Strategy & Innovation, Department of Surgery, Chief, Minimally Invasive Surgery, Chief, Surgical Endoscopy, The Guthrie Clinic, One Guthrie Square, Sayre, Pennsylvania, USA

ALIK FARBER, MD, Section Chief, Professor of Surgery, Division of Vascular and Endovascular Surgery, Boston University School of Medicine, Boston University, Boston, Massachusetts, USA

ROBERT E. GLASGOW, MBA, FACS, Professor and Interim Chair, Department of Surgery, University of Utah, Salt Lake City, Utah, USA

ELIZABETH M. GLEESON, MD, MPH, Hepatobiliary and Transplant Surgery Fellow, University of Edinburgh and Royal Infirmary of Edinburgh, Edinburgh, Scotland, United Kingdom

JESSICA KOLLER GORHAM, MD, FACS, DABOM, Staff Surgeon, Ochsner Clinic, New Orleans, Louisiana, USA

ELLIOTT R. HAUT, MD, PhD, FACS, Vice Chair of Quality, Safety and Service, Division of Acute Care Surgery, Department of Surgery, Department of Anesthesiology and Critical Care Medicine, Department of Emergency Medicine, Johns Hopkins School of Medicine, Core Faculty, The Armstrong Institute for Patient Safety and Quality, Johns Hopkins Medicine, Department of Health Policy and Management, Johns Hopkins Bloomberg School of Public Health, Baltimore, Maryland, USA

SHARON HENRY, MD, Professor of Trauma Surgery, University of Maryland School of Medicine, Director of the Wound Healing and Metabolism Service, R A Cowley Shock Trauma Center, Baltimore, Maryland, USA

HOWARD L. KAUFMAN, MD, Division of Gastrointestinal and Oncologic Surgery, Massachusetts General Hospital, Boston, Massachusetts, USA

ELIZABETH G. KING, MD, Assistant Professor of Surgery, Division of Vascular and Endovascular Surgery, Boston University School of Medicine, Boston University, Boston, Massachusetts, USA

TARI A. KING, MD, Chief, Division of Breast Surgery, Brigham and Women's Hospital, Dana-Farber/Brigham Cancer Center, Anne E. Dyson Professor of Surgery in the Field of Women's Cancers, Harvard Medical School, Boston, Massachusetts, USA

PATRIC LIANG, MD, Member of the Faculty of Surgery, Harvard Medical School, Division of Vascular and Endovascular Surgery, Boston, Massachusetts, USA

GUILHERME B. B. LIMA, MD, McGovern Medical School, The University of Texas Health Science Center at Houston, Houston, Texas, USA

NICOLE LUNARDI, MD, MSPH, General Surgery Resident, University of Texas Southwestern, Dallas, Texas, USA

THOMAS K. MAATMAN, MD, Chief Resident in General Surgery, Department of Surgery, Indiana University School of Medicine, Indianapolis, Indiana, USA

ANNE C. MOSENTHAL, MD, FACS, Chief Academic Officer, Academic Dean, Lahey Hospital and Medical Center, Burlington, Massachusetts, USA; Professor of Surgery, Tufts University School of Medicine, Boston, Massachusetts, USA

CHAITAN K. NARSULE, MD, FACS, Acute Care Surgeon and Surgical Intensivist, Department of Surgery, Lahey Hospital and Medical Center, Burlington, Massachusetts, USA; Assistant Professor of Surgery, Tufts University School of Medicine, Boston, Massachusetts, USA

NICOLE NEAL, MD, Resident, Ochsner Clinic, New Orleans, Louisiana, USA

GUSTAVO S. ODERICH, MD, McGovern Medical School, The University of Texas Health Science Center at Houston, Houston, Texas, USA

TIMOTHY M. PAWLIK, MD, MPH, MTS, PhD, Department of Surgery, The Ohio State University Wexner Medical Center and James Comprehensive Cancer Center, Columbus, Ohio, USA

SAMUEL J. PERA, MD, Assistant Professor, Hiram C. Polk Jr. Department of Surgery, University of Louisville, Louisville, Kentucky, USA

HENRY A. PITT, MD, Chief of Oncologic Quality, Rutgers Cancer Institute of New Jersey and Robert Wood Johnson University Hospital, New Brunswick, New Jersey, USA

VITALIY POYLIN, MD, FACS, FASCRS, Director, Section of Colon and Rectal Surgery, Associate Professor in Surgery, Feinberg School of Medicine, Northwestern Medical Group, Chicago, Illinois, USA

WILLIAM S. RICHARDSON, MD, FACS, FASMBS, Section Head, General Surgery, Ochsner Clinic, New Orleans, Louisiana, USA; Professor, University of Queensland, Brisbane, Australia

JOSEPH V. SAKRAN, MD, MPH, MPA, FACS, Director, Emergency General Surgery, Associate Professor of Surgery and Nursing, Associate Chief, Division of Acute Care Surgery, Vice Chair of Clinical Operations, Department of Surgery, Johns Hopkins Hospital, Baltimore, Maryland, USA; Senior Fellow, Satcher Health Leadership Institute at the Morehouse School of Medicine, Atlanta, Georgia, USA

MARC L. SCHERMERHORN, MD, George H.A. Clowes Jr. Professor of Surgery, Harvard Medical School, Chief, Division of Vascular and Endovascular Surgery, Boston, Massachusetts, USA

JESSICA SCHUCHT, MD, PhD, Clinical Instructor, Hiram C. Polk Jr. Department of Surgery, University of Louisville, Louisville, Kentucky, USA

KINJAL N. SETHURAMAN, MD, MPH, Associate Professor of Emergency Medicine, University of Maryland School of Medicine, Medical Director, Hyperbaric and Dive Medicine, University of Maryland Medical Center, Baltimore, Maryland, USA

ZAIN SHAHID, MD, Assistant Professor of Vascular Surgery and Endovascular Therapy, University of Florida College of Medicine, Division of Vascular Surgery and Endovascular Therapy, Gainesville, Florida, USA

SHANMUGAPPIRIYA SIVARAJAH, MD MPH, Department of Otolaryngology, Massachusetts Eye and Ear Infirmary, Boston, Massachusetts, USA

JASON W. SMITH, MD, PhD, MBA, FACS, Professor of Surgery and Physiology, Berel E. Abrams Endowed Professor in Surgery, Hiram C. Polk Jr. Department of Surgery, University of Louisville, Louisville, Kentucky, USA

RYAN SMOLIN, BS, MS, University of Maryland School of Medicine, Baltimore, Maryland, USA

ALTON SUTTER, MD, PhD, Wake Forest Baptist Hospital, Winston-Salem, North Carolina, USA

EMANUEL R. TENORIO, MD, PhD, McGovern Medical School, The University of Texas Health Science Center at Houston, Houston, Texas, USA

GILBERT R. UPCHURCH Jr, MD, Professor of Surgery and Department Chair, University of Florida College of Medicine, Department of Surgery, Gainesville, Florida, USA

ANNA WEISS, MD, Assistant Professor, Division of Breast Surgery, Brigham and Women's Hospital, Dana-Farber/Brigham Cancer Center, Harvard Medical School, Boston, Massachusetts, USA

MATTHEW J. WEISS, MD, MBA, Deputy Physician-in-Chief and Surgical Director, Northwell Health Cancer Institute, Professor of Surgery, Zucker School of Medicine at Hofstra University, Lake Success, New York, USA

NICHOLAS J. ZYROMSKI, MD, Professor of Surgery, Department of Surgery, Indiana University School of Medicine, Indianapolis, Indiana, USA

ADVANCES IN
Surgery

CONTENTS

VOLUME 56 • 2022

Necrotizing pancreatitis affects 10% to 15% of all patients with acute pancreatitis. Despite improved understanding of this complex disease, it is still attended by up to 15% mortality. Necrotizing pancreatitis provides the clinical challenges of working in a multi-disciplinary group, determining proper timing for intervention, and identifying appropriate intervention approaches. The step-up approach consists of supportive care initially. When there is documented infected necrosis, treatment begins with antibiotics, progressing to minimally invasive mechanical necrosis intervention, and reserving surgery as the final treatment modality. However, treatment must be tailored to the individual patient. This article provides an overview of necrotizing pancreatitis.

Should We Utilize Routine Cholangiography?
L. Michael Brunt

Intraoperative cholangiography (IOC) is an essential skill that surgeons need for the safe performance of cholecystectomy and intraoperative diagnosis and management of bile duct stones. Whether it should be performed routinely or selectively is an ongoing debate that goes back to the early days of laparoscopic cholecystectomy (LC). Benefits of IOC include ability to detect bile duct stones, recognition of aberrant anatomy, and, in some circumstances, mitigation of the risk of bile duct injury. In this review, key aspects of this debate, technical aspects of performing IOC, evidence regarding its benefits, and imaging alternatives to IOC during LC are presented.

Reducing Firearm Injury and Death in the United States

Joseph V. Sakran and Nicole Lunardi

Firearms injury is a major cause of American morbidity and mortality. Although the firearm is a common vector, the intentions with which it is used represent a wide array of social ills–suicide, community violence, domestic violence, mass shootings, legal intervention, and unintended injury. The political and social underpinnings of this epidemic are inseparable from its prevention measures. Surgeons have an important role in firearm policy, research, prehospital and hospital advances, trauma survivor networks, and hospital-based violence prevention programs. It is only through interdisciplinary, multilevel, evidence-based prevention measures that the tides will turn on American firearm injury.

Reducing Complications After Surgery for Benign Anorectal Conditions
Alton Sutter and Vitaliy Poylin

While generally perceived as mundane and low-risk procedures, anorectal surgeries by virtue of their anatomic real-estate–dense with nerves, blood supply, and structures critical to the quality of life–are fraught with the potential for complications. While these complications are generally not life-threatening, their impact to the quality of life can be severe. Furthermore, the sheer volume of anorectal procedures performed each year means that even low complication rates or less severe complications can have significant economic impact.

Private Equity and Its Increasing Role in US Healthcare
Kristen M. Beyer, Lyudmyla Demyan, and Matthew J. Weiss

Private equity investments in health care and surgery are on the rise. There are potential advantages and drawbacks of private equity investment in health care. However, if done under the right parameters, PE investment may have the potential to address some of the challenges and inefficiencies of the current health care system.

Facts and Fallacy of Benchmark Performance Indicators
James P. Byrne and Elliott R. Haut

Efforts to improve quality in healthcare have arisen from the recognition that the quality of care delivered and resulting outcomes are highly variable. Performance benchmarking using high-quality data to compare risk-adjusted outcomes between hospitals and surgeons has been widely adopted as one means for addressing this problem. In this article we discuss the history, current state, methodologies, and potential pitfalls of benchmarking efforts to improve quality of healthcare in the United States.

Transcarotid Artery Revascularization: Is It Better than Carotid Endarterectomy?

Patric Liang and Marc L. Schermerhorn

Transcarotid artery revascularization (TCAR) is a novel carotid stenting method that avoids the manipulation of the aortic arch and uses a flow-reversal neuroprotection system that effectively reduces the risk of embolic events during carotid intervention. Studies have shown a lower risk of stroke or death compared with the transfemoral carotid stenting approach, and an equivalent risk of stroke or death compared with traditional carotid endarterectomy. TCAR has added benefits of lower risk of myocardial infarction, cranial nerve injuries, and shorter operative times compared with endarterectomy. TCAR has become widely adopted by vascular surgeons in the United States for the treatment of patients with high-risk medical comorbidities and those with challenging surgical anatomy.

Endovascular Repair of Descending Thoracic Aortic Aneurysms

Michol A. Cooper, Zain Shahid, and Gilbert R. Upchurch Jr.

Descending thoracic aortic aneurysms (DTAAs) are an important cause of morbidity and mortality in the elderly. Once diagnosed, they should be surveilled and then repaired at a diameter of 5.5 to 6 cm, depending on the individual patient's physiologic and anatomic risk of repair. Thoracic endovascular aortic repair (TEVAR) is the preferred approach for repair and there are multiple procedural adjuncts that can expand indications for and use of TEVAR. Spinal cord injuries are an important and highly morbid complication after TEVAR and it is imperative to mitigate this risk.

What Surgeons Need to Know About Gene Therapy for Cancer

Shanmugappiriya Sivarajah, Kevin Emerick, and Howard L. Kaufman

The broad field of gene therapy offers numerous innovative approaches for cancer treatment. An understanding of the different modalities including gene replacement therapy, cancer vaccines, oncolytic viruses, cellular therapy, and gene editing is essential for managing patients with neoplastic disease. As in other areas of oncology, the surgeon plays a pivotal role in the diagnosis and treatment of the disease. This review focuses on what the clinical surgeon needs to know to optimize the benefit of gene therapy for patients with cancer.

Is There a Place for Hyperbaric Oxygen Therapy?
Kinjal N. Sethuraman, Ryan Smolin, and Sharon Henry

Hyperbaric oxygen therapy (HBOT) involves treating patients by providing 100% oxygen through inhalation while inside a treatment pressurized chamber. The oxygen acts as a drug and the hyperbaric chamber as the dosing device. The effect of hyperbaric hyperoxia is dose dependent and, therefore, treatment depth and duration are important when considering its use. HBOT can either be the primary method of treatment or used adjunctively to medications or surgical techniques. The underpinning physiology is to bring oxygen-rich plasma to hypoxic tissue, preventing reperfusion injury, strengthening immune responsiveness, and encouraging new collagen deposition as well as endothelial cell formation.

Endoscopic Treatment of Gastroesophageal Reflux Disease

William S. Richardson, Jessica Koller Gorham, Nicole Neal, and Robert D. Fanelli

Video content accompanies this article at http://www.advancessurgery.com

There have been many devices and ideas to treat reflux disease endoscopically. Several devices have been tried and even FDA approved but now are no longer used. The push for these therapies is to find effective reflux control with lower risk and faster recovery. In this article we describe an endoscopic suturing device (TIF), radiofrequency device (Stretta) and a newer technique that has a lot of promise called antireflux mucosectomy. All these procedures seem to help control reflux at a minimum of morbidity given current information. As reflux is so prevalent a shift to these techniques for appropriate patients is likely to improve patient care.

Direct Peritoneal Resuscitation for Trauma

Samuel J. Pera, Jessica Schucht, and Jason W. Smith

Direct peritoneal resuscitation (DPR) has been found to be a useful adjunct in the management of critically ill trauma patients. DPR is performed following damage control surgery by leaving a surgical drain in the mesentery, placing a temporary abdominal closure, and postoperatively running peritoneal dialysis solution through the surgical drain with removal through the temporary closure. In the original animal models, the peritoneal dialysate infusion was found to augment visceral microcirculatory blood flow reducing the ischemic insult that occurs following hemorrhagic shock. DPR was also found to minimize the aberrant immune response that occurs secondary to shock and contributes to multisystem organ dysfunction. In the subsequent human trials, performing DPR had significant effects in several key categories. Traumatically injured patients who received DPR had a significantly shorter time to definitive fascial closure, had a higher likelihood of achieving primary fascial closure, and experienced fewer abdominal complications. The use of DPR has been further expanded as a useful adjunct for emergency general surgery patients and in the pretransplant care of human cadaver organ donors.

What is the Best Inguinal Hernia Repair?
Jennwood Chen and Robert E. Glasgow

As the management of inguinal hernias have evolved over hundreds of years, so too has our paradigm of what constitutes the "best repair." To best answer what the ideal inguinal hernia repair is, the authors take an in-depth look at considerations to the patient, the provider, and the health care system.

Do all Patients Get the Same Care Across Hospitals?
Adrian Diaz and Timothy M. Pawlik

There is extensive research demonstrating significant variation in the utilization of surgery and outcomes from surgery, including differences in mortality, complications, readmission, and failure to rescue. Literature suggests that these variations exist across as well as within small area geographies in the United States. There is also significant evidence of variation in access and outcomes from surgery that is attributable to race. Emerging research is demonstrating that there may be some variation attributable to a patient's social determinants of health and their lived averment. Those affected must work together to determine rate of utilization and how much variation is acceptable.

What Is the Role of Neoadjuvant Endocrine Therapy for Breast Cancer?

Anna Weiss and Tari A. King

There is growing interest in neoadjuvant endocrine therapy (NET) for the treatment of hormone receptor-positive, human epidermal growth factor receptor 2 -negative (HR + HER2-) breast cancer. Expanding the use of genomic assays demonstrates that many patients with HR + HER2-breast cancer do not benefit from chemotherapy, leading to growing interest in NET as a less toxic alternative. Although NET's ability to downsize breast tumors and achieve breast conservation is well-known, axillary surgery algorithms are not well-defined. Here we review primary endocrine therapy, the landmark NET clinical trials, and management of residual nodal disease following NET.

What Is the Best Treatment for Acute Limb Ischemia?

Elizabeth G. King and Alik Farber

Acute limb ischemia (ALI) is a vascular emergency associated with high rates of limb loss and mortality. Management of these patients is challenging given the severe systemic illness resulting from tissue ischemia and the high incidence of preexisting comorbid conditions and underlying peripheral arterial disease. Expeditious diagnosis, anticoagulation, and revascularization are of utmost importance in reducing morbidity. Revascularization may be accomplished using open, endovascular, or hybrid techniques. Approach to revascularization depends on the severity of ischemia, location of occlusion, cause, chance of recovery, comorbidities, and available resources.

Endovascular Repair of Complex Aortic Aneurysms

Guilherme B.B. Lima, Marina Dias-Neto, Emanuel R. Tenorio, Aidin Baghbani-Oskouei, and Gustavo S. Oderich

Fenestrated-branched endovascular aortic repair (FB-EVAR) has gained widespread acceptance in patients

article aims to review the most recent and current reports for rib plating with respect to indications, preoperative evaluation and imaging, approaches, timing for intervention, outcomes in patients with flail chest and nonflail injuries, and the management of complications. From these data, it becomes clear that the surgical stabilization of rib fractures (SSRF) has a firm place in the management of thoracic trauma.

Advances in Surgery 56 (2022) 1–11
ADVANCES IN SURGERY

Failure to Rescue After the Whipple: What Do We Know?

Elizabeth M. Gleeson, MD, MPH[a,*], Henry A. Pitt, MD[b]

[a]University of Edinburgh and Royal Infirmary of Edinburgh, 51 Little France Crescent, Edinburgh EH16 4SA, Scotland UK; [b]Rutgers Cancer Institute of New Jersey and Robert Wood Johnson University Hospital, 195 Little Albany Street, ET 834, New Brunswick, NJ 09083, USA

Keywords

• Failure to rescue • Morbidity • Mortality • Pancreatoduodenectomy • Rescue

Key points

- Failure to rescue is defined as the percentage of patients who die postoperatively after developing a major complication.
- Patient-, postoperative-, surgeon-, and hospital-factors contribute to failure to rescue after pancreatoduodenectomy.
- Details of postoperative management play a key role in rescuing patients who develop a major postpancreatectomy complication.
- In stable patients, management of complications by interventional radiology is preferred over reoperation.

Abbreviations

ACS NSQIP	American College of Surgeons National Surgical Quality Improvement Program
ASA	American Society of Anesthesiology
CT	computed tomography
FTR	failure to rescue
ICU	intensive care unit
NQF	National Quality Forum
OR	odds ratio
POPF	postoperative pancreatic fistula
PPH	postpancreatectomy hemorrhage
SAQ	Safety Attitudes Questionaire
SES	socioeconomic status

*Corresponding author. *E-mail address:* elizabeth.gleeson@nhslothian.scot.nhs.uk

https://doi.org/10.1016/j.yasu.2022.02.001
0065-3411/22/

INTRODUCTION

Although mortality after pancreatoduodenectomy has improved dramatically over the past 50 years, approximately half of patients have a postoperative complication [1–4]. The improvement in mortality is likely a consequence of reductions in failure to rescue (FTR), or conversely, better rescue techniques [5]. First described in 1992, the FTR rate is defined as the number of patients who die after developing a major complication divided by the number of patients with a major complication [6]. Rather than compare unadjusted mortality rates, FTR has been used as a quality metric to compare hospitals. When hospitals have similar rates of major complications but different mortality, those with higher fatality rates are characterized as failing to rescue their patients. This semantic has led many to believe that hospital factors were the sole influencers of FTR.

Several other factors, however, have been shown to be associated with FTR. The patients themselves present with their own risk factors, and this issue was described in Silber's original work on the subject [6]. The surgeons and the hospitals to which the patients presented carry risk factors have long been thought of as the primary contributor to FTR. Other factors include monitoring of serum and drain amylase, serum C-reactive protein, vital signs, the threshold to perform imaging such as computed tomography (CT) scans and rescue techniques, such as the routine use of interventional radiology and reoperation, and geographic differences [7–15]. The following review seeks to outline factors that are known to be associated with FTR after pancreatoduodenectomy as well as describe areas of future research.

WHAT DO WE KNOW?

Patient Factors

Although the name FTR implies that a hospital or team is responsible for FTR, many factors contribute to this outcome. From the moment a patient presents with a clinical indication for pancreatoduodenectomy, they carry their own risk factors for FTR. In an ACS-NSQIP (American College of Surgeons National Surgical Quality Improvement Program) study of 14,993 patients, FTR occurred in 7.2%, 361 died among 5027 patients who developed a major complication. Preoperative risk factors associated with FTR included age $\geq$ 65 years (adjusted odds ratio [OR] 2.00, 95% confidence interval [CI; 1.45–2.74]) and albumin $\leq$ 3.5 g/dL (adjusted OR 1.46 [1.10–1.95]) [15]. Age $\geq$ 80 years also has been described as a significant predictor of FTR [9], and in another study, age $\geq$ 76 years had an OR of 2.46 for FTR [16].

In a study from Italy that reviewed patients undergoing pancreatoduodenectomy at 3 tertiary hospitals, sarcopenic obesity was found to be an independent risk factor for FTR (OR 5.7, 95% CI 1.6–20.7, $P = .008$). Sarcopenic obesity was defined as high visceral fat area-to-total abdominal muscle area ratio as measured on preoperative CT scans [17]. The only other preoperative patient-specific factor that was significant for FTR was American Society of Anesthesiology (ASA) score $\geq$3 (OR 4.1, 95% CI 1.2–14.3, $P = .025$) (Box 1).

Box 1: Patient risk factors for failure to rescue

Age ≥ 65 years

Albumin ≤ 3.5 g/dL

ASA ≥ 3

Sarcopenic obesity

Low SES

Abbreviations: ASA, American Society of Anesthesiology Score; dL, deciliter; g, grams; SES, Socio-Economic Status.

Socioeconomic status (SES) also has been studied in the context of FTR. Patients in the lowest quintile compared with the highest quintile of SES had increased in rates of FTR (26.7% vs 23.2%, $P = .007$) across 6 surgical procedures for cancer, including pancreatectomy. The OR of SES on FTR for the pancreatectomy subgroup was 1.45 (95% CI 1.21–1.73) [18]. However, patients in the highest quintile of SES treated at the lowest-SES hospitals (hospitals treating the highest volume of the lowest quintile-SES patients) experienced a higher rate of FTR than patients from the lowest quintile of SES being treated at high-SES hospitals. These results suggest that the hospital where patients with low SES are treated influences their outcome [18] (see Box 1).

Postoperative risk factors also play a role in predicting FTR. Factors identified in the large NSQIP study included postoperative development of shock, renal failure, and the need for reintubation [15]. Tamirisa and colleagues found the same postoperative factors to be significantly associated with FTR [9]. A risk score has been created from the NSQIP to predict FTR after pancreatoduodenectomy: 1*Albumin ≤ 3.5 g/dL + 2*Age ≥ 65 + 2*Shock + 5*Renal failure + 5*Reintubation. The risk of FTR increased with increasing score ($P < .001$) [15]. Pancreatic fistula (OR 3.2, 95% CI 1.0–10.2, $P = .045$) also was associated with FTR in the study focused on sarcopenic obesity [17] (Box 2). The development of these specific complications should trigger vigilance among surgeons caring for postpancreatoduodenectomy patients. Early CT scans and frequent monitoring should be conducted [19,20]. The finding of an intra-abdominal collection has been considered a surrogate for a pancreatic fistula [21] and, if amenable, requires drainage by interventional radiology.

Box 2: Postoperative risk factors for failure to rescue

Renal failure

Reintubation

Shock

Pancreatic fistula

Surgeon factors

Patients who underwent pancreatic resection at 5 low-volume and 2 high-volume centers in Italy demonstrated no difference in FTR from pancreatic fistula. The authors suggested that this observation was due to the same training of all the chiefs of pancreatic surgery at the respective hospitals. All chiefs were trained by the same mentor [13]. One group evaluated the effect of resident versus fellow involvement in pancreatoduodenectomy cases as documented by the NSQIP. No clinically or statistically significant difference in FTR was observed (residents 4% vs fellow 6%, $P = .68$) [22]. Confounding in this study is the fact that a supervising attending surgeon will always be present in the operating room. In a study that estimated the effects of physician variables on patient FTR, having a surgeon with board certification was associated with a reduction in FTR (adjusted OR 0.8, 95% CI 0.68–0.94 when taking other hospital factors into account) [23] (Table 1). Thus, FTR is multifactorial and more likely related to postoperative management than the surgeon's intraoperative care.

In a study of the national Medicare claims database from 1998 to 1999, mortality was examined for patients undergoing pancreatectomy. Surgeon volume was inversely associated with mortality with an adjusted odds ratio of 3.61 [24]. However, FTR was not specifically reported in this study. Likewise, a study using the State Inpatient Databases for Florida, Maryland, and New York, found that surgeon volume of pancreatectomy predicted mortality (OR 0.30, $P < .001$) [25]. When taking hospital volume into account, the effect of surgeon volume on mortality remained significant. These results suggest that surgeon volume may be more important than hospital volume for pancreatectomy [25]. In another study, frequency of pancreatectomy by the surgeon was studied. Surgeons with a frequent practice of pancreatectomy had a significantly lower risk of delayed gastric emptying (OR 0.56, 95% CI 0.38–0.83), postpancreatectomy hemorrhage (PPH; OR 0.64, 95% CI 0.42–0.98), and in-hospital mortality (OR 0.45, 95% CI 0.24–0.87) [26]. Another analysis from Indiana

Table 1
Surgeon risk factors studied for association with failure to rescue

Studies	Surgeon factors	Association
Aiken et al, [23]	American Board of Surgery Certification	Decreased FTR
Capretti et al, [13]	Mentorship from an Expert Pancreatic Surgeon	Decreased FTR
Carr et al, [22]	Resident vs Fellow Involvement	No difference in FTR
Krautz et al, [26]	Surgeon frequency[a] (≥3 pancreatectomies over last 6 wk)	Decreased morbidity and mortality
Birkmeyer et al, [24]	Surgeon volume[a] (≥11 pancreatectomies/y)	Decreased morbidity
Nathan et al, [25]	Surgeon volume[a] (>25 Whipples/y)	Decreased morbidity

Abbreviation: FTR, failure to rescue; vs, versus; wk, week; y, year.
[a]Study did not measure the outcome of failure to rescue.

University also supported the concept that both surgeon volume and surgeon experience influence the outcomes of pancreatoduodenectomy [27] (see Table 1).

Hospital Factors

Ghaferi and colleagues grouped hospitals from the Medicare Provider Analysis and Review files into quintiles with the very low-volume hospitals defined as performing ≤ 5 pancreatectomies per year and the very high-volume hospitals defined as performing ≥27 pancreatectomies per year. Significant differences were found in FTR rates between the very low and very high-volume hospitals (OR 3.21 95% CI [2.18–4.72]) [28] (Table 2). In the Netherlands, FTR decreased 560% from the lowest quartile of hospital volume of pancreatoduodenectomy to the highest quartile (0.9% vs 8.1%, respectively), with hospital volume categorized as less than 30, 30 to 39, and ≥40 pancreatoduodenectomies per year [29]. In Norway, all pancreatoduodenectomies performed from 2015 to 2016 were grouped into their respective high-volume (≥40 pancreatoduodenectomies per year) or medium-low-volume center. On multivariable analysis, high hospital volume was associated with lower 90-day mortality but not associated with differences in FTR [30].

Hospitals that complied with the full National Quality Forum (NQF) experienced a significant reduction in risk-adjusted 30-day mortality after pancreatectomy [31]. In a meta-analysis of increased nurse-to-patient ratios and patient outcomes, an increase of one registered nurse per patient day was associated with a lower risk of FTR (OR 0.84, 95% CI 0.79–0.90) [32]. This work was done across surgical and medical specialties. In a study of the American Hospital Association Annual Hospital Survey Data, differences in FTR after pancreatectomy were associated with decreasing nurse-patient ratio (OR 1.14, 95% CI 1.08–1.20), but also with hospital bed size less than 200 (OR 1.77, 95% CI 1.22–1.93), hospital occupancy less than 50% (OR 1.76, 95%

Table 2
Hospital risk factors for failure to rescue

Studies	Hospital factors	Association
Ghaferi et al,[28] 2011	Hospital volume >27 pancreatectomies/y	Decreased FTR
van Rijssen et al, [29]	Hospital volume ≥40 pancreatectomies/y	Decreased FTR
Nymo et al, [30]	Hospital volume >40 pancreatectomies/y	No difference in FTR
Brooke et al, [31]	National Quality Forum compliance	Decreased FTR
Sheetz et al, [33]	Hospital size <200 beds	Increased FTR
Sheetz et al, [33]	Teaching status	Decreased FTR
Sheetz et al, [33]	ICU beds <20	Increased FTR
Sheetz et al, [33]	Lack of hospital technology	Increased FTR
Sheetz et al, [33]	Hospital occupancy <50%	Increased FTR
Sheetz et al, [33]	Decreased nurse:patient ratios	Increased FTR
Aiken et al, [23]	Decreased nurse:patient ratios	Increased FTR
Aiken et al, [23]	Nurse bachelor degrees	Decreased FTR

Abbreviations: FTR, failure to rescue; ICU, intensive care unit; y, year.

CI 1.50–1.88), nonteaching status (OR 1.32, 95% CI 1.09–1.49), intensive care beds less than 20 (OR 1.58, 95% CI 1.38–1.71), and absence of high hospital technology (OR 1.48, 95% CI 1.27–1.63) [33]. In a study that estimated the effects of nurse variables on patient FTR, a 10% increase in the percentage of nurses with a bachelor's was associated with a 5% decrease in FTR (OR 0.95, 95% CI 0.91–0.99) [23]. Thus, hospital volume of pancreatic surgery clearly is associated with FTR rates.

Regional Factors

Several studies suggest that regional differences in FTR rates exist. In a transatlantic analysis, factors independently associated with FTR were age, ASA ≥3, Northern Europe (Fig. 1), postoperative pancreatic fistula (POPF), organ failure, life-threatening complication, and reoperation [15]. In comparison, percutaneous drainage by interventional radiology was protective. In another analysis, FTR in the Netherlands has been reported as 14.2% [30], compared

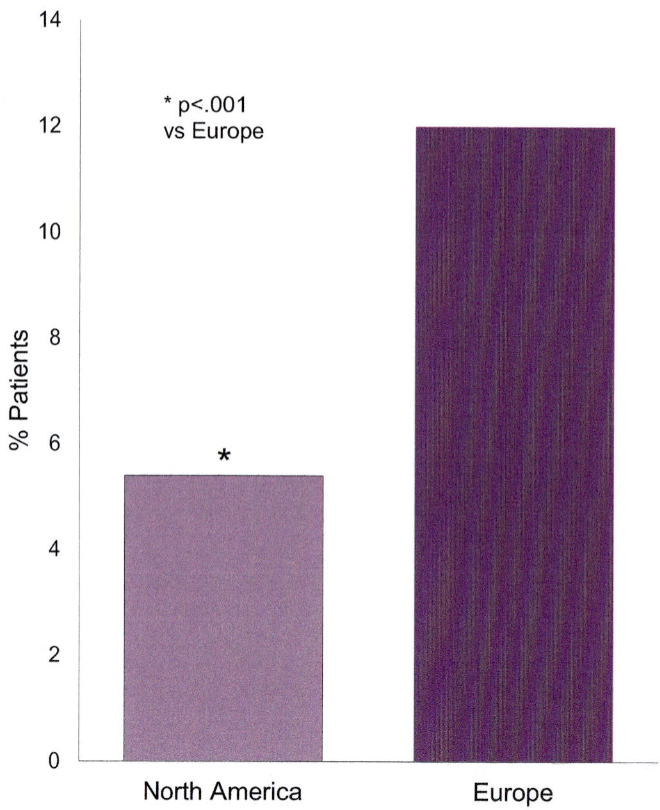

Fig. 1. Failure to rescue rates between North American and Northern European patients. (*Data from* [Gleeson EM, Pitt HA, Mackay TM, et al. Failure to rescue after pancreatoduodenectomy: A transatlantic analysis. *Ann Surg.* 2021; 1;274(3):459-466.].)

with 7.2% in the United States [10]. In a third international comparison, rates of FTR in the United States were 4.2% and in Japan were 1.1% [34]. These numbers are much less than expected, likely due to differences in the definition of FTR. In the Hurley study [34], FTR was defined as mortality after at least one complication, whereas the previous publications defined FTR as mortality after a major complication. These results underline the importance of consistent outcome definitions when comparing rates of complications and mortality.

Rescue Techniques

Operation-related complications (aspiration events, bleeding events, bowel obstruction, ischemic bowel, anastomotic leak exclusive of pancreatic fistula, vascular injuries, and graft thromboses) will require various interventions to rescue patients. However, after pancreatectomy, pancreatic fistula is the leading complication resulting in death with rates ranging between 3% and 45% [35,36]. The major techniques for rescuing or managing patients with pancreatic fistula include percutaneous drainage by interventional radiology and reoperation. In a transatlantic analysis of patients undergoing pancreatoduodenectomy, use of percutaneous drainage by interventional radiology was associated with a decreased risk of FTR (adjusted OR 0.46, 95% CI 0.31–0.67), whereas reoperation was associated with an increase in FTR (adjusted OR 1.58, 95% CI 1.14–2.18) [15] (Fig. 2).

In a study of 1524 patients undergoing pancreatic surgery, postpancreatectomy hemorrhage (PPH) was identified in 87 patients (5.7%) [37]. PPH-related mortality occurred in 14 patients or 16% of those with PPH. Pancreatic fistula was present in 13 of the 14 mortalities; 12 of 14 had vascular pseudoaneurysms or erosions; and all 14 mortalities had soft pancreas texture and delayed PPH occurrence [37]. Thus, the idea that early identification and treatment of pancreatic fistula could prevent mortality has evolved [38]. Simply admitting routinely to the intensive care unit (ICU) after pancreatectomy was not associated with decreased rates of FTR [38]. A Dutch group has conducted a nationwide stepped-wedge, cluster-randomized, superiority trial of an evidence- and consensus-based algorithm that provides daily multilevel advice compared to current care in the early detection and management of postoperative pancreatic fistula after pancreatectomy [39]. In this PORSCH trial, patients managed with early CT scans, antibiotics, and percutaneous drainage had a significant reduction in postoperative mortality and reduced FTR.

Safety Culture

Some evidence suggests that surgical culture around safety may improve outcomes. In a study by Babic and colleagues, an improvement in a single institution's Safety Attitudes Questionnaire (SAQ) was associated with improvement in ASC-NSQIP outcomes [40]. The study assessed complications across multiple operations and evaluated attitudes of the perioperative staff. Another study demonstrated that improvements with catheter-related bloodstream infection rates were correlated with improvements in safety attitudes among ICU staff [41]. Together,

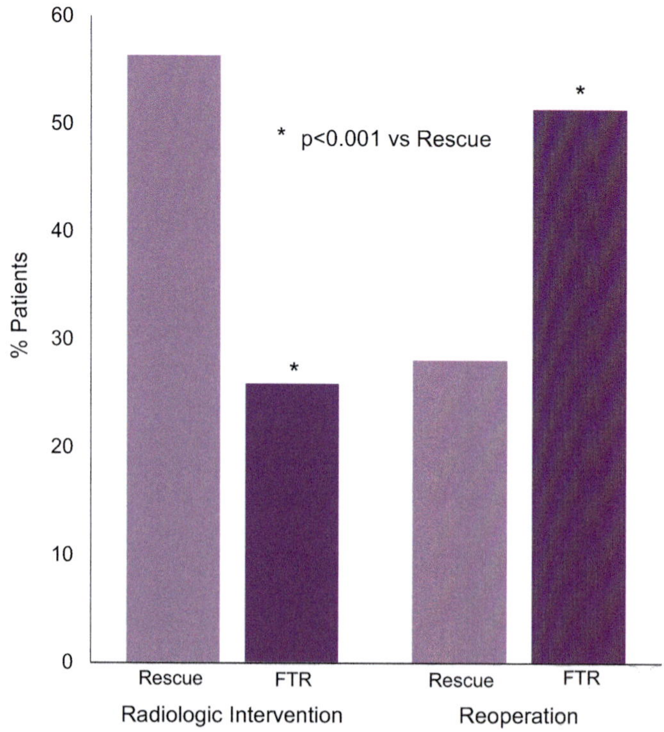

Fig. 2. Comparison of rescue (light purple) and failure to rescue (dark purple) rates among patients who had complications and were managed by percutaneous drainage (left) and reoperation (right). (*Data from* [Gleeson EM, Pitt HA, Mackay TM, et al. Failure to rescue after pancreatoduodenectomy: A transatlantic analysis. *Ann Surg.* 2021; 1;274(3):459-466.].)

these studies suggest that safety culture could improve outcomes through rescue in the perioperative and ICU settings.

DISCUSSION

Many of the studies include all pancreatectomies, not just pancreatoduodenectomy, which often carries a greater surgical risk than distal pancreatectomies. Additional limitations include varying definitions of FTR and retrospective analyses. Also, the authors included in this review defined major complications differently or simply defined FTR as death after any complication. Ideally, FTR should be defined consistently by all authors. Future research includes work in the early diagnosis of complications and culture surrounding patient safety after pancreatoduodenectomy.

SUMMARY

Mortality after pancreatoduodenectomy has improved greatly and, when compared with other highly morbid procedures, has a relatively low mortality rate (2.5% compared with 3.9% for trisegmentectomy, 2.9% for right hepatectomy, and 3% for esophagectomy) [42]. Despite improvements in mortality, morbidity after pancreatoduodenectomy still occurs in approximately one-half of patients. FTR, or mortality after the development of a major complication, is an important outcome to measure after pancreatoduodenectomy. Further studies should explore early diagnosis of complications and early interventions to prevent mortality [39]. Current evidence suggests that in stable patients, management of complications by interventional radiologists is preferred over reoperation.

CLINICS CARE POINTS

- Serum and drain fluid amylase should be measured in the early postoperative period to identify a pancreatic fistula.
- Drains should be removed by postoperative day 3 when postoperative day 1 drain fluid amylase is low.
- Broad-spectrum antibiotics should be used for perioperative prophylaxis and to escalate treatment of postoperative pancreatic fistula.
- Computed tomography (CT) should be performed (on postoperative days 5–7), if clinical and laboratory findings are suspicious for a pancreatic fistula.
- Patients with peripancreatic collections should be managed with early percutaneous drainage.
- Failure to rescue should be tracked by any center that performs pancreatoduodenectomy

Disclosure

The authors have nothing to disclose.

References

[1] Gleeson EM, Shaikh MF, Shewokis PA, et al. WHipple-ABACUS, a simple, validated risk score for 30-day mortality after pancreaticoduodenectomy developed using the ACS-NSQIP database. Surgery 2016;160(5):1279–87.

[2] van Roessel S, Mackay TM, van Dieren S, et al. Textbook outcome: Nationwide analysis of a novel quality measure in pancreatic surgery. Ann Surg 2020;271(1):155–62.

[3] Beane JD, Borrebach JD, Zureikat AH, et al. Optimal pancreatic surgery: Are we making progress in North America? Ann Surg 2021;274(4):e355–63.

[4] Mackay TM, Gleeson EM, Wellner UF, et al. Transatlantic registries of pancreatic surgery in the United States of America, Germany, the Netherlands, and Sweden: comparing design, variables, patients, treatment strategies, and outcomes. Surgery 2021;169(2):396–402.

[5] Pastrana Del Valle J, Mahvi DA, Fairweather M, et al. The improvement in post-operative mortality following pancreaticoduodenectomy between 2006 and 2016 is associated with an improvement in the ability to rescue patients after major morbidity, not in the rate of major morbidity. HPB (Oxford) 2021;23(3):434–43.

[6] Silber JH, Williams SV, Krakauer H, et al. Hospital and patient characteristics associated with death after surgery: a study of adverse occurrence and failure to rescue. Med Care 1992;30(7):615–29.

[7] Ghaferi AA, Osborne NH, Birkmeyer JD, et al. Hospital characteristics associated with failure to rescue from complications after pancreatectomy. J Am Coll Surg 2010;211(3): 325–30.
[8] Sheetz KH, Krell RW, Englesbe MJ, et al. The importance of the first complication: understanding failure to rescue after emergent surgery in the elderly. J Am Coll Surg 2014;219(3):365–70.
[9] Tamirisa NP, Parmar AD, Vargas GM, et al. Relative contributions of complications and failure to rescue on mortality in older patients undergoing pancreatectomy. Ann Surg 2016;263(2):385–91.
[10] Gleeson EM, Clarke JR, Morano WF, et al. Patient-specific predictors of failure to rescue after pancreaticoduodenectomy. HPB (Oxford) 2019;21(3):283–90.
[11] Staiger RD, Gerns E, Castrejon Subira M, et al. Can early postoperative complications predict high morbidity and decrease failure to rescue following major abdominal surgery? Ann Surg 2020;272(5):834–9.
[12] Krautz C, Nimptsch U, Weber GF, et al. Effect of hospital volume on in-hospital morbidity and mortality following pancreatic surgery in Germany. Ann Surg 2018;267(3):411–7.
[13] Capretti G, Balzano G, Gianotti L, et al. Management and outcomes of pancreatic resections performed in high-volume referral and low-volume community hospitals lead by surgeons who shared the same mentor: the importance of training. Dig Surg 2018;35(1): 42–8.
[14] Buchler MW, Wagner M, Schmied BM, et al. Changes in morbidity after pancreatic resection: toward the end of completion pancreatectomy. Arch Surg 2003;138(12):1310–4 [discussion: 1315].
[15] Gleeson EM, Pitt HA, Mackay TM, et al. Failure to rescue after pancreatoduodenectomy: A transatlantic analysis. Ann Surg 2021;274(3):459–66.
[16] Varley PR, Geller DA, Tsung A. Factors influencing failure to rescue after pancreaticoduodenectomy: a national surgical quality improvement project perspective. J Surg Res 2017;214:131–9.
[17] Pecorelli N, Capretti G, Sandini M, et al. Impact of sarcopenic obesity on failure to rescue from major complications following pancreaticoduodenectomy for cancer: Results from a multicenter study. Ann Surg Oncol 2018;25(1):308–17.
[18] Reames BN, Birkmeyer NJ, Dimick JB, et al. Socioeconomic disparities in mortality after cancer surgery: Failure to rescue. JAMA Surg 2014;149(5):475–81.
[19] Milgrom DP, Njoku VC, Fecher AM, et al. Unplanned intubation: When and why does this deadly complication occur? Surgery 2013;154:376–83.
[20] Johnston M, Arora S, King D, et al. Escalation of care and failure to rescue: A multicenter, multiprofessional qualitative study. Surgery 2014;155:989–94.
[21] Parikh JA, Beane JD, Kilbane EM, et al. Is American College of Surgeons NSQIP organ space infection a surrogate for pancreatic fistula? J Am Coll Surg 2014;219:1111–6.
[22] Carr RA, Chung CW, Schmidt CM 2nd, et al. Impact of fellow versus resident assistance on outcomes following pancreatoduodenectomy. J Gastrointest Surg 2017;21(6):1025–30.
[23] Aiken LH, Clarke SP, Cheung RB, et al. Educational levels of hospital nurses and surgical patient mortality. JAMA 2003;290(12):1617–23.
[24] Birkmeyer JD, Stukel TA, Siewers AE, et al. Surgeon volume and operative mortality in the United States. N Engl J Med 2003;349(22):2117–27.
[25] Nathan H, Cameron JL, Choti MA, et al. The volume-outcomes effect in hepato-pancreato-biliary surgery: hospital versus surgeon contributions and specificity of the relationship. J Am Coll Surg 2009;208(4):528–38.
[26] Krautz C, Haase E, Elshafei M, et al. The impact of surgical experience and frequency of practice on perioperative outcomes in pancreatic surgery. BMC Surg 2019;19(1):108.
[27] Schmidt CM, Turrini O, Parikh P, et al. Effect of hospital volume, surgeon experience and surgeon volume on patient outcomes after pancreatoduodenectomy: A single institution experience. Arch Surg 2010;145(7):634–40.

[28] Ghaferi AA, Birkmeyer JD, Dimick JB. Hospital volume and failure to rescue with high-risk surgery. Med Care 2011;49(12):1076–81.

[29] van Rijssen LB, Zwart MJ, van Dieren S, et al. Variation in hospital mortality after pancreatoduodenectomy is related to failure to rescue rather than major complications: A nationwide audit. HPB (Oxford) 2018;20:759–67.

[30] Nymo LS, Kleive D, Waardal K, et al. Centralizing a national pancreatoduodenectomy service: Striking the right balance. BJS Open 2020;4(5):904–13.

[31] Brooke BS, Dominici F, Pronovost PJ, et al. Variations in surgical outcomes associated with hospital compliance with safety practices. Surgery 2012;151(5):651–9.

[32] Kane RL, Shamliyan TA, Mueller C, et al. The association of registered nurse staffing levels and patient outcomes: Systematic review and meta-analysis. Med Care 2007;45(12): 1195–204.

[33] Sheetz KH, Dimick JB, Ghaferi AA. Impact of hospital characteristics on failure to rescue following major surgery. Ann Surg 2016;263(4):692–7.

[34] Hurley MP, Schoemaker L, Morton JM, et al. Geographic variation in surgical outcomes and cost between the United States and Japan. Am J Manag Care 2016;22(9):600–7.

[35] Vollmer CM Jr, Sanchez N, Gondek S, et al. A root-cause analysis of mortality following major pancreatectomy. J Gastrointest Surg 2012;16(1):89–102, ; discussion 102-3.

[36] Bassi C, Marchegiani G, Dervenis C, et al. The 2016 update of the International Study Group (ISGPS) definition and grading of postoperative pancreatic fistula: 11 Years After. Surgery 2017;161(3):584–91.

[37] Yekebas EF, Wolfram L, Cataldegirmen G, et al. Postpancreatectomy hemorrhage: diagnosis and treatment: an analysis in 1669 consecutive pancreatic resections. Ann Surg 2007;246(2):269–80.

[38] Cerullo M, Gani F, Chen SY, et al. Routine intensive care unit admission among patients undergoing major pancreatic surgery for cancer: No effect on failure to rescue. Surgery 2019;165(4):741–6.

[39] Smits FJ, Henry AC, van Eijck CH, et al. Care after pancreatic resection according to an algorithm for early detection and minimally invasive management of pancreatic fistula versus current practice (PORSCH-trial): design and rationale of a nationwide stepped-wedge cluster-randomized trial. Trials 2020;21(1):389.

[40] Babic B, Volpe AA, Merola S, et al. Sustained culture and surgical outcome improvement. Am J Surg 2018;216(5):841–5.

[41] Pronovost PJ, Berenholtz SM, Goeschel CA, et al. Creating high reliability in health care organizations. Health Serv Res 2006;41(4 Pt 2):1599–617.

[42] Foster JM, Sleightholm R, Patel A, et al. Morbidity and mortality rates following cytoreductive surgery combined with hyperthermic intraperitoneal chemotherapy compared with other high-risk surgical oncology procedures. JAMA Netw Open 2019;2(1):e186847.

Advances in Surgery 56 (2022) 13–35

ADVANCES IN SURGERY

Management of Necrotizing Pancreatitis

Thomas K. Maatman, MD, Nicholas J. Zyromski, MD*

Department of Surgery, Indiana University School of Medicine, 545 Barnhill Dr. EH 519, Indianapolis, IN 46202, USA

Keywords

• Pancreatitis acute necrotizing • Pancreatitis • Practice guideline

Key points

- Necrotizing pancreatitis is a complex, heterogeneous disease that requires multidisciplinary input to achieve optimal patient outcomes.
- Multiple interventions are available to treat infected or symptomatic necrosis.
- Experienced judgment is important in determining timing and type of intervention.
- Long-term care is essential, and ideally directed by a single physician.

INTRODUCTION

Necrotizing pancreatitis affects 10% to 15% of all patients with acute pancreatitis. Despite improved understanding of disease process and advances in therapeutic stagey, this complex disease is still attended by up to 15% mortality. Necrotizing pancreatitis provides the clinical challenges of working in a multidisciplinary group, determining proper timing for intervention, and identifying appropriate intervention approaches based on individual patient anatomy, physiology, and local expertise. The step-up approach consists of supportive care initially. When there is documented infected necrosis, treatment begins with antibiotics, stepping up to minimally invasive mechanical necrosis intervention, and reserving surgery as the final treatment modality. However, a one-size-fits-all approach does not apply to all patients with necrotizing pancreatitis and treatment must be tailored to the individual patient. This article

*Corresponding author. *E-mail address:* nzyromsk@iupui.edu

https://doi.org/10.1016/j.yasu.2022.02.010
0065-3411/22/

provides an overview of necrotizing pancreatitis, focusing on clinical care, intervention indications, and long-term sequelae of the disease.

INCIDENCE AND CAUSE

Worldwide, the prevalence of acute pancreatitis has doubled over the last 3 decades and is estimated to be more than 6 million cases annually [1]. Necrotizing pancreatitis develops in 10% to 15% of all acute pancreatitis cases, and, in the United States, necrotizing pancreatitis accounts for 30,000 to 60,000 cases per year [2–5]. The contemporary mortality in necrotizing pancreatitis ranges from 10% to 15%, despite an improved understand of the disease process and advances in therapeutic strategy [6–9]. The causes of necrotizing pancreatitis mirror that of acute pancreatitis, with the most common causes being biliary (20%–50% of cases) and alcohol (20%–40% of cases) [6,10,11]. Additional frequently seen causes, albeit less common, include hypertriglyceridemia, genetic mutations, medications, autoimmune, iatrogenic (ie, after endoscopic retrograde cholangiopancreatography), hypercalcemia, and trauma.

PATHOPHYSIOLOGY

Regardless of the cause or inciting event, the development of acute pancreatitis follows a common pathway. Abnormal activation of proteolytic enzymes within the pancreatic acinar cells results in pancreatic acinar cell injury and death [12]. Activation of trypsinogen to trypsin is thought to play a predominant role in this process, a model first proposed by Dr Hans Chiari in 1896 and supported in subsequent studies since that time [12,13]. Once released from damaged pancreatic acinar cells, trypsin activates digestive enzymes and additional trypsin leading to pancreatic parenchymal autodigestion, acinar cell injury, and damage to the vascular endothelium and surrounding interstitium [12]. An ensuing systemic inflammatory response and activation of the coagulation cascade play a key role in acute pancreatitis and are thought to be responsible for the progression from acute pancreatitis to necrotizing pancreatitis [14,15]. Why some patients progress to necrotizing pancreatitis but most develop mild acute pancreatitis is less clear; nonetheless, it likely stems from superfluous activation of the systemic inflammatory response and/or coagulation cascade.

The human immune system and its response to antigens requires a balance of proinflammatory and antiinflammatory mediators working in concert. A summary of the key proinflammatory and antiinflammatory mediators involved in acute pancreatitis is shown in Fig. 1. A self-limited and balanced inflammatory and antiinflammatory response is seen in mild acute pancreatitis [16–18]. The result is only mild systemic inflammation and resolution of disease with supportive care, and minimal or no long-term sequelae [17,19–21]. In stark contrast, severe acute pancreatitis develops when an imbalance in the inflammatory response develops and proinflammatory mediators are allowed to propagate unimpeded [14,16–18,22].

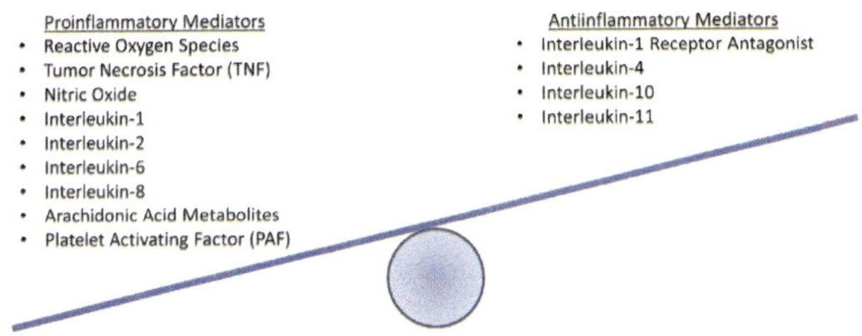

Fig. 1. Summary of the key inflammatory mediators in acute pancreatitis. An imbalance in the inflammatory response favoring proinflammatory mediators contributes to the progression of mild acute pancreatitis to severe acute pancreatitis.

In necrotizing pancreatitis, enzymatic autodigestion of the pancreatic parenchyma, vascular endothelium, and surrounding tissue results in focal or diffuse nonviable pancreatic and/or peripancreatic tissue [2]. Because the systemic inflammatory response is intimately associated with the coagulation cascade, the associated compromise of the pancreatic microcirculation, including arterioles, capillaries, and venules, results in ischemic changes and necrosis of the pancreas [23–25]. Pancreatic and peripancreatic necrosis further stimulates the systemic inflammatory response, amplifying the severity of the disease [14–18,22]. Thus, necrotizing pancreatitis is characterized by a profound systemic inflammatory response and organ failure is common, often with associated local pancreatic or peripancreatic complications. Not surprisingly, survivors of necrotizing pancreatitis frequently develop long-term complications that significantly affect their quality of life [26].

The impact of the systemic inflammatory response observed in necrotizing pancreatitis with respiratory, renal, and cardiovascular failure warrants further discussion. Progression from acute pancreatitis to necrotizing pancreatitis and its characteristic systemic inflammatory response plays a direct role in end-organ injury and the multiorgan dysfunction syndrome seen in patients with necrotizing pancreatitis. Inflammatory cytokines and chemokines released from the pancreatic parenchyma are disseminated to the respiratory, renal, and cardiovascular organ systems and lead to secondary inflammation and injury within these tissues [27–30]. An understanding of the consequence of concurrent injury to these organ systems and local peripancreatic inflammation/complications informs treatment, both in the early and late phases of disease. Associated organ failure and local complications contribute to a significant source of morbidity and mortality in treating patients who have necrotizing pancreatitis; thus, mitigating injury and avoiding further insult are critical to successfully treating this complex patient population.

DEFINITIONS

An expert international consensus survey in 2012 led to the publication of the revised Atlanta classification providing distinct definitions of acute pancreatitis and its associated complications, including necrotizing pancreatitis. Organ failure in necrotizing pancreatitis is defined according to the modified Marshall scoring system for organ dysfunction, with organ failure equating to a score of 2 or greater (Table 1) [2,31]. Necrotizing pancreatitis is diagnosed on contrast-enhanced cross-sectional imaging as the absence of pancreatic or peripancreatic enhancement [2]. In contrast, normal pancreatic parenchyma demonstrates homogeneous enhancement with contrast administration (Fig. 2).

Disease onset is defined by the timing of symptom onset and not by the presentation to the hospital or the diagnosis of necrotizing pancreatitis [2]. This distinction is critical, because the onset of necrotizing pancreatitis is a reference point for the disease course, the development of acute/subacute complications, the timing of intervention, and the development of complications after disease resolution. It is essential to realize that the degree of pancreatic necrosis will not be appreciated on imaging the first few days after the onset of symptoms; instead, parenchymal and peripancreatic necrosis begins to become apparent after 1 week [32,33]. Patterns of necrosis in necrotizing pancreatitis may involve a combination of pancreatic and peripancreatic parenchyma, isolated peripancreatic necrosis, or, less commonly, isolated pancreatic necrosis [34–37].

Local complications in necrotizing pancreatitis include acute necrotic collections (ANCs) and walled-off necrosis (WON). An ANC is a pancreatic or peripancreatic collection with liquid and/or solid necrosis within the first 4 weeks from symptom onset (Fig. 3A) [2]. After 4 weeks, the pancreatic and peripancreatic necrosis matures to WON, after a well-defined wall of inflammatory reactive tissue has developed (Fig. 3B) [2]. In interstitial edematous pancreatitis (nonnecrotizing pancreatitis), these terms must be differentiated from acute peripancreatic fluid collection (APFC; <4 weeks) and pancreatic pseudocyst (>4 weeks), respectively. It is of the utmost importance to understand the maturation phase of the pancreatic and peripancreatic necrosis, as well as the volume

Table 1
Modified Marshall scoring system for organ dysfunction in acute pancreatitis

	Score				
Organ system	0	1	2	3	4
Respiratory (PaO_2/FiO_2)	>400	301–400	201–300	101–200	≤100
Renal[a] (creatinine)	<1.4 mg/dL	1.4–1.8 mg/dL	1.9–3.6 mg/dL	3.6–4.9 mg/dL	>4.9 mg/dL
Cardiovascular[b] (systolic blood pressure)	>90 mm Hg	<90 mm Hg, fluid responsive	<90 mm Hg, not fluid responsive	<90 mm Hg, pH<7.3	<90 mm Hg, pH<7.2

Organ failure is defined as a score of 2 or greater.

Abbreviations: Fi O_2, fraction of inspired oxygen; Pa O_2, partial pressure of arterial oxygen.

[a]No formal correction exists for a baseline serum creatinine level ≥1.4 mg/dL.

[b]Off inotropes.

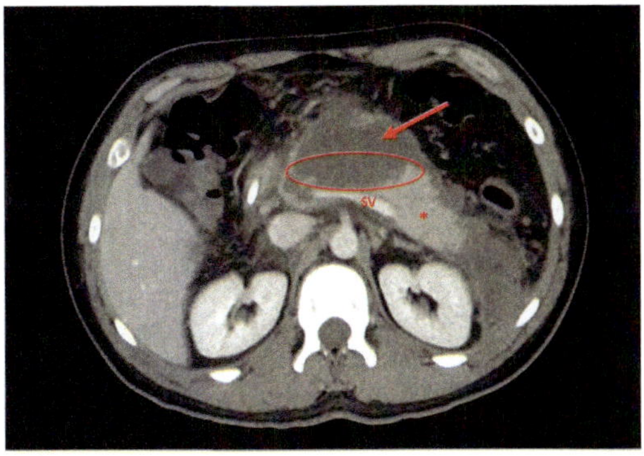

Fig. 2. Contrast-enhanced computed tomography 2-weeks after symptom onset showing pancreatic parenchymal necrosis of the neck and body of the gland (*oval*) compared with normal enhancement of the tail of the pancreas (*asterisk* [*]). Note the development of peripancreatic necrosis anterior to the gland and the development of an acute necrotic collection (*arrow*).SV, splenic vein.

of solid necrosis relative to liquid necrosis. The degree of solid necrosis is difficult to determine reliably on computed tomography scan and can be better assessed with MRI; however, the percentage of solid necrosis is best estimated with endoscopic or intraoperative ultrasonography [38]. Synonymous with the clinical picture of necrotizing pancreatitis, fluid collections in this disease are heterogeneous and dynamic. ANC and WON generally liquefy over time [38,39]. Therefore, intervention later in the disease process is warranted.

Infected necrosis can be presumed in the setting of extraluminal gas in the pancreatic and/or peripancreatic necrosis on cross-sectional imaging (Fig. 4) [2]. The diagnosis of infected necrosis is confirmed with positive bacteria and/or fungi on Gram stain and culture of aseptically obtained pancreatic

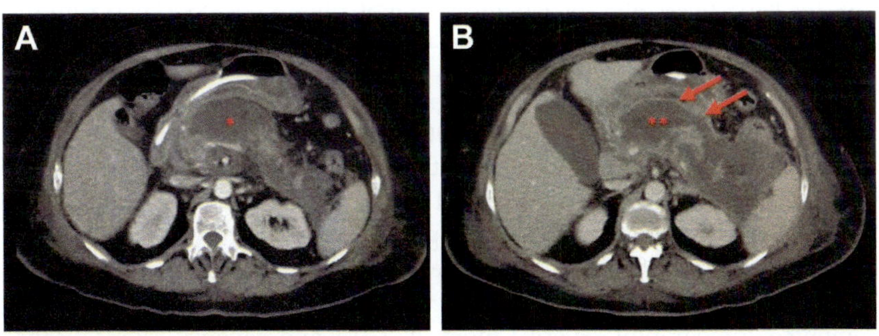

Fig. 3. Contrast-enhanced computed tomography at 2 weeks (*A*) and 2 months (*B*) in a patient with necrotizing pancreatitis. Note the transition from an acute necrotic collection (*asterisk* [*]) to WON (*double asterisk* [**]) characterized by the development of a well-defined inflammatory wall of reactive tissue (*arrows*).

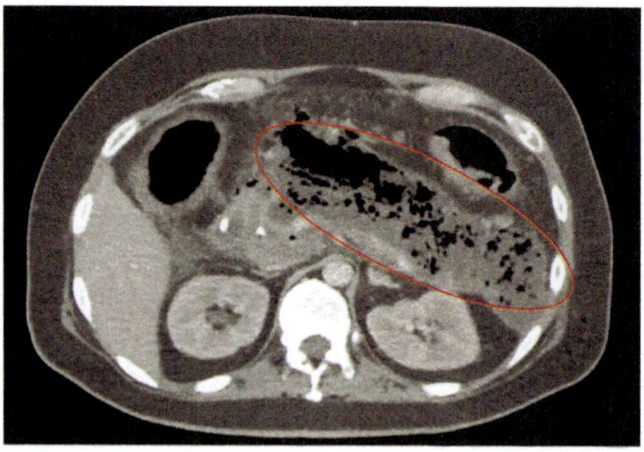

Fig. 4. Contrast-enhanced computed tomography showing an infected pancreatic necrosis with diffuse gas bubbles throughout the acute necrotic collection (*oval*).

necrosis specimens [2]. Routine percutaneous fine-needle aspiration (FNA) of pancreatic or peripancreatic fluid collections is only occasionally used in current practice [40,41]. The false-negative rate of FNA ranges from 12% to 25% and percutaneous aspiration has the small but real potential to introduce bacteria/fungus to an otherwise sterile ANC/WON [42,43].

An increasingly recognized complication of necrotizing pancreatitis is disconnected pancreatic duct syndrome, in which pancreatic parenchyma necrosis results in viable, upstream (left-sided) pancreatic tissue whose secretions are disconnected from the normal physiologic pancreatic duct drainage. This problem is diagnosed on endoscopic retrograde pancreatography or magnetic resonance pancreatography as extravasation of contrast or total cutoff of the main pancreatic duct (Fig. 5) [44–46].

Clinical course

Two overlapping phases are often described in acute and necrotizing pancreatitis: the early phase and the late phase. These phases are associated with the 2 peaks in mortality seen during the necrotizing pancreatitis clinical course.

Early phase

The early phase of necrotizing pancreatitis occurs during the first 1 to 2 weeks after disease onset and is associated with a profound activation of the systemic inflammatory response [2]. The initial symptoms associated with necrotizing pancreatitis are those typical of acute pancreatitis; however, the development of pancreatic and/or peripancreatic necrosis is often associated with clinical deterioration. A variety of clinical factors (C-reactive protein, procalcitonin, computed tomography severity index [CTSI]) and severity scores (Ranson criteria, Acute Physiology and Chronic Health Evaluation II [APACHE II] score, Bedside Index of Severity in Acute Pancreatitis, Japanese Severity Score) have been shown to predict the severity of pancreatitis [5,47–51]; regardless, treatment during the early phase is strictly supportive.

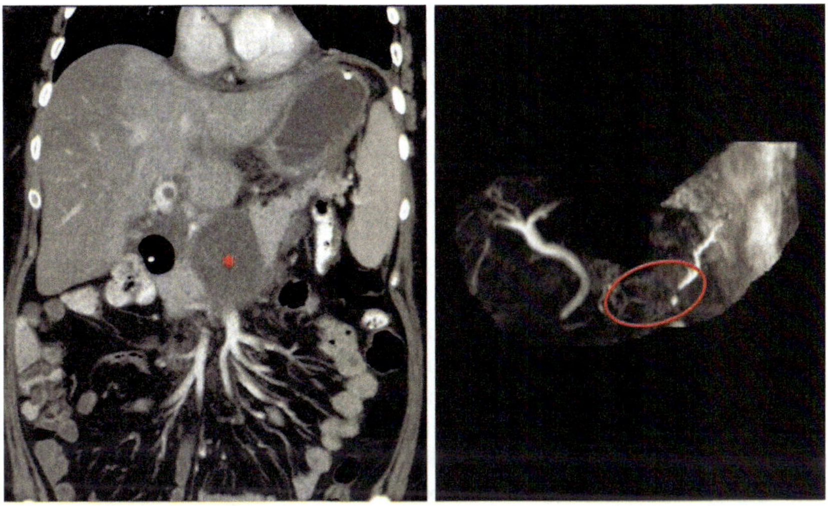

Fig. 5. Contrast-enhanced computed tomography showing necrosis involving the neck of the pancreas (*left, asterisk* [*]) resulting in cutoff of the main pancreatic duct on magnetic resonance pancreatography (*right, oval*).

Patients with necrotizing pancreatitis typically require aggressive fluid resuscitation because of substantial third-space loss and intravascular volume depletion. Goal-directed resuscitation with lactated Ringer solution is standard therapy, with the resuscitative phase tailored to the individual patient [41]. Supportive care in the intensive care unit is often warranted. Early organ failure (respiratory, renal, and or cardiovascular) is present in up to 25% to 35% of patients [7,52]. Early enteral nutrition is advocated in all pancreatitis patients, but clinicians must consider the discrete clinical scenario, because enteral nutrition may be poorly tolerated in necrotizing pancreatitis secondary to reactive ileus [40,41,53]. Patients not tolerating enteral nutrition warrant total parenteral nutrition because the catabolic state of necrotizing pancreatitis can rapidly produce malnutrition [40,41]. Many patients may tolerate partial enteral nutrition in the early course, and the remainder of their calories may be supplemented parenterally. Gastric ileus is common with inflammation in the lesser sac, and duodenal narrowing from extrinsic pressure develops in a small subset of patients with necrotizing pancreatitis [54]. Gastrojejunostomy feeding tubes are effective, permitting venting of the stomach and downstream enteral feeding, but may be associated with more severe complications compared with nasojejunal feeding tubes; thus, again, patient selection is critical [55].

The systemic inflammatory response associated with the early phase of necrotizing pancreatitis frequently results in fever and should not prompt prophylactic or empiric antibiotic usage because infection of necrosis during this phase is rare. Routine prophylactic antibiotic administration to prevent infection of pancreatic necrosis is not recommended [40,41]. Antibiotics should only be prescribed as treatment of documented infection or as empiric coverage during an infectious work-up in a patient with clinical deterioration [2,40,41]. In the early phase of necrotizing pancreatitis, mortality is predominately driven by multiple organ failure [7,8].

Late phase

The late phase in necrotizing pancreatitis begins a few weeks (>2 weeks) after disease onset and may last for several months, because overall disease duration is on average 5 to 6 months [35,56–58]. In the most severe cases, acute illness may persist up to or beyond 1 year. Ongoing intensive care may be required because persistent organ failure is common and present in 35% to 40% [7,8]. Attention to nutrition remains extremely important; critical illness and long-standing subacute inflammation can quickly result in nutritional depletion. As with the early phase, enteral nutrition is preferable to total parenteral nutrition. The route of administration (nasogastric, nasojejunal, percutaneous gastrostomy, percutaneous gastrojejunostomy) is less important and should be tailored to the individual patient, understanding the risks and benefits unique to each means of enteral access.

Several local and systemic complications may develop during the late phase. Critical illness, systemic inflammation, and infection predispose patients with necrotizing pancreatitis to an increased risk of venous thromboembolism (VTE), including deep vein thrombosis (DVT), which is observed in 16% to 38% of patients, and pulmonary embolism, documented in up to 6% of all patients with necrotizing pancreatitis [59,60]. Routine chemical VTE prophylaxis should be administered to all patients without clear contraindications, and strong consideration should be given to serial 4-extremity ultrasonography screening to promote early DVT detection, which allows for prompt initiation of full-dose anticoagulation and has been shown to decrease the development of symptomatic pulmonary embolism [60]. Splanchnic vein thrombosis is also extremely common and develops in about 50% of patients with necrotizing pancreatitis [26,60]. This problem is likely caused by a combination of mass effect and locoregional inflammation involving the portal, superior mesenteric, and/or splenic veins (Fig. 6). The ideal treatment strategy for pancreatitis-induced splanchnic vein thrombosis remains unknown. Anticoagulation may be required with thrombosis of the portal and/or superior mesenteric veins; however, anticoagulation for isolated splenic vein thrombosis is generally not warranted [61]. Left-sided (sinistral) portal hypertension may develop and can affect the selection of intervention, if warranted. Spontaneous bleeding in the setting of this sinistral portal hypertension is uncommon [61]. In contrast, bleeding from visceral artery pseudoaneurysms occurs in about 4% of patients with necrotizing pancreatitis and may involve virtually any visceral artery [62]. Clinicians must be aware of this potentially life-threatening problem and have a low index of suspicion to obtain arterial-phase cross-sectional imaging to secure this diagnosis. Visceral artery pseudoaneurysms are best treated with urgent/emergent percutaneous angioembolization (Fig. 7) [62].

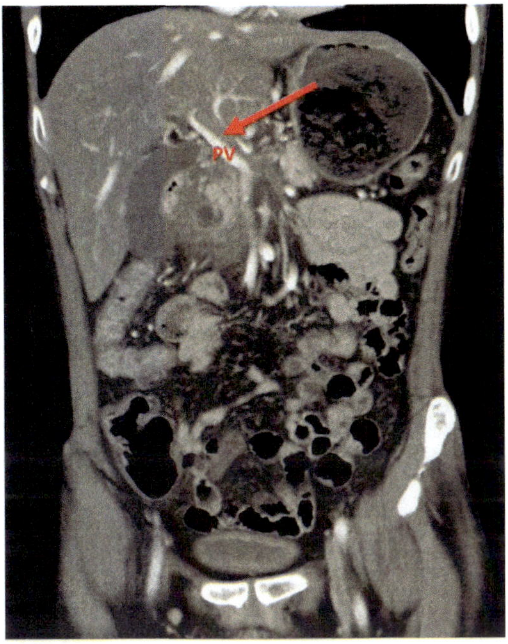

Fig. 6. Acute nonocclusive portal vein (PV) thrombosis (*arrow*) from necrotizing pancreatitis. In this case, thrombosis extended from the inferior mesenteric vein to the main portal vein, and into the left portal vein.

The impact of locoregional inflammation extends beyond vascular complications. Gastric outlet obstruction and biliary stricture can develop from regional inflammation and/or mass effect from necrosis [26,54,63]. Disconnected pancreatic duct syndrome can present with recurrent pancreatic pseudocysts, recurrent obstructive pancreatitis, and/or pancreaticocutaneous fistula and frequently requires multiple interventions to treat [35,64,65]. Furthermore, the presence of disconnected pancreatic duct syndrome may affect decision making when necrosis intervention is needed [35,64,66,67]. Colonic complications, with ischemia being the most common, are associated with considerable mortality and develop in up to 11% of patients with necrotizing pancreatitis [68]. Spontaneous gastrointestinal fistulae may occur or develop after necrosis intervention [26]. Fistulae involving the duodenum represent a particularly challenging problem associated with significant morbidity and mortality [54].

Nosocomial extrapancreatic infections are extremely common in patients with necrotizing pancreatitis. In the setting of clinical concern for infection, confirmatory testing should direct the appropriate duration of antibiotics. When infection is ruled out, empiric antibiotic therapy should be halted [69]. Tailoring empiric antibiotic therapy based on culture is critically important given the high incidence of antimicrobial resistance and *Clostridioides difficile* infection [70]. Infected pancreatic necrosis develops in 20% to 40% of patients

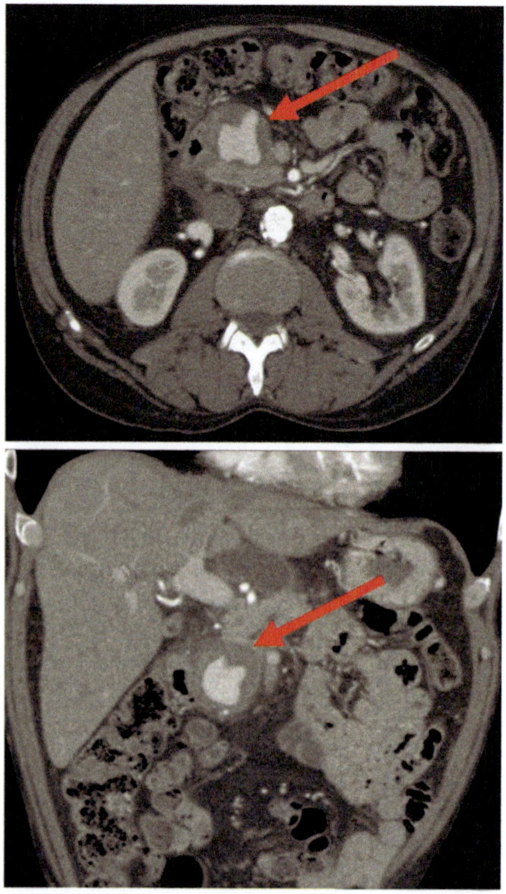

Fig. 7. Representative axial (*top*) and coronal (*bottom*) computed tomography images showing visceral artery pseudoaneurysm in necrotizing pancreatitis arising from a branch of the anterior pancreaticoduodenal artery (*arrows*).

and is the primary indication for intervention in necrotizing pancreatitis (which is discussed in detail later) [6–8,69,71]. Pancreatic necrosis has an unclear impact but tends to develop in patients with more severe disease, a prolonged disease course, and frequent and/or prolonged antibiotic therapy, further highlighting the importance of judicious antibiotic therapy [72].

When patients are suitable for discharge from inpatient treatment, several outpatient goals of care must be achieved. Nutritional optimization and physical rehabilitation should be continued to promote recovery and return to baseline. Communication between the patient, the patient's outpatient care team, and the responsible pancreatologist must be readily available to monitor clinical improvement, allow early detection of developing complications, and minimize hospital readmission [52]. Unplanned hospital readmission is extremely common in this patient population, and the tenets of frequent communication and early detection of impending treatable problems decreases the need for hospital readmission [6,52]. In addition, reprieve from inpatient treatment can decrease the risk of nosocomial infection and exposure to multidrug-resistant organisms. In addition, routine, short-interval follow-up should be scheduled to evaluate progress and plan for appropriate intervention, if required.

INTERVENTION IN NECROTIZING PANCREATITIS

Evolution in treating necrotizing pancreatitis

Pancreatic and peripancreatic necrosis was traditionally treated by operative surgical debridement, a strategy that often included multiple debridements and, in some cases, laparostomy to facilitate planned reoperations [73,74]. Historical reports of operative pancreatic debridement were associated with high perioperative morbidity, including enteral and pancreatic fistula, as well as high postoperative mortalities, often in the 25% to 40% range [75,76]. With improved understanding of the disease process and accumulated operative experience, mortality after pancreatic debridement has decreased substantially over time [57,77].

The past 20 years have witnessed a remarkable change in the treatment of pancreatic necrosis [9,78]. With application of contemporary step-up strategies, most patients are managed successfully using minimally invasive treatment approaches, including percutaneous therapy, endoscopic directed therapy, and often some combination of the two [56,58,71,78–81].

Indications and goals of intervention

The principles of intervention to address pancreatic necrosis are (1) to control infection, (2) evacuate fluid and solid necrotic debris, (3) drain pancreatic fistula (typically the result of disconnected pancreatic duct syndrome) either internally or externally, (4) prevent recurrent pancreatitis (by cholecystectomy in the setting of biliary pancreatitis), and (5) establish enteral access. It is ideal to accomplish these goals with minimal physiologic disruption in a uniformly frail patient population. A one-size fits all approach does not apply in necrotizing pancreatitis, a fundamental general principle is that a single debridement technique does not apply widely to all patients. Care of patients with necrotizing pancreatitis requires dedicated physicians to lead multidisciplinary teams providing closely monitored care during this long-term acute/subacute illness. Selection of type and timing of intervention requires expert clinical judgment; the ideal treatment approach is individualized to the patient's unique clinical circumstance and depends highly on local experience and expertise.

Additional important selection considerations include the patient physiology: no patient with necrotizing pancreatitis is ever physiologically perfect for intervention. Residual necrosis is a catabolic situation and good judgment is required to identify the appropriate window for intervention. This point speaks

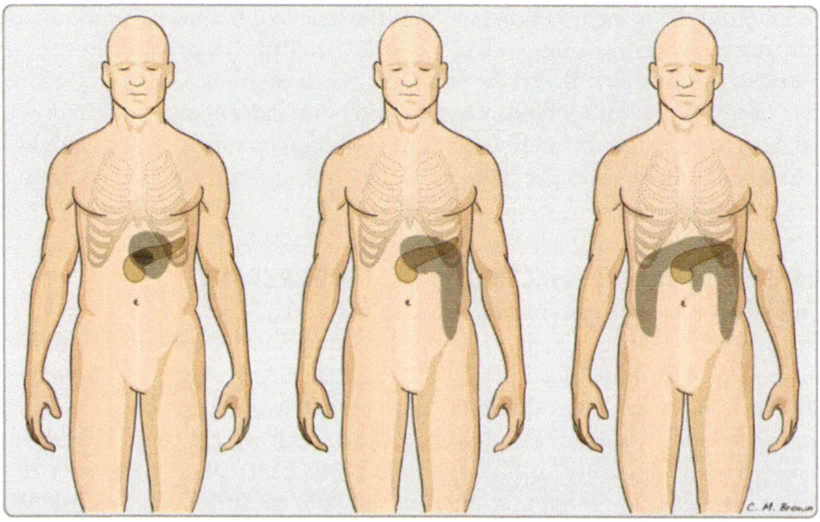

Fig. 8. Patterns of necrosis in necrotizing pancreatitis. Necrosis confined to the lesser sac (*left*) may be best for a transgastric approach, either endoscopic or surgical. Patients with necrosis tracking down 1 paracolic gutter (*middle*) are suitable for percutaneous drainage and subsequent videoscopic-assisted retroperitoneal debridement, if needed. Multiple fields of retroperitoneal necrosis (*right*) may be best served with operative pancreatic debridement. (*Illustration reprinted from* "Transgastric Pancreatic Necrosectomy: How I Do It" by Zyromski and colleagues (2016)) [89].

to the need to have at least 1 physician involved in a patient's care longitudinally to evaluate changes in progress. Necrosis distribution plays perhaps an equally important role in decision making. A patient with necrosis consolidated in the lesser sac with or without (usually with) a disconnected pancreatic tail is ideally suited for a transgastric approach (either endoscopic or surgical) (Fig. 8, left), whereas a patient with necrosis tracking down 1 paracolic gutter may be approached with percutaneous drainage with aggressive drain management (frequent drain exchanges/repositioning, or additional drain placement) followed by videoscopic-assisted retroperitoneal debridement (VARD), if necessary (see Fig. 8, middle). A patient with multiple retroperitoneal fields involved with necrosis may be best served with operative debridement as a first treatment step (see Fig. 8, right).

Natural history of pancreatic necrosis

Fig. 9 shows the natural history of pancreatic and peripancreatic necrosis. A small proportion of patients with necrotizing pancreatitis resolve their necrosis without any specific intervention. This number is approximately 5% to 10% in large series, but may be as high as 20% in select populations [9,26]. A second group of patients develop infected necrosis, documented either by cross-sectional imaging with gas bubbles or by directly sampling and culturing the

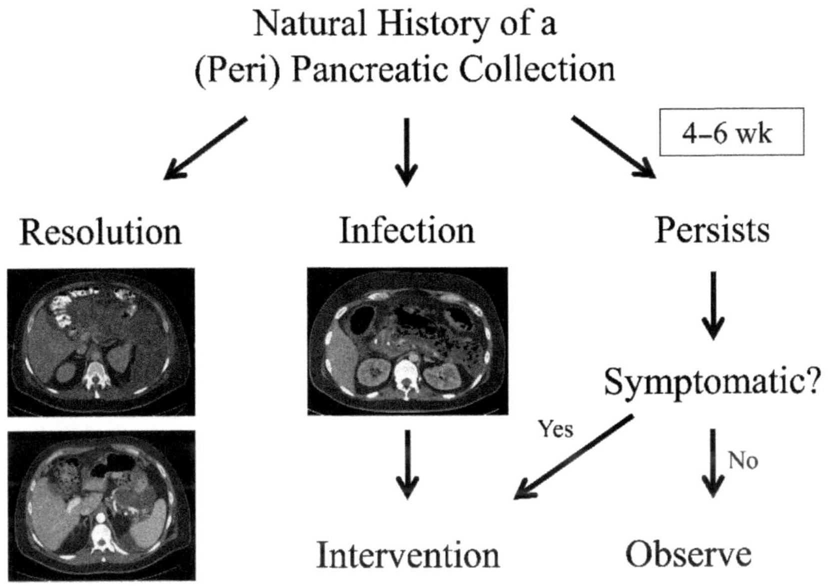

Fig. 9. Natural history of pancreatic and peripancreatic necrosis.

necrosis. A third group of patients have persistent necrosis, which, if asymptomatic, may be observed. Patients with persistent sterile necrosis may develop unremitting symptoms without resolution over time, including gastric outlet obstruction, abdominal pain, or persistent unwellness. These patients with symptomatic (presumed sterile) necrosis should be considered for debridement. It is notable in this latter category of presumed sterile necrosis that a significant percentage (up to 40%) are found to have occult infection [82]. Infected necrosis rarely resolves with antibiotic therapy alone and is the most common indication for intervention in necrotizing pancreatitis. Infected necrosis develops in 50% to 60% of patients and the subsequent clinical course is extremely heterogeneous [6–8,26]. Treatment may require few interventions over the course of weeks to months; in contrast, repeated intervention over months to years is common.

Percutaneous drainage

Percutaneous drainage has become the first mechanical interventional step in the step-up approach for most patients with necrotizing pancreatitis, because most institutions have the resources to perform percutaneous drainage safely. It was observed in the PANTER trial that nearly one-third of patients resolved their pancreatic/peripancreatic collections with percutaneous drainage alone [78]. This finding has been validated in subsequent studies, although no published data exist to identify accurate predictors of success or failure of percutaneous drainage alone [35,56,83]. Once treatment begins by any approach (percutaneous, endoscopic, or otherwise), the clock is ticking, and efforts should be directed toward evacuating the infected solid necrosis expediently. Most institutions favor a strategy of fairly short-interval (3–5 days) imaging with frequent upsizing or repositioning of percutaneous drains or placement of additional drains [35,84]. Although labor intensive, this aggressive approach to percutaneous drainage of pancreatic necrosis effectively evacuates residual necrosis, minimizes recurrent bouts of sepsis from undrained infected necrosis, and accelerates recovery. Percutaneous drains by themselves do not provide definitive treatment in two-thirds of patients with pancreas necrosis, and clinical judgment is critically important once treatment has begun. In the situation where treatment by percutaneous drainage stalls, the next step in the approach may include endoscopic dual-modality drainage, sinus tract endoscopy, or operative surgical debridement.

Transgastric debridement

Endoscopic transgastric debridement was first described in 1996, and, over the next 2 decades, sporadic small case reports emerged in both the medical and surgical literature [85]. More recently, enthusiasm has grown significantly for endoscopic transgastric debridement, and many institutions with advanced endoscopic experience use an endoscopic step-up approach as initial intervention in necrotizing pancreatitis. Patients with necrosis confined to the lesser sac are ideal candidates; however, with accumulating experience, aggressive endoscopists have pushed the envelope in terms of which necrosis morphology to approach endoscopically [86,87]. An important consideration is the available local expertise; even in the most skilled hands, endoscopic evacuation of peripancreatic necrosis requires multiple debridement sessions, each under a general anesthetic. Patient selection is critical and still becoming better delineated, but may be best suited for patients with nonbiliary causes of pancreatitis. The long-term success of endoscopic debridement in patients with disconnected pancreatic duct syndrome is incompletely delineated, but this treatment seems to be durable in most patients (~70%), with about 30% of patients treated surgically for recurrent symptoms from disconnected pancreatic duct syndrome after endoscopic transgastric debridement [67].

Surgical transgastric debridement provides the ability to address pancreatic necrosis as well as perform cholecystectomy with cholangiography in the same setting. Several surgical groups have reported excellent results with increasingly large series of transgastric debridement [67,88]. The authors' opinion is that surgical transgastric debridement should be the treatment of choice with patients with biliary pancreatitis and appropriate necrosis morphology [89]. This approach may be ideal for patients with disconnected pancreatic duct syndrome, because the transgastric approach drains the disconnected tail into the stomach. These patients experience recurrent pancreatitis and fluid collections approximately 20% of the time and should be counseled accordingly [67].

Minimally invasive approaches include VARD as well as sinus tract endoscopy/necrosectomy. VARD was studied prospectively by the Dutch group in the PANTER trial [78]. A small incision permits insertion of an operating nephroscope or video endoscope to guide debridement. This approach may be performed by left or right flank; occasionally bilateral VARD is used to treat extensive necrosis. Sinus tract necrosectomy involves a similar technical approach and uses endoscopy to guide debridement through a small incision; however, this approach is typically performed along established drain tracts in a transperitoneal orientation.

A fundamental principle of either the retroperitoneal or transperitoneal minimally invasive approach is allowing an appropriate period of time for the necrosis cavity to mature. This window permits adequate debridement with minimal disruption of surrounding tissue.

Open pancreatic debridement

Open pancreatic debridement has traditionally served as the gold standard for evacuation of infected or symptomatic solid necrosis. No contemporary minimally invasive approach has ever been compared with open debridement in a randomized fashion; this comparison in current time is not practical. Open pancreatic debridement provides the advantage of addressing multiple necrosis fields, biliary disorder, and potentially a small pancreatic tail remnant in a single procedure. The safety of this procedure is established and, in experienced hands, mortality is less than 2% [57,77,90]. Safety is a particularly important consideration in the setting of superior mesenteric or splenic vein thrombosis. In this circumstance, resultant gastric varices may lead to major hemorrhage during transgastric approaches. Open pancreatic necrosectomy is time tested and widely applicable to well-trained surgeons familiar with basic surgical principles. In current times, open pancreatic debridement is often relegated to the last effort when other percutaneous and endoscopic approaches have unsuccessfully resolved pancreatic necrosis [57,90].

From a technical standpoint, it is important to review recent cross-sectional imaging to understand the pattern of residual necrosis distribution. Intraoperative ultrasonography is useful to localize collections. Adhesions from the small bowel to the underside of the transverse colon are common. A safe approach to necrosis is obtained via lateral paracolic gutters. Perhaps the most effective debridement tool is the "educated" finger of the surgeon. A ring forceps works well too; however, only freely mobile necrosis should be debrided. Large-caliber closed suction drains are placed in the necrosis bed after vigorous irrigation. Gastrojejunostomy feeding tubes facilitate postoperative management because many patients have gastric ileus (may vent gastrostomy ports) but tolerate small bowel feeding [55].

Contemporary series of pancreatic debridement in experienced hands document excellent outcomes. To reiterate, judgment regarding timing of operation and extent of operation is critically important. In some circumstances, damage-control debridement is necessary [90].

In summary, important considerations in necrotizing pancreatitis intervention include the cause of pancreatitis; necrosis distribution (including percentage of solid necrosis), parenchymal involvement, presence of disconnected pancreatic duct syndrome, splanchnic vein thrombosis, infection, patient physiology, and local expertise. One technique does not fit all patients. A dedicated physician taking "ownership" of patient care is required ideally to promote interface among a multidisciplinary team through the duration of this long-term acute illness.

OUTCOMES, INCLUDING LONG-TERM SEQUELAE

The modern mortality in all patients with necrotizing pancreatitis is about 10% to 15% [6–9]. Mortalities are higher in patients with organ failure, those with infected necrosis, or those who require intervention, ranging from 10% to 30% [7,8,56,71,77,78,91]. Organ failure and infected necrosis are the two strongest influencing factors associated with mortality [7,8]. Patients who survive an episode of acute necrotizing pancreatitis generally required about 5 to 6 months for acute/subacute disease resolution [26,52,57,67]. Emerging research has identified a variety of long-term disease sequelae in necrotizing pancreatitis survivors (Table 2) [26].

Table 2
Long-term sequelae of necrotizing pancreatitis

Long-term sequelae	Incidence (%)
Endocrine insufficiency	40–60
Exocrine insufficiency	10–40
Splanchnic vein thrombosis	50
Disconnected pancreatic duct syndrome	45
Recurrent acute pancreatitis	20
Chronic pancreatitis	10–20
Biliary stricture	16
Duodenal stricture	5
Uncommon sequelae	—
Tracheal stenosis	—
Ureteral stricture	—
Colonic stricture	—
Progressive renal failure	—
Pancreatic ductal adenocarcinoma	—
Gastrointestinal failure requiring transplant	—
Male impotence	—
Metabolic peripheral polyneuropathy	—
Pericardial effusion	—
Deafness	—
Blindness	—

Pancreatic endocrine and exocrine insufficiency after acute pancreatitis are common; the risk of pancreatic function loss is directly correlated with the disease severity and volume of parenchymal necrosis [20,21,26,92]. In patients with necrotizing pancreatitis, endocrine (type 3c diabetes mellitus) and exocrine insufficiency develop in 40% to 60% and 10% to 40% of survivors, respectively [21,26,83,92,93]. One in 5 patients (20%) may experience recurrent acute pancreatitis during long-term follow-up, and chronic pancreatitis is reported to develop in 10% to 20% [26,83,94]. Pancreatic duct stricture after necrotizing pancreatitis contributes to the development of recurrent acute pancreatitis and chronic pancreatitis [26,95,96].

Several less commonly reported complications are noteworthy. Splanchnic vein thrombosis develops in up to 50% of patients, with infrequent recanalization [26,59,96,97]. This situation often results in either left-sided or generalized portal hypertension. Disconnected pancreatic duct syndrome is an increasingly recognized complication of necrotizing pancreatitis. Disconnected pancreatic duct syndrome is diagnosed in 45% of patients and commonly manifests after acute disease resolution [26,35,65]. The treatment of disconnected pancreatic duct syndrome and its associated recurrent pancreatitis and/or pseudocyst frequently require endoscopic and/or surgical intervention. Biliary stricture and duodenal stricture may form as a result of the local inflammatory process in necrotizing pancreatitis and frequently require interventional therapy [54,63]. Gastric, duodenal, enteric, and colonic fistulae may develop during necrotizing pancreatitis or as a result of its treatment; these fistulae often persist after disease resolution [26,68]. Incisional hernia is more common in patients requiring laparotomy for necrotizing pancreatitis compared with laparotomy for other indications [26,98]. Rare complications from necrotizing pancreatitis or its treatment that are reported as case reports or as anecdotes include tracheal stenosis, ureteral stricture, colonic stricture, progressive renal failure, pancreatic ductal adenocarcinoma, irreversible gastrointestinal failure requiring multivisceral transplant, male impotence, metabolic peripheral polyneuropathy, pericardial effusion, deafness, and blindness [26].

Clinicians should be aware that necrotizing pancreatitis has a significant impact on patients' mental health both during the acute phase and long-term after disease resolution. The disease elicits posttraumatic stress disorder, anxiety, and depression. Several studies have evaluated a variety of quality-of-life metrics after acute necrotizing pancreatitis resolution and the theme is a long-term impairment in quality of life regardless of treatment strategy; however, the exact impact remains difficult to quantify [93,99–101]. Of significance, these studies report that, during follow-up, 40% to 75% of patients reported disability that prevented return to baseline, pre–necrotizing pancreatitis function. Clearly, long-term follow-up of necrotizing pancreatitis survivors is important.

After acute disease resolution, routine follow-up should include focused history, physical examination, and laboratory screening for the development of these long-term sequelae in survivors of necrotizing pancreatitis.

SUMMARY

The past 2 decades have witnessed considerable evolution in our understanding of both the disease process and technical approaches to managing pancreatic necrosis. Patients requiring interventions should uniformly be treated by the step-up approach. This approach starts with antibiotics, stepping up to percutaneous drainage or endoscopic therapy and progressing to surgical therapy. A combination of these approaches is often necessary to expedite disease resolution. Objective metrics in determining the optimal timing for step-up are needed. It is unknown which subset of patients may benefit from operative pancreatic debridement as first-line therapy. An unmet need is the investigation, discovery, and development of therapy directed toward treating the disease itself, because current therapy simply addresses complications of the disease.

CLINICS CARE POINTS

- Support of organ failure is the primary goal in the first phase of necrotizing pancreatitis
- During the second phase (1–4 months) of necrotizing pancreatitis, clinicians should be aware of the potential for venous thromboembolism, visceral arterial pseudoaneurysm, and ischemic viscera.
- Timing and type of intervention to treat necrosis should be addressed in a multidisciplinary fashion; once an intervention has been initiated, progression should continue with regular assessment of efficacy and step-up as indicated.
- Long-term follow-up is necessary to identify and treat disease complications, which occur in more than 80% of patients with necrotizing pancreatitis.

DISCLOSURE

The authors have nothing to disclose.

References

[1] Ouyang G, Pan G, Liu Q, et al. The global, regional, and national burden of pancreatitis in 195 countries and territories, 1990-2017: a systematic analysis for the Global Burden of Disease Study 2017. BMC Med 2020;18:388.

[2] Banks PA, Bollen TL, Dervenis C, et al. Classification of acute pancreatitis–2012: revision of the Atlanta classification and definitions by international consensus. Gut 2013;62:102–11.

[3] van Dijk SM, Hallensleben NDL, van Santvoort HC, et al. Acute pancreatitis: recent advances through randomised trials. Gut 2017;66:2024–32.

[4] Buter A, Imrie CW, Carter CR, et al. Dynamic nature of early organ dysfunction determines outcome in acute pancreatitis. Br J Surg 2002;89:298–302.

[5] Bollen TL, Singh VK, Maurer R, et al. A comparative evaluation of radiologic and clinical scoring systems in the early prediction of severity in acute pancreatitis. Am J Gastroenterol 2012;107:612–9.

[6] Maatman TK, Mahajan S, Roch AM, et al. High rates of readmission in necrotizing pancreatitis: natural history or opportunity for improvement? J Gastrointest Surg 2019;23: 1834–9.
[7] Guo Q, Li A, Xia Q, et al. The role of organ failure and infection in necrotizing pancreatitis: a prospective study. Ann Surg 2014;259:1201–7.
[8] Petrov MS, Shanbhag S, Chakraborty M, et al. Organ failure and infection of pancreatic necrosis as determinants of mortality in patients with acute pancreatitis. Gastroenterology 2010;139:813–20.
[9] Roch AM, Maatman T, Carr RA, et al. Evolving treatment of necrotizing pancreatitis. Am J Surg 2018;215:526–9.
[10] Yasuda H, Horibe M, Sanui M, et al. Etiology and mortality in severe acute pancreatitis: a multicenter study in Japan. Pancreatology 2020;20(3):307–17.
[11] Portelli M, Jones CD. Severe acute pancreatitis: pathogenesis, diagnosis and surgical management. Hepatobiliary Pancreat Dis Int 2017;16:155–9.
[12] Lankisch PG, Apte M, Banks PA. Acute pancreatitis. Lancet 2015;386:85–96.
[13] Saluja A, Dudeja V, Dawra R, et al. Early intra-acinar events in pathogenesis of pancreatitis. Gastroenterology 2019;156:1979–93.
[14] Mayerle J, Sendler M, Hegyi E, et al. Genetics, cell biology, and pathophysiology of pancreatitis. Gastroenterology 2019;156:1951–1968 e1.
[15] Hall JC, Crawford HC. The conspiracy of autophagy, stress and inflammation in acute pancreatitis. Curr Opin Gastroenterol 2014;30:495–9.
[16] Makhija R, Kingsnorth A. Cytokine storm in acute pancreatitis. J Hepatobiliary Pancreat Surg 2002;9:401–10.
[17] Kylanpaa L, Rakonczay Z Jr, O'Reilly DA. The clinical course of acute pancreatitis and the inflammatory mediators that drive it. Int J Inflam 2012;2012:360685.
[18] Bhatia M, Wong FL, Cao Y, et al. Pathophysiology of acute pancreatitis. Pancreatology 2005;5:132–44.
[19] Takeyama Y. Long-term prognosis of acute pancreatitis in Japan. Clin Gastroenterol Hepatol 2009;7:S15–7.
[20] Vipperla K, Papachristou GI, Slivka A, et al. Risk of new-onset diabetes is determined by severity of acute pancreatitis. Pancreas 2016;45:e14–5.
[21] Hollemans RA, Hallensleben NDL, Mager DJ, et al. Pancreatic exocrine insufficiency following acute pancreatitis: systematic review and study level meta-analysis. Pancreatology 2018;18:253–62.
[22] Beger HG, Rau BM. Severe acute pancreatitis: clinical course and management. World J Gastroenterol 2007;13:5043–51.
[23] Sunamura M, Yamauchi J, Shibuya K, et al. Pancreatic microcirculation in acute pancreatitis. J Hepatobiliary Pancreat Surg 1998;5:62–8.
[24] Bassi D, Kollias N, Fernandez-del Castillo C, et al. Impairment of pancreatic microcirculation correlates with the severity of acute experimental pancreatitis. J Am Coll Surg 1994;179:257–63.
[25] Cuthbertson CM, Christophi C. Disturbances of the microcirculation in acute pancreatitis. Br J Surg 2006;93:518–30.
[26] Maatman TK, Roch AM, Ceppa EP, et al. The continuum of complications in survivors of necrotizing pancreatitis. Surgery 2020;168:1032–40.
[27] De Campos T, Deree J, Coimbra R. From acute pancreatitis to end-organ injury: mechanisms of acute lung injury. Surg Infect (Larchmt) 2007;8:107–20.
[28] Zhang XP, Wang L, Zhou YF. The pathogenic mechanism of severe acute pancreatitis complicated with renal injury: a review of current knowledge. Dig Dis Sci 2008;53: 297–306.
[29] Greer SE, Burchard KW. Acute pancreatitis and critical illness: a pancreatic tale of hypoperfusion and inflammation. Chest 2009;136:1413–9.

[30] Wilson PG, Manji M, Neoptolemos JP. Acute pancreatitis as a model of sepsis. J Antimicrob Chemother 1998;41(Suppl A:):51–63.
[31] Marshall J, Cook D, Christou N, et al. Multiple organ dysfunction score: a reliable descriptor of a complex clinical outcome. Crit Care Med 1995;23:1638–52.
[32] Spanier BW, Nio Y, van der Hulst RW, et al. Practice and yield of early CT scan in acute pancreatitis: a Dutch observational multicenter study. Pancreatology 2010;10:222–8.
[33] Balthazar E, Robinson D, Megibow A, et al. Acute pancreatitis: value of CT in establishing prognosis. Radiology 1990;174:331–6.
[34] Sakorafas G, Tsiotos G, Sarr M. Extrapancreatic necrotizing pancreatitis with viable pancreas: a previously under-appreciated entity. J Am Coll Surg 1999;188:643–8.
[35] Maatman TK, Mahajan S, Roch AM, et al. Disconnected pancreatic duct syndrome predicts failure of percutaneous therapy in necrotizing pancreatitis. Pancreatology 2020;20:362–8.
[36] Bakker OJ, Van Santvoort HC, Besselink MG, et al. Extrapancreatic necrosis without pancreatic parenchymal necrosis: a separate entity in necrotising pancreatitis? Gut 2013;62:1475–80.
[37] Wang M, Wei A, Guo Q, et al. Clinical outcomes of combined necrotizing pancreatitis versus extrapancreatic necrosis alone. Pancreatology 2016;16:57–65.
[38] Dhaka N, Samanta J, Kochhar S, et al. Pancreatic fluid collections: what is the ideal imaging technique? World J Gastroenterol 2015;21:13403–10.
[39] Rana SS, Bhasin DK, Reddy YR, et al. Morphological features of fluid collections on endoscopic ultrasound in acute necrotizing pancreatitis: do they change over time? Ann Gastroenterol 2014;27:258–61.
[40] Working Group IAP/APA Acute Pancreatitis Guidelines. IAP/APA evidence-based guidelines for the management of acute pancreatitis. Pancreatology 2013;13:e1–15.
[41] Baron TH, DiMaio CJ, Wang AY, et al. American gastroenterological association clinical practice update: management of pancreatic necrosis. Gastroenterology 2020;158: 67–75 e1.
[42] Rau B, Pralle U, Mayer JM, et al. Role of ultrasonographically guided fine-needle aspiration cytology in the diagnosis of infected pancreatic necrosis. Br J Surg 1998;85:179–84.
[43] Rodriguez JR, Razo AO, Targarona J, et al. Debridement and closed packing for sterile or infected necrotizing pancreatitis: insights into indications and outcomes in 167 patients. Ann Surg 2008;247:294–9.
[44] Sandrasegaran K, Tann M, Jennings G, et al. Disconnection of the Pancreatic Duct: an important but overlooked complication of severe acute pancreatitis. Radiographics 2007;27:1389–400.
[45] Kozarek R, Traverso L. Pancreatic fistulas: etiology, consequences, and treatment. Gastroenterologist 1996;4:239–44.
[46] Kozarek R. Endoscopic therapy of complete and partial pancreatic duct disruptions. Gastrointest Endosc Clin N Am 1998;8:39–53.
[47] Forsmark CE, Vege SS, Wilcox CM. Acute pancreatitis. N Engl J Med 2016;375: 1972–81.
[48] Stirling AD, Moran NR, Kelly ME, et al. The predictive value of C-reactive protein (CRP) in acute pancreatitis - is interval change in CRP an additional indicator of severity? HPB (Oxford) 2017;19:874–80.
[49] Staubli SM, Oertli D, Nebiker CA. Laboratory markers predicting severity of acute pancreatitis. Crit Rev Clin Lab Sci 2015;52:273–83.
[50] Mortele KJ, Wiesner W, Intriere L, et al. A modified CT severity index for evaluating acute pancreatitis: improved correlation with patient outcome. AJR Am J Roentgenol 2004;183: 1261–5.
[51] Ranson JH, Rifkind KM, Roses DF, et al. Prognostic signs and the role of operative management in acute pancreatitis. Surg Gynecol Obstet 1974;139:69–81.

[52] Maatman TK, McGreevy KA, Sood AJ, et al. Improved outpatient communication decreases unplanned readmission in necrotizing pancreatitis. J Surg Res 2020;253: 139–46.
[53] Moran RA, Jalaly NY, Kamal A, et al. Ileus is a predictor of local infection in patients with acute necrotizing pancreatitis. Pancreatology 2016;16:966–72.
[54] Banter LR, Maatman TK, McGuire SP, et al. Duodenal complications in necrotizing pancreatitis: Challenges of an overlooked complication. Am J Surg 2021;221:589–93.
[55] Roch AM, Carr RA, Watkins JL, et al. Percutaneous Gastrostomy in Necrotizing Pancreatitis: Friend or Foe? J Gastrointest Surg 2020;24(12):2800–6.
[56] Horvath K, Freeny P, Escallon J, et al. Safety and efficacy of video-assisted retroperitoneal debridement for infected pancreatic collections: a multicenter, prospective, single-arm phase 2 study. Arch Surg 2010;145:814–25.
[57] Maatman TK, Flick KF, Roch AM, et al. Operative pancreatic debridement: contemporary outcomes in changing times. Pancreatology 2020;20:968–75.
[58] Gluck M, Ross A, Irani S, et al. Dual modality drainage for symptomatic walled-off pancreatic necrosis reduces length of hospitalization, radiological procedures, and number of endoscopies compared to standard percutaneous drainage. J Gastrointest Surg 2012;16: 248–56 [discussion: 256-7].
[59] Roch AM, Maatman TK, Carr RA, et al. Venous thromboembolism in necrotizing pancreatitis: an underappreciated risk. J Gastrointest Surg 2019;23:2430–8.
[60] Maatman TK, McGuire SP, Lewellen KA, et al. Prospective analysis of the mechanisms underlying ineffective deep vein thrombosis prophylaxis in necrotizing pancreatitis. J Am Coll Surg 2021;232:91–100.
[61] Butler JR, Eckert GJ, Zyromski NJ, et al. Natural history of pancreatitis-induced splenic vein thrombosis: a systematic review and meta-analysis of its incidence and rate of gastrointestinal bleeding. HPB (Oxford) 2011;13:839–45.
[62] Maatman TK, Heimberger MA, Lewellen KA, et al. Visceral artery pseudoaneurysm in necrotizing pancreatitis: incidence and outcomes. Can J Surg 2019;63:E272–7.
[63] Maatman TK, Ceppa EP, Fogel EL, et al. Biliary stricture after necrotizing pancreatitis: an underappreciated challenge. Ann Surg 2020 doi:[Epub ahead of print].
[64] Bang J, Wilcox C, Hasan M, et al. Impact of disconnected pancreatic duct syndrome on the endoscopic management of pancreatic fluid collections. Ann Surg 2018;267:561–8.
[65] Maatman TK, Roch AM, Heimberger MA, et al. Disconnected pancreatic duct syndrome: spectrum of operative management. J Surg Res 2020;247:297–303.
[66] Lawrence C, Howell DA, Stefan AM, et al. Disconnected pancreatic tail syndrome: potential for endoscopic therapy and results of long-term follow-up. Gastrointest Endosc 2008;67:673–9.
[67] Maatman TK, McGuire SP, Flick KF, et al. Outcomes in endoscopic and operative transgastric pancreatic debridement. Ann Surg 2021;274:516–23.
[68] Maatman TK, Nicolas ME, Roch AM, et al. Colon involvement in necrotizing pancreatitis: incidence, risk factors, and outcomes. Ann Surg 2022;275(3):568–75 [online ahead of print].
[69] Lim CL, Lee W, Liew YX, et al. Role of antibiotic prophylaxis in necrotizing pancreatitis: a meta-analysis. J Gastrointest Surg 2015;19:480–91.
[70] Maatman TK, Westfall-Snyder JA, Nicolas ME, et al. The morbidity of C. difficile in necrotizing pancreatitis. Am J Surg 2019;219:509–12.
[71] van Santvoort HC, Bakker OJ, Bollen TL, et al. A conservative and minimally invasive approach to necrotizing pancreatitis improves outcome. Gastroenterology 2011;141: 1254–63.
[72] Singh RR, Mitchell W, David Y, et al. Pancreatic fungal infection in patients with necrotizing pancreatitis: a systematic review and meta-analysis. J Clin Gastroenterol 2021;55: 218–26.

[73] Sarr MG, Nagorney DM, Mucha P Jr, et al. Acute necrotizing pancreatitis: management by planned, staged pancreatic necrosectomy/debridement and delayed primary wound closure over drains. Br J Surg 1991;78:576–81.
[74] Tsiotos GG, Luque-de León E, Söreide JA, et al. Management of necrotizing pancreatitis by repeated operative necrosectomy using a zipper technique. Am J Surg 1998;175:91–8.
[75] Warshaw AL, Jin GL. Improved survival in 45 patients with pancreatic abscess. Ann Surg 1985;202:408–17.
[76] Rau B, Bothe A, Beger HG. Surgical treatment of necrotizing pancreatitis by necrosectomy and closed lavage: changing patient characteristics and outcome in a 19-year, single-center series. Surgery 2005;138:28–39.
[77] Howard TJ, Patel JB, Zyromski N, et al. Declining morbidity and mortality rates in the surgical management of pancreatic necrosis. J Gastrointest Surg 2007;11:43–9.
[78] Van Santvoort H, Besselink M, Bakker O, et al. A step-up approach or open necrosectomy for necrotizing pancreatitis. N Engl J Med 2010;362:1491–502.
[79] van Brunschot S, Hollemans RA, Bakker OJ, et al. Minimally invasive and endoscopic versus open necrosectomy for necrotising pancreatitis: a pooled analysis of individual data for 1980 patients. Gut 2018;67:697–706.
[80] Hyun JJ, Sahar N, Singla A, et al. Outcomes of infected versus symptomatic sterile walled-off pancreatic necrosis treated with a minimally invasive therapy. Gut Liver 2019;13: 215–22.
[81] Ross AS, Irani S, Gan SI, et al. Dual-modality drainage of infected and symptomatic walled-off pancreatic necrosis: long-term clinical outcomes. Gastrointest Endosc 2014;79: 929–35.
[82] van Baal MC, Bollen TL, Bakker OJ, et al. The role of routine fine-needle aspiration in the diagnosis of infected necrotizing pancreatitis. Surgery 2014;155:442–8.
[83] Hollemans RA, Bakker OJ, Boermeester MA, et al. Superiority of step-up approach vs open necrosectomy in long-term follow-up of patients with necrotizing pancreatitis. Gastroenterology 2019;156:1016–26.
[84] van Grinsven J, Timmerman P, van Lienden KP, et al. Proactive versus standard percutaneous catheter drainage for infected necrotizing pancreatitis. Pancreas 2017;46:518–23.
[85] Baron TH, Thaggard WG, Morgan DE, et al. Endoscopic therapy for organized pancreatic necrosis. Gastroenterology 1996;111:755–64.
[86] Nemoto Y, Attam R, Arain MA, et al. Interventions for walled off necrosis using an algorithm based endoscopic step-up approach: outcomes in a large cohort of patients. Pancreatology 2017;17:663–8.
[87] Trikudanathan G, Tawfik P, Amateau SK, et al. Early (<4 Weeks) Versus Standard (>/= 4 Weeks) endoscopically centered step-up interventions for necrotizing pancreatitis. Am J Gastroenterol 2018;113:1550–8.
[88] Driedger M, Zyromski NJ, Visser BC, et al. Surgical transgastric necrosectomy for necrotizing pancreatitis: a single-stage procedure for walled-off pancreatic necrosis. Ann Surg 2018;271:163–8.
[89] Zyromski NJ, Nakeeb A, House MG, et al. Transgastric pancreatic necrosectomy: how I do it. J Gastrointest Surg 2016;20:445–9.
[90] Maatman TK, Roch AM, Ceppa EP, et al. Damage control pancreatic débridement: salvaging the most severely ill. JOP 2019;20:37–43.
[91] Parikh PY, Pitt HA, Kilbane M, et al. Pancreatic necrosectomy: North American mortality is much lower than expected. J Am Coll Surg 2009;209:712–9.
[92] Das SL, Singh PP, Phillips AR, et al. Newly diagnosed diabetes mellitus after acute pancreatitis: a systematic review and meta-analysis. Gut 2014;63:818–31.
[93] Umapathy C, Raina A, Saligram S, et al. Natural history after acute necrotizing pancreatitis: a large US Tertiary care experience. J Gastrointest Surg 2016;20:1844–53.

[94] Ahmed Ali U, Issa Y, Hagenaars JC, et al. Risk of recurrent pancreatitis and progression to chronic pancreatitis after a first episode of acute pancreatitis. Clin Gastroenterol Hepatol 2016;14:738–46.
[95] Howard TJ, Moore SA, Saxena R, et al. Pancreatic duct strictures are a common cause of recurrent pancreatitis after successful management of pancreatic necrosis. Surgery 2004;136:909–16.
[96] Nealon WH, Bhutani M, Riall TS, et al. A unifying concept: pancreatic ductal anatomy both predicts and determines the major complications resulting from pancreatitis. J Am Coll Surg 2009;208:790–9 [discussion: 799-801].
[97] Easler J, Muddana V, Furlan A, et al. Portosplenomesenteric venous thrombosis in patients with acute pancreatitis is associated with pancreatic necrosis and usually has a benign course. Clin Gastroenterol Hepatol 2014;12:854–62.
[98] Al-Azzawi HH, Kuhlenschmidt H, Howard TJ, et al. The burden of incisional hernia in necrotizing pancreatitis: how can we improve? Am J Surg 2010;199:310–4 [discussion: 314].
[99] Cinquepalmi L, Boni L, Dionigi G, et al. Long-term results and quality of life of patients undergoing sequential surgical treatment for severe acute pancreatitis complicated by infected pancreatic necrosis. Surg Infect (Larchmt) 2006;7(Suppl 2):S113–6.
[100] Hochman D, Louie B, Bailey R. Determination of patient quality of life following severe acute pancreatitis. Can J Surg 2006;49:101–6.
[101] Wright SE, Lochan R, Imrie K, et al. Quality of life and functional outcome at 3, 6 and 12 months after acute necrotising pancreatitis. Intensive Care Med 2009;35:1974–8.

Advances in Surgery 56 (2022) 37–48

ADVANCES IN SURGERY

Should We Utilize Routine Cholangiography?

L. Michael Brunt, MD

Section of Minimally Invasive Surgery, Department of Surgery, Washington University School of Medicine, 660 S Euclid Avenue, St. Louis, MO 63110, USA

Keywords

• Cholecystectomy • Cholangiography • Bile duct injury • Common bile duct stones • Near-infrared cholangiography

Key points

- Intraoperative cholangiography is a unique and essential component of cholecystectomy and management of patients with gallstone disease.
- Intraoperative cholangiography should be used liberally in patients who are at increased risk for having common bile duct stones.
- In patients with acute cholecystitis and uncertainty of biliary anatomy, intraoperative cholangiography may mitigate the risk of bile duct injury.
- Alternatives to IOC are laparoscopic intraoperative ultrasound and near-infrared cholangiography but the latter does not allow assessment for bile duct stones.
- All general surgery trainees should become facile with performing intraoperative cholangiography and interpreting cholangiogram images during training.

Intraoperative cholangiography (IOC) has been an integral component of performing cholecystectomy for almost 90 years. The ability to carry out real-time fluoroscopic imaging of the biliary tree has many advantages that include accurate assessment and understanding of biliary anatomy and detection of common bile duct (CBD) stones. Whether cholangiography should be performed routinely or selectively has been a matter of considerable debate, with no consensus on this topic. However, there should be no debate that surgeons (and trainees) who perform cholecystectomy should be facile in performing IOC and be able to accurately interpret cholangiogram images. In this review, various aspects of the indications for IOC, technique of cholangiography, and its role in prevention and detection of bile duct injury (BDI) will

E-mail address: bruntm@wustl.edu

https://doi.org/10.1016/j.yasu.2022.02.002
0065-3411/22/

be discussed. Alternatives and adjuncts to IOC for intraoperative biliary imaging will also be presented.

HISTORY OF CHOLANGIOGRAPHY

The era of biliary imaging was ushered in with the development of the oral cholecystogram by Graham and Cole in 1925. The next major advance was high-resolution ultrasound, which became the preferred imaging modality for the diagnosis of gallstones in the 1980s. The first series of intraoperative cholangiograms was reported by Pablo Mirrizzi in 1932. His many contributions to biliary surgery included defining anatomy and function of the sphincter of Oddi and the first use of a T-tube after performing CBD exploration [1]. For the first few decades of use, IOC was performed using static plain x-rays, which was cumbersome as the films had to be developed and processed in a film room and then returned to the operating room for viewing. The technique was time-consuming and often required repeat imaging if there was inadequate ductal filling or other abnormalities. Fluoroscopic cholangiography developed by George Berci and others eventually replaced static imaging early in the laparoscopic cholecystectomy era and is now the standard method of intraoperative radiographic visualization of the biliary tree. With the advent of laparoscopic cholecystectomy, techniques were developed for laparoscopic ultrasound imaging, which were soon applied to the biliary tree. More recently, near-infrared imaging techniques have been applied to the biliary tree with applications both in cholecystectomy and liver surgery.

RATIONALE FOR IOC

Whether to perform IOC routinely or selectively has been an area of controversy almost since the beginnings of laparoscopic cholecystectomy over 30 years ago. Regardless of one's position in this debate, there are several reasons why surgeons should be skilled in performing IOC so they can do it reliably when the indications are compelling: (1) it is an essential and unique skill component of managing patients with gallstone disease and performing cholecystectomy that requires facility to perform reliably; (2) experience with IOC enables accurate interpretation of the various cholangiogram findings and alterations in biliary anatomy; (3) IOC is an important component of training for general surgery trainees in order for them to become facile with it before entering surgical practice; (4) it is a prerequisite to performing laparoscopic CBD exploration and avoiding missed CBD stones in at-risk patients; and (5) it may reduce the risk of BDI in some circumstances (as discussed below) and/or prevent a higher level injury from occurring if the CBD has been misidentified as the cystic duct.

INDICATIONS FOR CHOLANGIOGRAPHY

The classic indications for performing IOC are listed in Box 1 and include suspicion of possible CBD stones, the risk of which is greater in patients with any of several preoperative variables such as abnormal liver function tests, a history

Box 1: Indications for intraoperative cholangiography

Preoperative:

- Abnormal liver function tests
- Dilated common bile duct on preoperative imaging (>7-8 mm)
- Suspected CBD stone on ultrasound/CT scan or MRCP
- History of pancreatitis/gallstone pancreatitis
- Acute cholecystitis of history of acute cholecystitis
- Jaundice of history of jaundice
- History of prior Roux-en-Y gastric bypass
- History of ERCP for CBD stones

Intraoperative:

- Dilated common bile duct
- Stones in the cystic duct
- Unclear anatomy
- Suspicion of possible bile duct injury

or presence of jaundice, dilated CBD on ultrasound, and a history of gallstone pancreatitis. Multiple small gallstones have also been associated with an increased risk of passing stones into the CBD. A recent large institutional series of laparoscopic cholecystectomies with IOC in patients with gallstone pancreatitis operated within 7 days of onset of symptoms found the incidence of persistent CBD stones to be 19.9% [2]. In addition, a history of prior Roux-en-Y gastric bypass should be considered a compelling reason to do IOC because of the likely inability to access the duodenum and bile duct by endoscopic retrograde cholangiopancreatography (ERCP) postoperatively. Intraoperatively, the finding of a stone in the cystic duct increases somewhat the risk of finding a CBD stone as well and should be considered an indication. In cases of uncertainty of anatomy or any suspicion of a BDI, cholangiography can be critical in defining the anatomy, avoiding further injury, and determining how to proceed.

The reported technical success rate of performing IOC has been in the 82% to 97% range and in most series has been over 90% [1]. The reported sensitivity of IOC for detection of bile duct stones has been between 75% and 100% with overall accuracy rates for stone detection of 92% to 99%. (Reviewed in Ref. 2.) In the laparoscopic era, utilization rates of IOC have varied considerably, ranging from 2.4% to 98.4% in one Medicare claims database study [3] to not at all in some reported institutional series [4].

TECHNIQUE

Performance of IOC is carried out after confirmation of achieving the critical view of safety. Typically, the cystic artery is clipped and divided although it can be left intact and a clip is placed on the upper cystic duct/neck of the gallbladder. In some cases, it may be necessary to tie the neck of the gallbladder if a clip does not adequately occlude it. A cystic ductotomy is then made in the upper cystic duct and the duct is dilated with microscissors to disrupt any cystic duct valves. A 4 French cholangiocatheter (ureteral catheter) is then inserted through a cholangioclamp and secured in place with the clamp (Fig. 1). Alternatively, the catheter may be secured by a partially occluding clip or a disposable balloon occluding catheter may be used. Contrast is then injected (typically 50:50 mix of Conray 60% and saline) under fluoroscopy. The initial injection should be slow to visualize details in the distal duct and then more rapidly to fill the entire ductal system. Fluoroscopy time can be minimized by starting with still shots until adequate contrast begins to fill the distal duct before using continuous fluoroscopy. A complete cholangiogram should include visualization of the common bile and hepatic ducts, the right and left hepatic ducts, cystic duct, and presence of contrast entering the duodenum (Fig. 2). It must be emphasized that both the right anterior and posterior hepatic ducts should be seen. If no contrast enters the duodenum, glucagon 1 mg intravenously can be given to relax the sphincter of Oddi and reinjection performed 3 to 4 minutes later. The images should be carefully viewed for filling defects and aberrant anatomy. Common variants include a separate right hepatic or right posterior hepatic duct that enters the common hepatic duct below the left hepatic duct, a cystic duct that joins the right hepatic duct (Figs. 3), and a cystic duct that runs parallel to the CBD or spirals and enters the CBD on the left side. Some experience with cholangiography is necessary to ensure accurate interpretation of the images acquired. Failure to visualize the proximal common hepatic or right hepatic ducts should raise concern for a possible injury and further assessment. One should never presume that failure of proximal duct visualization is acceptable, as it could mean a clip has been placed on the CBD above the catheter insertion site. Maneuvers that may be carried out if only the distal duct is seen include putting the patient in Trendelenberg position, repositioning the catheter, and giving morphine to cause the sphincter of Oddi to contract.

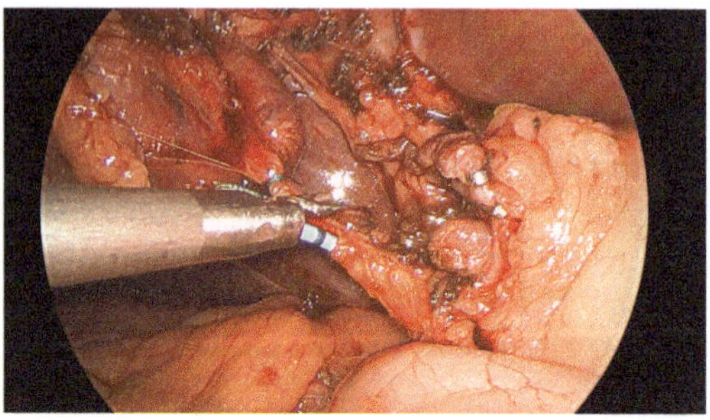

Fig. 1. Cystic duct cannulation for intraoperative cholangiography. A 4 French ureteral catheter is used placed through a cystic ductotomy and the catheter is secured through a cholangioclamp.

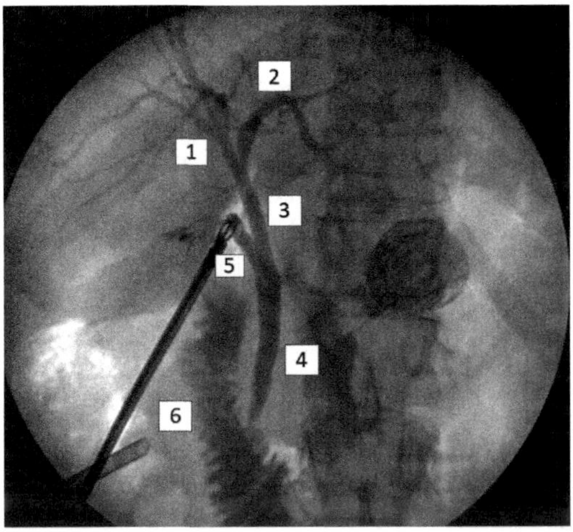

Fig. 2. Normal intraoperative cholangiogram. Ductal structures visualized are: 1—right hepatic ducts; 2—left hepatic duct; 3—common hepatic duct; 4—common bile duct; 5—cystic duct; and 6—duodenum.

If stones are found in the CBD, management options include administration of glucagon and flushing with saline, transcystic CBD exploration, laparoscopic choledochotomy (if the CBD is dilated over 8–10 mm and the stone(s) is larger than 6-7 mm), or postoperative ERCP according to the circumstances and surgeon experience with CBD exploration. One of the aforementioned minimally invasive options is almost always possible, and open CBD exploration should

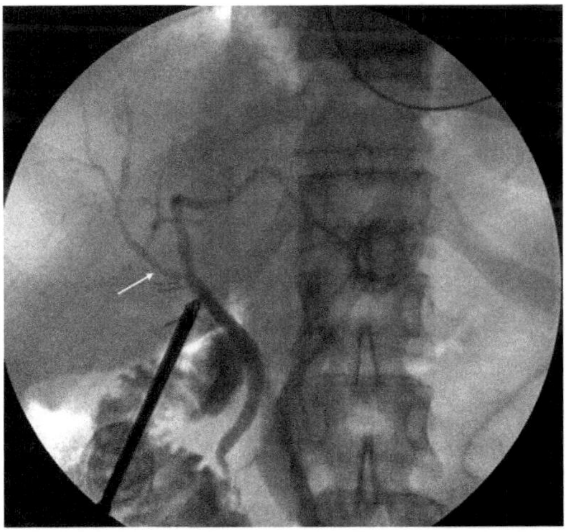

Fig. 3. Intraoperative cholangiogram in a patient with a separate right hepatic duct (*arrow*) that enters into the common hepatic duct.

be rarely needed unless multiple large stones or an impacted stone are found in the bile duct.

In some cases, it may not be possible to cannulate the cystic duct adequately due to cystic duct valves, but the success rate should be over 90% with experience. The time to do IOC should be 7 to 10 minutes in most cases. An alternative to IOC via the cystic duct is direct gallbladder (GB) puncture or use of a specialized device (Kumar clamp) with installation of contrast. This approach takes additional time for contrast to enter the biliary tree and may fail in cases in which there is occlusion of the cystic duct by a stone.

PREVENTION OF BDI

Controversy exists on whether the use of IOC can prevent bile duct injuries during cholecystectomy. The Society of American Gastrointestinal Surgeons (SAGES) has addressed this issue as a part of the Safe Cholecystectomy program. A Delphi expert consensus was undertaken to identify the factors most critical for the safe performance of cholecystectomy [5]. Thirty-nine factors were rated by 160 SAGES committee members using a nominal group consensus process. This process led to the development of the SAGES Six-Step program for safe cholecystectomy (https://www.sages.org/safe-cholecystectomy-program/). One of the 6 steps was to make liberal use of cholangiography or other methods to image the biliary tree intraoperatively.

Subsequently, a multisociety consensus conference and clinical practice guideline addressed the question of whether IOC versus other means of imaging the biliary tree should be used to mitigate the risk of BDI during cholecystectomy in a detailed review of the evidence on this topic [6]. Prospective, randomized trials have been underpowered to examine this issue. Fourteen studies mostly of large administrative type databases found some association of IOC with a reduced BDI incidence: odds ratio (OR) 0.78 (95% confidence interval [CI] 0.63–0.96) unadjusted and 0.81 (95% CI, 0.62–1.07) adjusted. These studies were at moderate to high risk of bias because of the nature of the administrative data. The best data on this question come from the Swedish National GallRiks data, which captures over 90% of all cholecystectomies performed in that country. They found that the intent to use IOC was associated with a lower risk of death [7]. A further Gallriks analysis found that the use of IOC significantly decreased the occurrence of BDI in patients with acute cholecystitis (OR 0.44, 95% CI 0.30–0.63) or a history of acute cholecystitis (OR 0.57, 95% CI 0.35–1.02) but not in patients who did not have acute cholecystitis (OR 1.06, 95% CI 0.75–1.49) [8]. Based on these data, the guideline panel suggested that in patients with acute cholecystitis or a history of acute cholecystitis, IOC be performed to mitigate the risk of BDI. No recommendation was made for patients with uncomplicated biliary colic.

Other groups have argued that IOC may not protect against BDI during laparoscopic cholecystectomy. Sheffield and colleagues [9] studied all Medicare claims in Texas from 2000 through 2009 that included 92,932 patients who underwent cholecystectomy. IOC was performed in 37,533 cases (40.4%). The rate of BDI was 0.21% in patients who had IOC versus 0.36% in patients who did not undergo IOC. A logistic regression model that controlled for surgeon, hospital, and patient characteristics found an increased odds of BDI in cholecystectomies in which IOC was not performed versus those in which IOC was done (OR 1.79, 95% CI 1.35–2.36, $P<.01$). When confounding was controlled for using instrumental variable analysis, the association of IOC and a reduction in BDI was no longer present (OR 1.26, 85% CI 0.81–1.96, $P = .31$). An interesting aspect of the Sheffield study is that hospitals that used IOC more frequently had higher BDI rates when they *did not use it* (0.12% with IOC, 0.76% without IOC); conversely, hospitals that used IOC infrequently had higher BDI rates when *they did use it* (0.96% with IOC vs 0.25% without IOC), the latter implying perhaps that it was used when there was a concern of a potential problem.

Another question regarding IOC considered by the guideline panel was its role in cases in which there is intraoperative suspicion of a possible BDI or uncertainty of biliary anatomy. An analysis of 8 studies of 1256 BDI cases was done that compared IOC versus no IOC and the intraoperative recognition of injury [6]. Most studies strongly favored IOC for intraoperative detection (OR 2.92, 95% CI 1.55–5.68). Although there was low certainty of evidence, because of the considerably higher risk to patients in this situation, the panel made a strong recommendation for use of IOC to mitigate the risk of further BDI. In one of the largest studies examining this issue, Alvarez and associates successfully performed IOC in 95.7% of 11,432 consecutively laparoscopic cholecystectomies [10]. Twenty patients had a BDI and the diagnosis was made intraoperatively in 18 of those patients (90%). Importantly, all of the injuries diagnosed during surgery were repaired at the time of the initial procedure. It is important to emphasize the point that if the bile duct is mistaken for the cystic duct and is cannulated during cholangiography, proper interpretation of the images should prevent one from proceeding with dissection and resection of a portion of the bile duct, creating a higher level injury that is more complex to repair. One should never proceed with removal of the gallbladder when there is no filling/visualization of the proximal bile ducts on cholangiography for this reason. Rather, one should call for help from another surgeon, move the dissection higher up on the neck of the gallbladder, or if a BDI is confirmed, stop, place a drain and refer/transfer the patient to a tertiary institution with expertise in BDI repair.

ALTERNATIVES TO IOC

Laparoscopic ultrasound has also been shown to be effective in defining intraoperative anatomy and detection of bile duct stones. Whether it can reduce the incidence of BDI is unclear but it should be considered an acceptable alternative for surgeons who have developed the skill and facility with this modality. It has the advantage of no radiation exposure and not requiring cannulation of the cystic duct. The disadvantages of ultrasound are that surgeons are not widely trained in it and it has not been studied as extensively as cholangiography.

Near-infrared fluorescent cholangiography (NIRC) has gained much attention recently as an alternative or supplement to IOC during cholecystectomy.

NIRC has the advantage of allowing biliary mapping throughout the procedure at various time points in the dissection both before and after the critical view of safety has been reached and avoids radiation exposure. It does not allow examination of the bile duct for stones and has not been studied widely in obese patients (Fig. 4) or conditions of biliary inflammation where the risk of BDI is

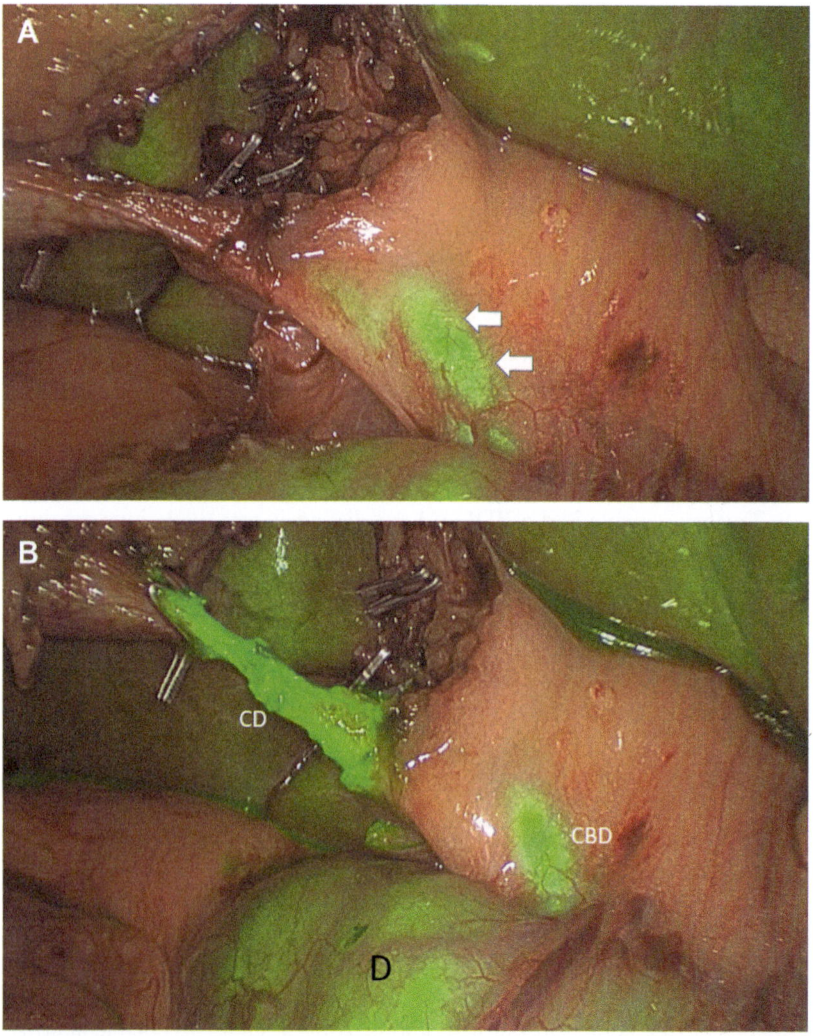

Fig. 4. Near-infrared cholangiography in a patient with a BMI of 41 kg/m^2. (*A*) Fluorescence can be seen in the common bile duct (*arrows*) with background fluorescence in the liver and also in the duodenum but the common hepatic duct is not visualized due to overlying fat. Note there is also no fluorescence of the cystic duct. (*B*) After opening the cystic duct and clearing sludge from it, fluorescence is now seen in the cystic duct (CD), the common bile duct (CBD), and the duodenum (D).

greatest. It also requires specialized imaging equipment, which may not be readily available in many operating rooms.

Dip and colleagues [11] carried out a prospective randomized trial of 640 patients that compared white light alone (N = 318 to white light plus NIRC [N = 321]). They found that visualization rates of biliary ducts were significantly better before dissection in the NIRC group versus white light alone. Similar differences were observed postdissection except no differences were seen for identification of the cystic duct and cystic duct/gallbladder junction. Two patients, both in the white light group, suffered a minor biliary injury. In a recent meta-analysis that compared NIRC with IOC, 7 studies that included 481 patients were analyzed [12]. Overall, visualization rates were higher for the cystic duct, cystic duct-CBD junction, and common hepatic duct for the majority of studies. However, the lower visualization rates with IOC were largely due to technical failures to successfully cannulate the cystic duct in the IOC group rather than limitations of this modality.

The consensus conference guideline panel reviewed all available evidence on NIRC and observed that most studies were small, and the data were insufficient to address the question of impact on BDI. Data were also inconclusive to make a recommendation regarding its comparison to IOC. However, based on data from Dip and others using identification of biliary anatomy as a surrogate for risk of BDI, the panel posited that near-infrared imaging may be used as an adjunct to white light alone for identification of biliary anatomy during LC. However, it should not be a substitute for good dissection technique and use of the critical view of safety. The author has found NIRC to be most useful in difficult gallbladder cases and such as cases of elective remnant cholecystectomy after prior subtotal or incomplete cholecystectomy (Fig. 5).

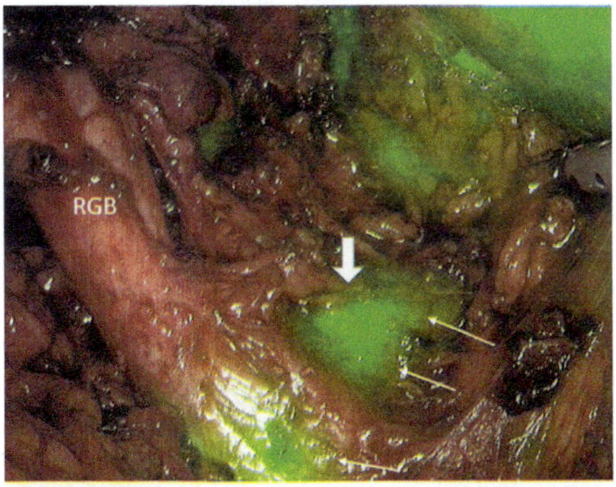

Fig. 5. Remnant cholecystectomy with near-infrared cholangiography after previous remote subtotal cholecystectomy. Note the fluorescence in the common bile duct (*arrows*) but not in the remnant gallbladder (RGB).

CBD STONES

Preoperative suspicion that a patient may have a CBD stone should be raised if a dilated duct (>8 mm) is seen on ultrasound, there is a history of jaundice or persistently abnormal liver function tests, or a stone is seen in the bile duct on ultrasound or CT scan. Additional studies that may be performed preoperatively that may impact the management algorithm include magnetic resonance cholangiopancreatography (MRCP). The sensitivity of MRCP for the detection of CBD stones is over 90% and the specificity approaches 100% [13]. However, it is expensive to perform, but may lower costs if it avoids a preoperative ERCP. Endoscopic ultrasound also has high sensitivity and specificity for the detection of CBD stones and may be superior to MRCP. Another advantage of EUS is that it could be performed in conjunction with ERCP, but it is an invasive procedure that requires anesthesia.

The most direct and cost-effective approach to the management of choledocholithiasis is laparoscopic cholecystectomy with IOC and laparoscopic CBD exploration (Fig. 6). IOC is a prerequisite to performing CBD exploration. It is beyond the scope of this review to delve into CBD exploration technique, but suffice it to say that facility with cannulation of the cystic duct is the first step toward laparoscopic CBD exploration, which most often is performed using a transcystic approach. In addition to lower costs, advantages of laparoscopic CBD exploration over postoperative ERCP include one-stage management of the problem, potentially shorter hospitalization, and avoidance of the risk of post-ERCP pancreatitis [14].

A clinical spotlight review from SAGES on the management of choledocholithiasis provides a recent evidence-based literature summary on approaches to the management of CBD stones [13]. They note 2 prior systematic reviews, which found

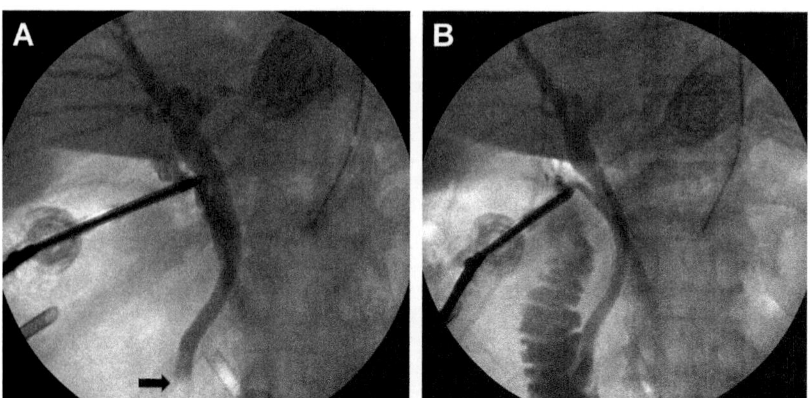

Fig. 6. (*A*) Intraoperative cholangiogram that shows a dilated bile duct with a meniscus in the distal duct (*arrow*) and no contrast entering the duodenum. Laparoscopic transcystic common bile duct exploration was performed with removal of 3 small stones and sludge. (*B*) Cholangiogram after stone clearance that shows no filling defects and good flow of contrast into the duodenum.

similar efficacy rates between a 2-stage procedure with ERCP and single-stage laparoscopic (Lap) cholecystectomy/CBD exploration with no significant differences in patient morbidity or mortality [15,16]. The single-stage approach was associated with longer operative times but resulted in fewer interventions and was, therefore, a more cost-effective strategy. Two other recent meta-analyses have addressed this topic. Pan and colleagues [17] analyzed 13 studies that were either prospective randomized trials or observational cohort and case-controlled studies. The 13 studies involved 1757 patients (872 LC + Lap CBD exploration vs 885 LC + ERCP). They found a higher stone clearance rate with Lap CBD exploration (94.1% vs 90.0%, $P = .012$). Other variables of perioperative complications, conversion to other procedure, retained stones rates, length of hospital stay, and total hospital charges all favored laparoscopic CBD exploration as well. Most recently, a meta-analysis of 5 randomized trials involving 860 patients was published [18]. No differences between LC/Lap CBDE versus ERCP + LC were found regarding technical success rates, morbidity, and conversion rates. Bile leaks (2.6% vs 0.5%) and retained stones (8.5% vs 3.6%) occurred more often in the LC + Lap CBDE group, whereas postoperative pancreatitis was more common in the ERCP + LC group (2.0% vs 8.4%).

SUMMARY

IOC is an important aspect of the safe performance of cholecystectomy, and all surgeons who do this procedure should be adept at performing it. This author does not presume to recommend that IOC should be done routinely, but it should be used liberally for the indications discussed in this review. Evidence also suggests that in some circumstances such as acute cholecystitis, difficult cholecystectomy, or unclear anatomy, it may mitigate the risk or severity of BDI. Learning how to perform cholangiography and interpret cholangiogram images should be a key component of every general surgery training program.

CLINICS CARE POINTS

- When performing intraoperative cholangiography, ensure that the entire biliary tree is visualized, that there is contrast emptying into the duodenum, and be aware of the potential for aberrant ductal anatomy.
- In the setting of uncertainty of anatomy or concern for possible bile duct injury during cholecystectomy, perform intraoperative cholangiography to help define the anatomy and avoid a higher level of injury.
- When undertaking cholecystectomy in patients with a prior gastric bypass, always perform intraoperative cholangiography to avoid missed common bile duct stones, which would be more difficult to manage once the gallbladder is out.
- Recognize that the most efficient and cost-effective approach to the management of common bile duct stones is intraoperative cholangiography and laparoscopic common bile duct exploration with stone extraction.

DISCLOSURE

Dr Brunt has no commercial relationships to disclose.

References

[1] Hope WW, Fanelli R, Walsh DS, et al. SAGES clinical spotlight review: Intraoperative cholangiography. Surg Endosc 2017;31:2007–16.
[2] Fratantoni ME, Giuffrida P, Menno J, et al. Prevalence of persistent common bile duct stones and acute biliary pancreatitis remains stable within the 1st week of symptoms. J Gastrointest Surg 2021;25:3178–87.
[3] Sheffield KM, Han Y, Kuo Y-F, et al. Variation in the use of intraoperative cholangiography during cholecystectomy. J Am Coll Surg 2012;214:668–81.
[4] Ammori MB, Al-Dabbagh AK. Laparoscopic cholecystectomy without intraoperative cholangiography. J Laparoendosc Adv Surg Tech A 2012;22:146–51.
[5] Pucher PH, Brunt LM, Fanelli RD, et al. SAGES expert Delphi consensus: critical factors for safe surgical factors in cholecystectomy. Surg Endosc 2015;29:3074–85.
[6] Brunt LM, Deziel DJ, Telem DA, et al. Safe cholecystectomy multi-society practice guideline and state of the art consensus conference on prevention of bile duct injury during cholecystectomy. Ann Surg 2020;272:3–23, co-publication Surg Endosc 2020; 34: 2827-2855.
[7] Tornqvist B, Stromberg C, Persson G, et al. Effect of intraoperative cholangiographic and early detection of bile duct injury on survival after cholecystectomy: Population based cohort study. BMJ 2012;345:e6457.
[8] Tornqvist B, Stromberg C, Akre O, et al. Selective intraoperative cholangiography and risk of bile duct injury during cholecystectomy. Br J Surg 2015;102:952–8.
[9] Sheffield KM, Riall TS, Han Y, et al. Association between cholecystectomy with verses without intraoperative cholangiography and risk of common duct injury. JAMA 2013;310:812–20.
[10] Alvarez FA, deSantibanies M, Palaveccino M, et al. impact of routine intraoperative cholangiography during laparoscopic cholecystectomy on bile duct injury. Br J Surg 2014;101: 677–84.
[11] Dip F, LoMenzo E, Sarotto L, et al. Randomized trial of near-infrared incisionless fluorescent cholangiography. Ann Surg 2019;270:992–9.
[12] Lim SH, Tan HTA, Shelat VG. Comparison of indocyanine green dye fluorescent cholangiography with intra-operative cholangiography in laparoscopic cholecystectomy: a meta-analysis. Surg Endosc 2021;35:1511–20.
[13] Narula VK, Fung EC, Overby DW, et al. Clinical spotlight review for the management of choledocholithiasis. Surg Endosc 2020;34:1482–91.
[14] Berci G, Hunter J, Morgenstern L, et al. Laparoscopic cholecystectomy: 1st, do no harm; 2nd, take care of bile duct stones. Surg Endosc 2013;27:1051–4.
[15] Dasari BV, Tan CJ, Gurusamy KS, et al. Surgical verses endoscopic treatment of bile duct stones. Cochrane Database Syst Rev 2013;12:1–126.
[16] Urbach DR, Khajanchee YS, Jobe BA, et al. Cost-effective management of common bile duct stones: A decision analysis of the use of endoscopic retrograde cholangiopancreatography (ERCP), intra-operative cholangiography, and laparoscopic bile duct exploration. Surg Endosc 2001;15:4–13.
[17] Pan L, Chen M, Ji L, et al. The safety and efficacy of laparoscopic common bile duct exploration combined with cholecystectomy for the management of cholecysto-choledocholithiasis: An up to date meta-analysis. Ann Surg 2018;268:247–53.
[18] Zhu J, Li G, Zhou X, et al. Laparoscopic common bile duct exploration versus intraoperative endoscopic retrograde cholangiopancreatography in patients with gallbladder and common bile duct stones: a meta-analysis. Surg Endosc 2021;35:997–1005.

Advances in Surgery 56 (2022) 49–67

ADVANCES IN SURGERY

Reducing Firearm Injury and Death in the United States

Joseph V. Sakran, MD, MPH, MPA[a,*], Nicole Lunardi, MD, MSPH[b]

[a]Emergency General Surgery, Division of Acute Care Surgery, Department of Surgery, Johns Hopkins Hospital, 1800 Orleans Street, Sheikh Zayed Tower / Suite 6107B, Baltimore, MD 21287, USA; [b]Department of Surgery, UT Southwestern Medical Center, 5323 Harry Hines Boulevard, Dallas, TX 75390-9159, USA

Keywords

• Firearm injury • Suicide • Homicide • Prevention • Firearm policy
• Prehospital care • Trauma systems • Hospital-based violence prevention programs

Key points

- In 2019, there were nearly 40,000 firearm fatalities. Most of these deaths were suicides followed by homicides.
- Firearm injuries cost approximately $280 billion annually.
- The political and social determinants of firearm injury must be addressed in prevention efforts.
- Primary prevention includes evidence-based policy and furthering firearm research.
- Secondary and tertiary prevention include improvements in prehospital and hospital care, trauma systems, survivors' networks, and hospital-based violence prevention programs.

Internationally, there were an estimated 251,000 firearm deaths in 2016. The preponderance of these deaths was among civilians unrelated to armed conflict. More than 50% of all firearm deaths occurred in countries that account for less than 10% of the total global population: the United States, Brazil, Mexico, Venezuela, and Guatemala [1]. How is it that American lives have become a major contributor to the number of firearm deaths worldwide? This

*Corresponding author. *E-mail address:* jsakran1@jhmi.edu
Twitter: @JosephSakran (J.V.S.)

https://doi.org/10.1016/j.yasu.2022.03.001
0065-3411/22/

article aims to explore firearm morbidity and mortality, an American public health crisis, and we will explore the burden, causes, and opportunities for prevention.

Americans own more guns per capita than any other country, with 120.5 firearms per 100 residents [2]. Between 2001 and 2019, there were 634,221 firearm-related deaths accounting for more than 15 million years of potential life lost in the United States. During the same time frame, there were more than 1.5 million nonfatal firearm injury emergency department (ED) visits [3] (Fig. 1). This translates to more than 300 gun-related incidents per day. Ninety-three percent of these injuries required treatment in the ED, of which 50% were hospitalized and 43% subsequently discharged from the ED. If the human toll is not enough, there is a significant economic burden of these injuries that is staggering, with a price tag estimated at $280 billion annually (Fig. 2). American taxpayers pay $12.7 billion for medical, police, and criminal justice costs annually: $270,399 per fatality and $53,000 per nonfatal incident [4]. The average cost of firearm ED and inpatient visits are $5000 and $96,000, respectively [5].

BURDEN OF DISEASE

Data on the demographics and circumstances of fatal and nonfatal firearm injuries are readily available via the Center for Disease Control National Center for Injury Prevention and Control's Web-based Injury Statistics Query and Reporting System. These data sources track injuries including, but not limited, to those caused by firearm. The nonfatal firearm injury data, as will be described

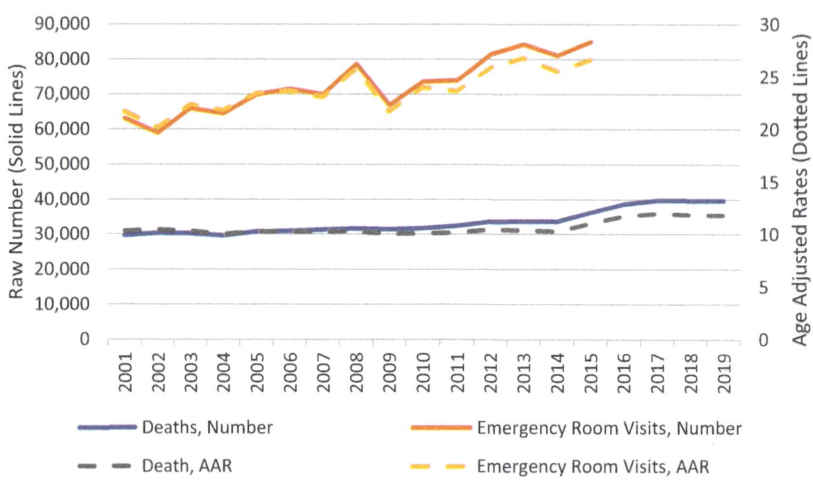

Fig. 1. Firearm-Related Deaths and Emergency Room Visits 2001 to 2019, Number and Age Adjusted Rates Cdc.gov. 2021. *WISQARS (Web-based Injury Statistics Query and Reporting System) I Injury Center I CDC.* [online] Available at: <https://www.cdc.gov/injury/wisqars/index.html>.

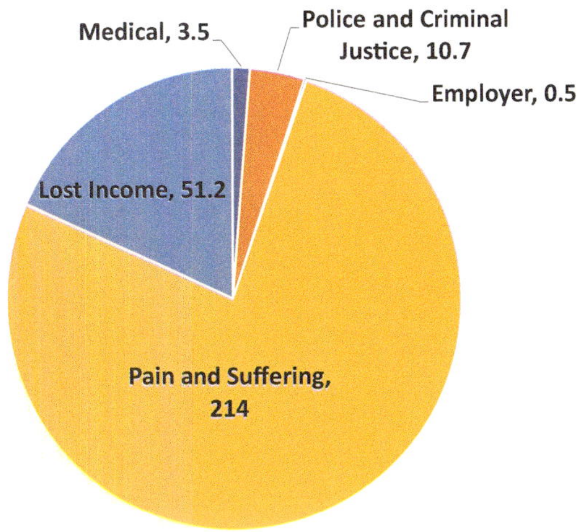

Fig. 2. Annual Economic Burn of Firearm Injury, Billions of US Dollars. Everytown Research & Policy. The economic cost of gun violence. https://everytownresearch.org/report/the-economic-cost-of-gun-violence/#lost-quality-of-life. Published February 18, 2021.

below, is far less robust compared with the data available for fatal injuries. In addition to demographic data regarding the victims, this resource also describes the cost, years of potential life lost, and intent of injury (suicide, homicide, unintentional, legal intervention, and not determined) as coded by the International Classification of Disease-10. Among the firearm-related deaths between 2001 and 2019, only 5089 (<1%) were of undetermined intent [3].

Suicide

Suicides account for most firearm deaths (59.2%) in the United States (Table 1). The suicide rate has been steadily increasing during the last decade and is highest in the Western states (Figs. 3 and 4). These deaths are majority white (92% age adjusted rate [AAR] 7.01), non-Hispanic (94%) men (87%) (see Fig. 4, Table 1) [3]. The age-adjusted firearm suicide rate increases with age (see Fig. 4, Table 1). Veterans, in particular, are at higher risk of firearm suicide than the civilian population [6]. Very few suicide attempts with a firearm survive due to the lethality of the weapon. In fact, there are so few nonfatal self-harm firearm injuries that the absolute number is not reported [3].

Homicide

Homicides account for 37% of all firearm deaths (see Table 1) [3]. The homicide rate has been increasing nationally, with notable rise in large American urban cities (see Fig. 4) [7]. The concentration of interpersonal, community violence has been well documented. Most of homicide victims are African American (56%, AAR 15.49), non-Hispanic (82%) men (84%) between the ages of 20 and 40 years (61%) (Fig. 5, see Table 1). In fact, homicide is the leading cause of death in this demographic (see Fig. 5). Seventy-three percent of all

Table 1
Firearm-related deaths by intent, sex, race, ethnicity, and age 2001-2019

	Suicide	Homicide	Unintentional	Legal Intervention	Undetermined
Total (%[a])	375,569 (59.2%)	234,397 (37%)	11,379 (1.8%)	7787 (1.2%)	5089 (0.8%)
Sex (%[a])					
Men	325,988 (87%)	197,973 (84%)	9940 (87%)	7460 (96%)	4038 (79%)
Women	49,581 (13%)	36,424 (16%)	1439 (13%)	327 (4%)	1051 (21%)
Race (AAR[b])					
African American	22,044 (2.8)	131,251 (15.49)	2225 (0.26)	1924 (0.23)	897 (0.11)
American Indian	3378 (4.48)	2385 (2.93)	196 (0.24)	205 (0.25)	125 (0.15)
Asian	4671 (1.37)	4089 (1.18)	133 (0.04)	200 (0.06)	69 (0.02)
White	345,476 (7.01)	96,672 (2.13)	8825 (0.19)	5458 (0.12)	3998 (0.08)
Ethnicity (%[a])					
Hispanic	19,857 (5%)	40,703 (17%)	1071 (9%)	1595 (20%)	522 (10%)
Non-Hispanic	354,689 (94%)	192,688 (82%)	10,280 (90%)	6171 (79%)	4530 (89%)
Unknown	1023 (<1%)	1006 (<1%)	26 (0%)	21 (0%)	37 (1%)
Age (AAR[b])					
0–4	0 (0.00)	1067 (0.28)	426 (0.11)	1 (0.00)	48 (0.01)
5–9	8 (0.00)	1083 (0.28)	254 (0.07)	0 (0.00)	44 (0.01)
10–14	2065 (0.52)	2446 (0.62)	476 (0.12)	0 (0.00)	145 (0.04)
15–19	15,300 (3.77)	30,109 (7.43)	1377 (0.34)	458 (0.11)	573 (0.14)
20–24	27,758 (6.78)	49,851 (12.17)	1491 (0.36)	1159 (0.28)	784 (0.19)
25–29	26,655 (6.66)	40,563 (10.13)	1064 (0.27)	1237 (0.31)	578 (0.14)
30–34	25,063 (6.38)	30,070 (7.76)	804 (0.20)	1139 (0.29)	402 (0.10)
35–39	26,410 (6.70)	22,226 (5.63)	775 (0.20)	1031 (0.26)	394 (0.10)
40–44	29,808 (7.38)	16,998 (4.21)	751 (0.19)	815 (0.20)	368 (0.09)
45–49	33,999 (8.26)	13,019 (3.16)	763 (0.19)	671 (0.16)	344 (0.08)
50–54	36,446 (9.09)	9473 (2.36)	764 (0.19)	495 (0.12)	322 (0.08)
55–59	34,501(9.41)	6497 (1.77)	638 (0.17)	337 (0.09)	338 (0.09)
60–64	27,848 (9.02)	4114 (1.33)	442 (0.14)	207 (0.07)	218 (0.07)

65–69	22,623 (9.13)	2568 (1.04)	416 (0.17)	106 (0.04)	188 (0.08)
70–74	20,107 (10.42)	1701 (0.88)	308 (0.16)	56 (0.03)	127 (0.07)
75–79	18,430 (12.39)	1157 (0.78)	259 (0.17)	32 (0.02)	89 (0.06)
80–84	14,886 (13.7)	774 (0.71)	230 (0.21)	17 (0.02)	73 (0.07)
85+	13,624 (13.06)	566 (0.54)	138 (0.13)	11 (0.01)	45 (0.04)
Unknown	38 (0.00)	115 (0.00	3 (0.00)	-	9 (0.00)

[a]%, percent of total.
[b]AAR, Age Adjusted Rate, Cdc.gov. 2021. *WISQARS (Web-based Injury Statistics Query and Reporting System)|Injury Center|CDC*. [online] Available at: <https://www.cdc.gov/injury/wisqars/index.html>.

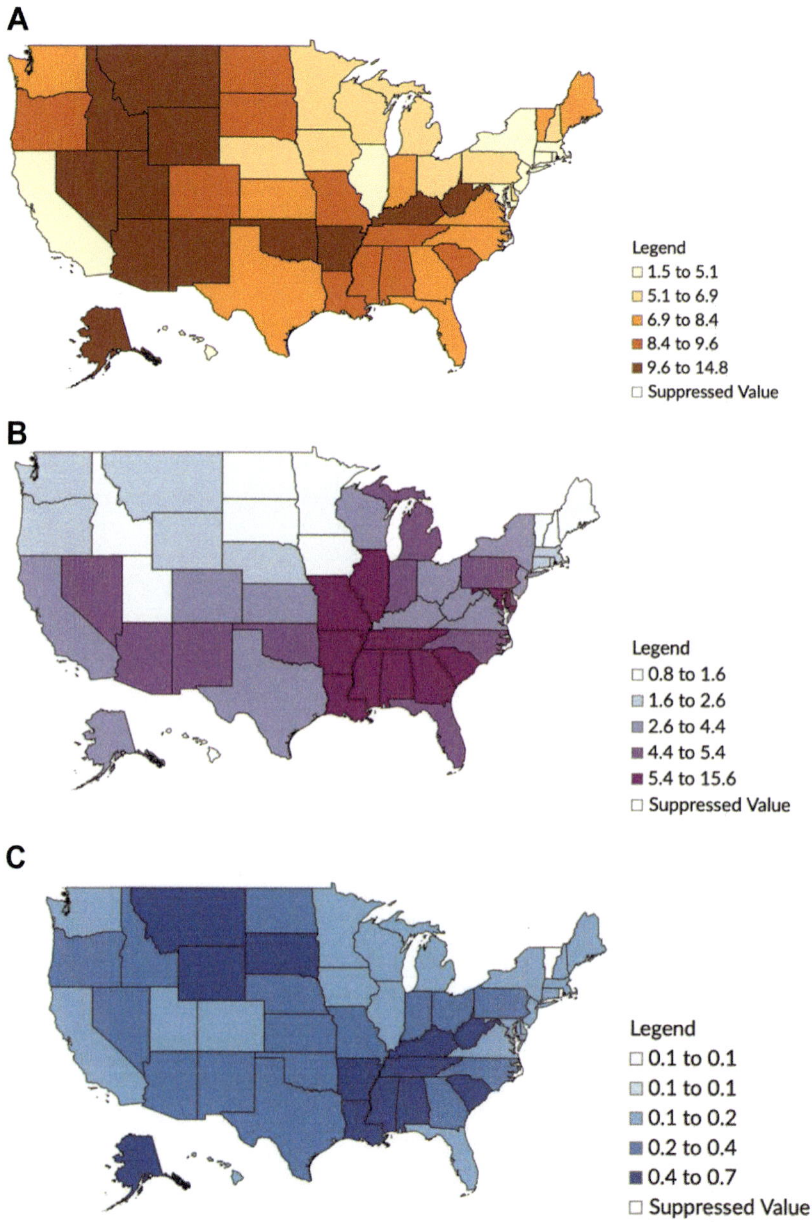

Fig. 3. Age adjusted Firearm death Density Maps by mechanism 2001 to 2019: (*A*) Suicide, (*B*) Homicide, (*C*) Unintended. Centers for disease control and prevention, national center for injury prevention and control. Web-based injury statistics Query and reporting system (wisqars) [online]. (2021) available from URL: www.cdc.gov/injury/wisqars.

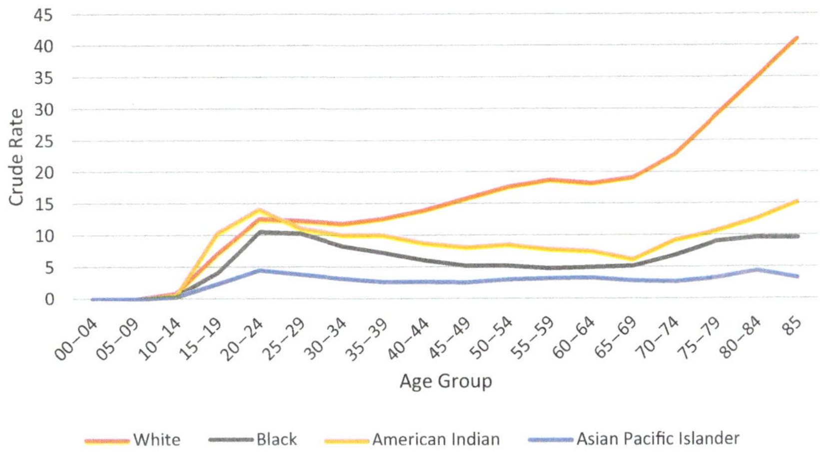

Fig. 4. Crude Rates of Suicides with Firearm among Men by Age Group and Race 2001 to 2019 CDC.gov. 2021. *WISQARS (Web-based Injury Statistics Query and Reporting System) | Injury Center | CDC.* [online] Available at: <https://www.cdc.gov/injury/wisqars/index.html>.

nonfatal firearm injuries are assault victims. Most of these individuals are also young (aged 10–40 years: 86%) men (89%). Race and ethnicity data are not well reported, with the only reported metric being 48% of these victims are African American (Table 2) [3].

Mass shootings victims are captured within the homicide and assault data. These events, by definition, include 4 or more victims that occur in a public

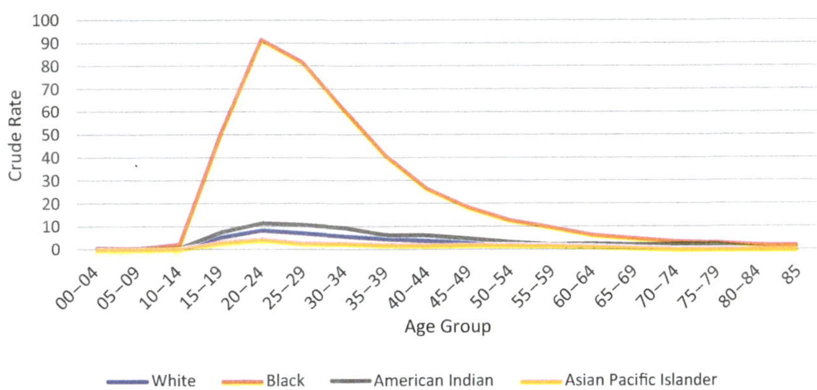

Fig. 5. Crude Rates of Homicides with Firearm among Men by Age Group and Race 2001 to 2019 CDC.gov. 2021. *WISQARS (Web-based Injury Statistics Query and Reporting System) | Injury Center | CDC.* [online] Available at: <https://www.cdc.gov/injury/wisqars/index.html>.

Table 2
Firearm-related nonfatal injuries by intent, sex, race, ethnicity and age 2001-2019

	Assault	Unintentional
	1,167,659 (73.4%)	330,102 (20.8%)
Sex (%[a])		
Men	1,041,045 (89%)	292,005 (88%)
Women	126,509(11%)	37,947 (11%)
Race (%[a])		
African American	557,129 (48%)	161,277 (49%)
American Indian	-	-
Asian	-	-
White	-	72,694 (22%)
Age (AAR[b])		
0–4	1675 (0.44)	-
5–9	-	-
10–14	11,878 (3.00)	9718 (2.45)
15–19	210,144 (51.83)	48,151 (11.88)
20–24	303,089 (74.00)	69,987 (17.09)
25–29	220,491 (55.05)	45,693 (11.41)
30–34	141,328 (35.95)	31,434 (8.00)
35–39	98,660 (25.01)	22,890 (5.80)
40–44	61,706 (15.27)	21,571 (5.34)
45–49	41,216 (10.01)	20,338 (4.94)
50–54	29,034 (7.25)	16,193 (4.04)
55–59	17,541 (4.78)	11,461 (3.13)
60–64	-	9232 (2.99)
65–69	-	-
70–74	2605 (1.35)	4632 (2.40)
75–79	-	3379 (2.27)
80–84	-	-
85+	-	-

[a]%, percent of total.
[b]AAR, Age Adjusted Rate Cdc.gov. 2021. *WISQARS (Web-based Injury Statistics Query and Reporting System) I Injury Center I CDC.* [online] Available at: <https://www.cdc.gov/injury/wisqars/index.html>.

setting. They account for less than 1% of all shooting victims. In 2021, for example, only 51 of the 6850 firearm deaths were related to mass shootings. Many more nonfatal injuries occurred, but there is no reliable reported estimate. These events are becoming more frequent, with one event every 47 days on average between 2015 and 2019. Among the 189 mass shooting events that occurred between 1966 and 2021, there were 202 shooters (98% men) using 360 firearms. Fifty-two percent of the firearms were acquired illegally [8–10].

Unintentional

There were 11,379 unintentional firearm deaths between 2001 and 2019, primarily among white (76%) men (87%) (see Table 1). The rate of these injuries has been decreasing during the past several decades. There were far more nonfatal unintentional injuries, with just more than 330,000 in the same time frame. These injuries, from the data available, were majority African American (49%) men (88%) (see Table 2) [3].

Legal intervention

Injuries inflicted by on-duty law enforcement are captured in WISQARS under the "legal intervention" mechanism. There were 7787 firearm-related deaths due to legal intervention between 2001 and 2019. Ninety-six percent of these victims were men. Although most of the victims were white (70%, AAR 0.12), the age adjusted mortality rate was higher among African American (0.23) and American Indians (0.25) (see Table 1) [3]. There are data to suggest these deaths are underreported, particularly among minorities [11,12].

CAUSE OF FIREARM INJURY

The unprecedented morbidity and mortality caused by firearms in the United States is not a new public health problem. In fact, it was first recognized as such in the 1980s [13]. How is it that 40 years later the country is still among the major contributors of firearm deaths worldwide? An understanding of the social and political determinants of firearm injury is necessary in order to truly engage in a discussion regarding prevention.

Political determinants of firearm injury

Structural racism

The burden of homicides is carried by a small fraction of American communities. It is an undeniable fact that the preponderance of homicide victims is black men. As previously mentioned, it is the number one leading cause of death in this demographic between the ages of 15 and 34 years [3].

For hundreds of years, structural racism, or race-based systems and policies, has shaped American communities [14]. Contrary to what contemporary political dialog would suggest, the systematic separation of wealth and resources by race has been perpetuated by both sides of the political aisle. The effects are, as a result, deeply rooted across housing, education, criminal justice, health care, etc. Policies of the Jim Crow era overtly segregated communities while policies after desegregation covertly kept neighborhoods segregated by differential housing values, mortgage lending, and prohibiting interracial marriage. More recently, the War on Drugs and Tough on Crime political agendas have resulted in the mass incarceration of men of color through racial profiling, mandatory minimum sentencing, and harsher punishments for petty crimes and cheaper street drugs. It is ultimately the concentration of poverty within American communities and paucity of opportunities that contribute to rates of crime and violence, which further drives resources (jobs, competitive housing prices, and so forth) from communities [15,16].

The centuries of policy and social constructs that have contributed the unequal distribution of wealth and resources in America fill entire sections of a library. The purpose here is not to be comprehensive, rather to shed light on the disgraceful political and social underpinnings of firearm violence

Table 3
The social and political determinants of Firearm injury

Individual	• Problem-solving skills • Impulsivity, anger management • Learning disorders • Mental health problems • Substance abuse • Prior adverse childhood events • Severe/chronic emotional distress • Witnessing or experiencing violence • Education, employment • Access to firearms
Interpersonal	• Social support (family, peers, school, place of worship) • Behaviors of family/peers (violence, substance abuse, delinquency)
Community	• Poverty/unemployment level • Concentration of liquor stores, vacant/abandoned lots, green space • Resource availability (mental health, primary care, substance abuse programs) • Relationship with law enforcement • Crime levels
State/National	• Firearm, health, economic, and education policy • Structural racism • Research and evidence-based programming

[17,18]. If these are not acknowledged as such, future policy and prevention will not succeed and only continue to perpetuate the problem.

Access to firearms

As previously mentioned, Americans own more guns per capita than any country in the world. There are approximately 55-million gun owners in the United States, translating to 30% of Americans living with a firearm in their household [19]. The right to bear arms is a Constitutional Right that Americans value highly. Gun ownership, in itself, is not to be viewed as intrinsically good or bad. It is important, however, to recognize that the wide accessibility of firearms is an important contributing factor to firearm morbidity and mortality.

Access to a firearm increases suicide risk among adult men and women (increase in 3 to 7× risk) [20,21]. Access to unlocked and loaded firearms increases the risk of both suicide and unintentional firearm injury among children and adolescents [22]. Access to firearms also increases the lethality of interpersonal violence. This has been shown among domestic violence disputes, with firearms being involved in most women killed by their partner [23]. High-capacity magazine assault weapons have been associated with the lethality of mass shootings. As a corollary, states with more permissive gun laws have higher rates of mass shootings [24–26].

Firearm research

The relationship between access to firearm homicide and suicide was first described by federally funded violence prevention research in the 1990s [27,28]. There was resulting controversy that government funds were being used to promote gun control. This ultimately resulted in Representative Jay Dickey's 1996 Omnibus Appropriations Act, which effectively halted the use of CDC funding for gun violence prevention research. This "ban" was later extended to NIH funding. The moratorium on firearm research recently ended in 2019 when Congress appropriated $25 million for gun violence prevention research that was divided between the NIH and the CDC. Although this is a cause for celebration, the paucity of research during the past 2 decades has stalled progress on firearm morbidity and mortality prevention [29]. The amount of funding that is needed based on the proportional burden on disease is upward of $1.4 Billion annually [30].

Social determinants of firearm injury

The social determinants that moderate the risk of firearm injury span individual, interpersonal, community, and state/national levels (Table 3). These risk and protective factors interact with one another and are dynamic over time. Thus, they provide insight in opportunities of intervention.

FIREARM INJURY PREVENTION

The outcome of firearm injury, be it suicide, homicide, unintended, or legal intervention, has deep-seated social and political underpinnings. As such, its prevention requires a diverse group of stakeholders including community members and organizations, educators, social workers, law enforcement, health professionals, researchers, and politicians (local, state, and national).

Surgeons have an important and unique role in firearm injury prevention because we are charged with the task of preventing mortality and minimizing morbidity of patients who have sustained gunshot wounds. Thus, the surgical community has a personal connection with this patient population. This was recently brought into the public arena via the @ThisIsOurLane campaign. It demonstrated the surgeon's role in firearm injury prevention is not to infringe on American liberties, but it is about saving American lives [31].

Surgeons and surgical associations have vocalized support for patient education, federally funded research, evidence-based policy change, interdisciplinary collaboration, and trauma center community engagement to prevent injury and promote safe gun ownership [32–36]. Importantly, this consensus has occurred among gun-owning and nongun-owning surgeons across the political spectrum.

In general, prevention initiatives are designed to minimize risk and bolster protective factors in order to prevent the event from ever occurring (primary prevention), minimizing the severity of the event (secondary prevention), or reducing its long-term sequelae (tertiary prevention). The following discussion will outline several strategies to which we, as individual surgeons and as a surgical community, can contribute to preventing firearm injury and death.

Primary prevention

Safe gun ownership

As previously outlined, access to a firearm is an independent risk factor for homicide, suicide, and unintended injuries [19–23]. Firearm storage practices, therefore, are an important strategy for risk reduction. The goal is to keep unlocked and loaded firearms out of the reach of high-risk individuals–that is, adults with cognitive impairment, mental illness, or a history of violence and all children. There is a substantial need for education and behavior change regarding storage practices in the United States. Less than half of gun-owners store their firearms unloaded, locked with ammunition stored separately. This translates to approximately 5 million American children living in a home with an accessible firearm [19,37].

Community and hospital-based education programs have demonstrated increase in safe storage knowledge and behavior [38,39]. However, the most effective education interventions with sustained changes in safe storage practices also provide a gun storage safety device [40,41]. Surgeons have an important role in safe gun ownership patient screening and counseling given the unique access to individuals at high risk for firearm injury [34–36]. However, individual physician knowledge and comfort engaging patients in these conversations is a barrier to implementation.

The American College of Surgeons Committee on Trauma has education materials available in Spanish and English to guide these conversations regarding firearm ownership, storage practices, and suicidal/homicidal ideation [42]. Other medical associations have created similar education materials for physicians and their patients. These efforts can be augmented by providing patients with gun safety devices, through the hospital or local partnerships. Any suicidal or homicidal ideation expressed in these conversations should prompt formal psychiatric evaluation. This may prompt emergency detention of the individual or temporary removal of the firearm from the home depending on the local laws and circumstances [43].

Policy and research

Surgeons can serve as influential advocates that can influence policy makers by sharing experiences, data, and solutions through a variety of platforms whether it's social media or personal visits to members of Congress on Capitol Hill [31,44]. The American College of Surgeons has extensive federal and state advocacy resources for those interested in learning practical ways to get involved [45]. Firearm legislature is not ubiquitous–in fact, states have anywhere from less than 10 to 100s of these laws. Statewide firearm injury rates have been shown to be inversely proportional to the number of their own laws in addition to the laws of the its surrounding states [46–49]. Although the nuances of firearm policy are beyond the scope of this article, there are several types of firearm legislation with data to support their efficacy.

Background checks aim to prevent firearm sales to individuals at high risk of harming themselves or others, examples are those with history of violent crime, domestic violence, severe psychiatric disorder, dishonorable discharge from military, and so forth. Currently, federal law does not require background checks when purchasing from a private firearm dealer. States laws range from requiring no background check, to a point-of-sale background check, to a gun license before purchase. Twenty-nine states do not require any formal background check. These laws, when properly enforced, have demonstrated a reduction in firearm morbidity and mortality related to homicides, domestic violence, and suicide [23,50].

These laws, however, are not equally efficacious. A study published in 2020 suggested gun licensing laws may be superior to point of sales background checks [51]. Furthermore, although these laws have been shown to decrease homicides in large urban centers, homicides and assaults using firearms purchased illegally or passed along in informal networks will not be affected by such laws [52]. Ultimately, legislation to reduce community violence will need to address its root causes namely the systemic racism resulting in profound social, health, and political disparities discussed previously.

Background checks and licenses will not identify all individuals with suicidal or homicidal ideation. These individuals, however, may be identified by family, health professions (ie, on health screening and counseling as outlined above), law enforcement, and so forth. Several states have passed *Extreme Risk Protective Orders*; these laws allow temporary firearm removal based on filed petitions expressing concern for the safety of an individual or those around them [53]. These laws are associated with lower suicide rates and confiscation of weapons from individuals threatening mass shootings [51,54].

After the *federal ban on assault weapons* ended in 2004, less than 10 states have imposed new restrictions. Highly lethal weapons are designed to cause severe injury in a short time frame. These include weapons such as semiautomatic firearms, bump stocks, and high-capacity magazines [55]. States without restrictions on such weapons not only have more mass shootings but also have more fatalities per mass shooting when compared with other states [26]. Legislation can and should be used to keep firearms, including highly lethal weapons, out of the hands of those who are at increased risk of harming themselves and others.

The recent end to the nearly 25-year moratorium on federal funding for firearm research is a humbling reminder to vocalize ardent support for ongoing funding legislation [29]. There is ample opportunity for surgeon scientists to push firearm morbidity and mortality prevention research forward [56]. The National Trauma Database and the Trauma Quality Improvement program collect national trauma data and have been invaluable in outcomes and quality improvement research, respectively [57,58]. These resources, however, capture hospital data only. As the cause of firearm injury is multifactorial, there is a paucity of high-quality data that spans public health, criminal justice, and the health sectors. Such data sets may improve quality of background checks to health equity driven community-based initiatives.

Secondary prevention

Interventions of this type aim to prevent morbidity and mortality after an injury occurs. It is estimated that 20% of firearm deaths could have been prevented. Many of these deaths occur before hospital arrival, highlighting the importance in prehospital care and organized trauma systems [59,60]. Clinical improvements in the operative and nonoperative care of patients are also part of secondary prevention, but they are beyond the scope of this article.

The Stop the Bleed campaign, modeled after the military's Tactical Combat Casualty Care program, was designed to address this need. The program targets nonmedical bystanders in the application of tourniquets. Its participants have been shown to have increased knowledge and skills as a result of the training [61,62].

In addition to hemorrhage control, expeditious transport to the hospital saves lives. Odds of death increase between 2% and 4% for each additional minute of transport [63]. This is thought to be the reason why survival is increased among victims transported by private vehicle compared with EMS. This is referred to as "Scoop and Run" in the literature [64]. Quality improvement measures can be made by working with EMS to minimize interventions that delay transport to definitive care, which, in certain circumstances, may include intubation, IV access, and thoracostomies.

There are prehospital systems equipped for more advanced trauma life support, including the administration of blood products. Data have demonstrated patients in hemorrhagic shock who receive red blood cells as well as plasma have a mortality benefit. Thus, the role of prehospital interventions should be tailored to the experience of the providers, transportation time, and resources available. Once en route, EMS then has the task of appropriately triaging the patient, or determining the correct level of care. Undertriaged patients have a 30% increase in mortality [65–67]. Regionalized Trauma Networks, particularly those in which multiple hospitals provide level appropriate care, reduce mortality as soon as 2 years of their establishment [68–70]. Thus, systems coordination between EMS and trauma centers has important implications for improving survival.

Tertiary prevention

Tertiary prevention aims to reduce the long-term sequelae of firearm injury—namely increase survivorship and decrease recidivism. A firearm injury may occur in one single moment, but its effects on the individual, family, and community are long lasting. The life-long social, mental, and physical repercussions of such an injury are well documented [71,72]. Community, hospital, and national-based survivor networks exist for this very reason [73]. These resources should be shared with trauma patients.

Furthermore, firearm injury survivors are at increased risk of either perpetrating or falling victim to future violent acts. Hospital-based violence prevention programs work with high-risk individuals to identify and eliminate barriers to behavior change. These programs have been shown to increase service utilization, change attitude and behaviors, and reduce recidivism. They have also been shown to be cost beneficial. The Health Alliance for Violence Interventions, a national network of hospital and community-based programs, and the American College of Surgeons Committee on Trauma provide resources for initiating and sustaining a hospital-based violence prevention programs [74–78].

SUMMARY

Firearms injury is a major cause of death and disability to Americans. Although the firearm is a common vector, the intentions with which it is used represent a wide array of social ills–suicide, community violence, domestic violence, mass shootings, legal intervention, and unintended injury. The political and social underpinnings of this public health crisis are inseparable from its prevention measures. Surgeons have an important role in firearm policy, research, prehospital and hospital advances, trauma survivor networks, and hospital-based violence prevention programs. There is no one solution. It is only through interdisciplinary, multilevel, evidence-based prevention measures that the tides will turn on American firearm injury.

Disclosure

The authors have nothing to disclose.

References

[1] Global Burden of Disease 2016 Injury Collaborators, Naghavi M, Marczak LB, et al. Global Mortality From Firearms, 1990-2016. JAMA 2018;320(8):792–814; https://doi.org/10.1001/jama.2018.10060, 2018 Sep 25;320(12):1288.

[2] Karp A. Estimating Global Civilian- Held Firearms Numbers. Small Arms Survey. 2018. Available at: http://www.smallarmssurvey.org/about-us/highlights/2018/highlight-bp-firearms-holdings.html. Accessed September 18, 2021.

[3] gov CDC. Web-based Injury Statistics Query and Reporting System. 2020. Available at: https://www.cdc.gov/injury/wisqars/index.html. Accessed September 15, 2021.

[4] Everytown Research & Policy. The Economic Cost of Gun Violence. 2021. Available at: https://everytownresearch.org/report/the-economic-cost-of-gun-violence/#lost-quality-of-life. Accessed April 17, 2021.

[5] Gani F, Sakran JV, Canner JK. Emergency Department Visits For Firearm-Related Injuries In The United States, 2006-14. Health Aff (Millwood) 2017;36(10):1729–38; https://doi.org/10.1377/hlthaff.2017.0625.

[6] U.S. Department. of Veteran Affairs Office of Mental Health and Suicide Prevention. 2019 National Veteran Suicide Prevention Annual Report. 2019. https://tinyurl.com/y534tthe. Accessed September 20, 2021.

[7] Major Cities Chiefs Police Association. Reducing Violent Crime in American Cities Report. 2017. Available at: https://www.majorcitieschiefs.com/pdf/news/reducing_violent_crime_in_American_cities_pressre-lease_final.pdf/. Accessed June 15, 2020.

[8] Berkowitz B, Alcantara C. The Terrible Numbers That Grow with Each Mass Shooting. 2019 The Washington Post Available at: https://www.wash-ingtonpost.com/graphics/2018/national/mass-shootings-in-america/. Accessed June 26, 2020.

[9] Gun Violence Archive. Gun Violence Archive. 2020. Available at: https://www.gun-violencearchive.org/. Accessed June 27, 2020.

[10] Duwe G. Patterns and prevalence of lethal mass violence. Criminology & Public Policy 2019;19(1):17–35; https://doi.org/10.1111/1745-9133.12478.

[11] Feldman JM, Gruskin S, Coull BA, et al. Quantifying underreporting of law-enforcement-related deaths in United States vital statistics and news-media-based data sources: A capture-recapture analysis. Plos Med 2017;14(10):e1002399; https://doi.org/10.1371/journal.pmed.1002399 [published correction appears in PLoS Med. 2017;14(10):e1002449].

[12] Mooney AC, McConville S, Rappaport AJ, et al. Association of Legal Intervention Injuries With Race and Ethnicity Among Patients Treated in Emergency Departments in California.

JAMA Netw Open 2018;1(5):e182150; https://doi.org/10.1001/jamanetworkopen.2018.2150.

[13] Department of Health and Human Services, Department of Justice. Surgeon General's Workshop on violence in public health Report. Leesburg, VA: Health Resources and Services Administration; 1985.

[14] Boeck MA, Strong B, Campbell A. Disparities in Firearm Injury: Consequences of Structural Violence. Curr Trauma Rep 2020;6(1):10–22; https://doi.org/10.1007/s40719-020-00188-5.

[15] Benns M, Ruther M, Nash N, et al. The impact of historical racism on modern gun violence: Redlining in the city of Louisville. KY Inj 2020;51(10):2192–8; https://doi.org/10.1016/j.injury.2020.06.042.

[16] Irvin-Erickson Y, Lynch M, Gurvis A, et al. Gun violence Affects the economic health of communities. Washington, DC: Urban Institute; 2017. Available at: https://www.urban.org/sites/default/files/publication/90666/eigv_brief_3.pdf. Accessed June 30, 2021.

[17] Knopov A, Rothman EF, Cronin SW, et al. The Role of Racial Residential Segregation in Black-White Disparities in Firearm Homicide at the State Level in the United States, 1991-2015. J Natl Med Assoc 2019;111(1):62–75; https://doi.org/10.1016/j.jnma.2018.06.002.

[18] Rowhani-Rahbar A, Quistberg DA, Morgan ER, et al. Income inequality and firearm homicide in the US: a county-level cohort study. Inj Prev 2019;25(Suppl 1):i25–30; https://doi.org/10.1136/injuryprev-2018-043080.

[19] Azrael D, Cohen J, Salhi C, et al. Firearm Storage in Gun-Owning Households with Children: Results of a 2015 National Survey. J Urban Health 2018;95(3):295–304; https://doi.org/10.1007/s11524-018-0261-7.

[20] Anglemyer A, Horvath T, Rutherford G. The accessibility of firearms and risk for suicide and homicide victimization among household members: a systematic review and meta-analysis [published correction appears in Ann Intern Med. Ann Intern Med 2014;160(9):658–9; https://doi.org/10.7326/M13-1301, 2014;160(2):101-110.

[21] Studdert DM, Zhang Y, Swanson SA, et al. Handgun Ownership and Suicide in California. N Engl J Med 2020;382(23):2220–9; https://doi.org/10.1056/NEJMsa1916744.

[22] Monuteaux MC, Azrael D, Miller M. Association of Increased Safe Household Firearm Storage With Firearm Suicide and Unintentional Death Among US Youths [published correction appears in JAMA Pediatr. 2019 Jul 1;173(7):704]. JAMA Pediatr 2019;173(7):657–62; https://doi.org/10.1001/jamapediatrics.2019.1078.

[23] Vigdor ER, Mercy JA. Do laws restricting access to firearms by domestic violence offenders prevent intimate partner homicide? Eval Rev 2006;30(3):313–46; https://doi.org/10.1177/0193841X06287307.

[24] Mass Shootings in America. Everytown Research & Policy. 2021. Available at: https://everytownresearch.org/maps/mass-shootings-in-america-2009-2019/. Accessed October 14, 2021.

[25] Webster DW, McCourt AD, Crifasi CK, et al. Evidence concerning the regulation of firearms design, sale, and carrying on fatal mass shootings in the United States. Criminology & Public Policy 2020;19(1):171–212; https://doi.org/10.1111/1745-9133.12487.

[26] Klarevas L, Conner A, Hemenway D. The Effect of Large-Capacity Magazine Bans on High-Fatality Mass Shootings, 1990-2017. Am J Public Health 2019;109(12):1754–61; https://doi.org/10.2105/AJPH.2019.305311.

[27] Kellermann AL, Rivara FP, Rushforth NB, et al. Gun ownership as a risk factor for homicide in the home [published correction appears in N Engl J Med. 1998 Sep 24;339(13):928-9]. N Engl J Med 1993;329(15):1084–91; https://doi.org/10.1056/NEJM199310073291506.

[28] Kellermann AL, Rivara FP, Somes G, et al. Suicide in the home in relation to gun ownership. N Engl J Med 1992;327(7):467–72; https://doi.org/10.1056/NEJM199208133270705.

[29] Strong BM, Sangji NF, Barrera K. Gun violence and firearm policy in the U.S.: A brief history and the current status. The Bulletin American College of Surgeons. 2018. Available at:

https://bulletin.facs.org/2018/07/gun-violence-and-firearm-policy-in-the-u-s-a-brief-history-and-the-current-status/. Accessed June 27, 2020.
[30] Stark DE, Shah NH. Funding and Publication of Research on Gun Violence and Other Leading Causes of Death. JAMA 2017;317(1):84–5; https://doi.org/10.1001/jama.2016.16215.
[31] Sakran JV, Maa J, Masiakos PT. Turning experience into action: this is our lane. Curr Trauma Rep 2020;6(1):5–9; https://doi.org/10.1007/s40719-020-00187-6.
[32] Streib E, Blake D, Christmas AB, et al. American Association for the Surgery of Trauma statement on firearm injuries. J Trauma Acute Care Surg 2016;80(6):849; https://doi.org/10.1097/TA.0000000000001090.
[33] Eastern Association for the Surgery of Trauma. Eastern Association for the Surgery of Trauma firearm injury prevention statement. Trauma Surg Acute Care Open 2019;4(1):e000294; https://doi.org/10.1136/tsaco-2018-000294.
[34] Kuhls DA, Stewart RM, Bulger EM. Building consensus to decrease firearm injuries and death in the USA: engaging medical and public health organizations to find common ground. Curr Trauma Rep 2020;6(1):56–61; https://doi.org/10.1007/s40719-020-00190-x.
[35] Kuhls DA, Campbell BT, Burke PA, et al. Survey of American College of Surgeons Committee on trauma members on firearm injury: Consensus and opportunities. J Trauma Acute Care Surg 2017;82(5):877–86; https://doi.org/10.1097/TA.0000000000001405.
[36] Puls MW, Kuhls DA, Campbell BT, et al. Survey of the American College of Surgeons Board of governors on firearm injury prevention: consensus and opportunities. Bull Am Coll Surg 2017;102(10):30–6.
[37] Crifasi CK, Doucette ML, McGinty EE, et al. Storage Practices of US Gun Owners in 2016. Am J Public Health 2018;108(4):532–7; https://doi.org/10.2105/AJPH.2017.304262.
[38] Bradyunited.org. End Family Fire. 2019. Available at: https://www.bradyunited.org/program/end-family-fire. Accessed December 8, 2021.
[39] Miller M, Salhi C, Barber C, et al. Changes in Firearm and Medication Storage Practices in Homes of Youths at Risk for Suicide: Results of the SAFETY Study, a Clustered, Emergency Department-Based, Multisite, Stepped-Wedge Trial. Ann Emerg Med 2020;76(2):194–205; https://doi.org/10.1016/j.annemergmed.2020.02.007.
[40] Violano P, Bonne S, Duncan T, et al. Prevention of firearm injuries with gun safety devices and safe storage: An Eastern Association for the Surgery of Trauma Systematic Review. J Trauma Acute Care Surg 2018;84(6):1003–11; https://doi.org/10.1097/TA.0000000000001879.
[41] Rowhani-Rahbar A, Simonetti JA, Rivara FP. Effectiveness of Interventions to Promote Safe Firearm Storage. Epidemiol Rev 2016;38(1):111–24; https://doi.org/10.1093/epirev/mxv006.
[42] Firearm Injury Prevention Activities. Gun Safety and Your Health: A Proactive Guide to Protect You and Those Around You. American College of Surgeons. Available at: https://www.facs.org/quality-programs/trauma/advocacy/ipc/firearm-injury. Accessed October 14, 2021.
[43] Swanson JW, Norko MA, Lin HJ, et al. Implementation and effectiveness of Connecticut's risk-based gun removal law: does it prevent suicides. L Contemp. Probs 2017;80:179.
[44] Rubin R. Physicians Are Steering the Conversation About Gun Violence. JAMA 2019;321(2):133–5; https://doi.org/10.1001/jama.2018.20385.
[45] Advocacy. American College of Surgeons. Available at: https://www.facs.org/advocacy. Accessed October 1, 2021.
[46] Zeoli AM, Webster DW. Firearm Policies That Work. JAMA 2019;321(10):937–8; https://doi.org/10.1001/jama.2019.0706.

[47] Jehan F, Pandit V, O'Keeffe T, et al. The burden of firearm violence in the United States: stricter laws result in safer states. J Inj Violence Res 2018;10(1):11–6; https://doi.org/10.5249/jivr.v10i1.951.
[48] Crandall M, Eastman A, Violano P, et al. Prevention of firearm-related injuries with restrictive licensing and concealed carry laws: An Eastern Association for the Surgery of Trauma systematic review. J Trauma Acute Care Surg 2016;81(5):952–60; https://doi.org/10.1097/TA.0000000000001251.
[49] Olson EJ, Hoofnagle M, Kaufman EJ, et al. American firearm homicides: The impact of your neighbors. J Trauma Acute Care Surg 2019;86(5):797–802; https://doi.org/10.1097/TA.0000000000002212.
[50] Kalesan B, Mobily ME, Keiser O, et al. Firearm legislation and firearm mortality in the USA: a cross-sectional, state-level study. Lancet 2016;387(10030):1847–55; https://doi.org/10.1016/S0140-6736(15)01026-0.
[51] McCourt AD, Crifasi CK, Stuart EA, et al. Purchaser Licensing, Point-of-Sale Background Check Laws, and Firearm Homicide and Suicide in 4 US States, 1985-2017. Am J Public Health 2020;110(10):1546–52; https://doi.org/10.2105/AJPH.2020.305822.
[52] Crifasi CK, Merrill-Francis M, McCourt A, et al. Association between Firearm Laws and Homicide in Urban Counties [published correction appears in J Urban Health. J Urban Health 2018;95(3):383–90; https://doi.org/10.1007/s11524-018-0273-3, 95(5):773-776.
[53] Gondi S, Pomerantz AG, Sacks CA. Extreme Risk Protection Orders: An Opportunity to Improve Gun Violence Prevention Training. Acad Med 2019;94(11):1649–53; https://doi.org/10.1097/ACM.0000000000002935.
[54] Wintemute GJ, Pear VA, Schleimer JP, et al. Extreme Risk Protection Orders Intended to Prevent Mass Shootings: A Case Series. Ann Intern Med 2019;171(9):655–8; https://doi.org/10.7326/M19-2162.
[55] de Jager E, Goralnick E, McCarty JC, et al. Lethality of Civilian Active Shooter Incidents With and Without Semiautomatic Rifles in the United States [published correction appears in JAMA. 2018 Nov 27;320(20):2154. JAMA 2018;320(10):1034–5; https://doi.org/10.1001/jama.2018.11009.
[56] 100 Critical Questions for Gun Violence Research. The Joyce Foundation; 2020. Available at: https://www.joycefdn.org/research-reports/insights-research-reports-100-critical-questions-for-gun-violence-research. Accessed November 14, 2021.
[57] Shafi S, Nathens AB, Cryer HG, et al. The Trauma Quality Improvement Program of the American College of Surgeons Committee on Trauma. J Am Coll Surg 2009;209(4):521–30.e1; https://doi.org/10.1016/j.jamcollsurg.2009.07.001.
[58] Hashmi ZG, Kaji AH, Nathens AB. Practical Guide to Surgical Data Sets: National Trauma Data Bank (NTDB). JAMA Surg 2018;153(9):852–3; https://doi.org/10.1001/jamasurg.2018.0483.
[59] Gedeborg R, Chen LH, Thiblin I, et al. Prehospital injury deaths–strengthening the case for prevention: nationwide cohort study. J Trauma Acute Care Surg 2012;72(3):765–72; https://doi.org/10.1097/TA.0b013e3182288272.
[60] National Trauma Care System A. Integrating Military and Civilian Trauma Systems to Achieve Zero Preventable Deaths After Injury. Mil Med 2017;182(5):1563–5; https://doi.org/10.7205/MILMED-D-17-00043.
[61] Smith AA, Ochoa JE, Wong S, et al. Prehospital tourniquet use in penetrating extremity trauma: Decreased blood transfusions and limb complications. J Trauma Acute Care Surg 2019;86(1):43–51; https://doi.org/10.1097/TA.0000000000002095.
[62] Schroll R, Smith A, Martin MS, et al. Stop the Bleed Training: Rescuer Skills, Knowledge, and Attitudes of Hemorrhage Control Techniques. J Surg Res 2020;245:636–42; https://doi.org/10.1016/j.jss.2019.08.011.
[63] Brown JB, Rosengart MR, Forsythe RM, et al. Not all prehospital time is equal: Influence of scene time on mortality. J Trauma Acute Care Surg 2016;81(1):93–100; https://doi.org/10.1097/TA.0000000000000999.

[64] Zafar SN, Haider AH, Stevens KA, et al. Increased mortality associated with EMS transport of gunshot wound victims when compared to private vehicle transport. Injury 2014;45(9): 1320–6; https://doi.org/10.1016/j.injury.2014.05.032.
[65] Williamson K, Ramesh R, Grabinsky A. Advances in prehospital trauma care. Int J Crit Illn Inj Sci 2011;1(1):44–50; https://doi.org/10.4103/2229-5151.79281.
[66] Choi J, Carlos G, Nassar AK, et al. The impact of trauma systems on patient outcomes. Curr Probl Surg 2021;58(1):100849; https://doi.org/10.1016/j.cpsurg.2020.100849.
[67] Haas B, Stukel TA, Gomez D, et al. The mortality benefit of direct trauma center transport in a regional trauma system: a population-based analysis. J Trauma Acute Care Surg 2012;72(6):1510–7; https://doi.org/10.1097/TA.0b013e318252510a.
[68] Guyette FX, Sperry JL, Peitzman AB, et al. Prehospital Blood Product and Crystalloid Resuscitation in the Severely Injured Patient: A Secondary Analysis of the Prehospital Air Medical Plasma Trial. Ann Surg 2021;273(2):358–64; https://doi.org/10.1097/SLA.0000000000003324.
[69] Schechtman D, He JC, Zosa BM, et al. Trauma system regionalization improves mortality in patients requiring trauma laparotomy. J Trauma Acute Care Surg 2017;82(1):58–64; https://doi.org/10.1097/TA.0000000000001302.
[70] Claridge JA, Allen D, Patterson B, et al. Regional collaboration across hospital systems to develop and implement trauma protocols saves lives within 2 years. Surgery 2013;154(4):875–84; https://doi.org/10.1016/j.surg.2013.07.013.
[71] Herrera-Escobar JP, Rivero R, Apoj M, et al. Long-term social dysfunction after trauma: What is the prevalence, risk factors, and associated outcomes? Surgery 2019;166(3):392–7; https://doi.org/10.1016/j.surg.2019.04.004.
[72] Joseph B, Hanna K, Callcut RA, et al. The Hidden Burden of Mental Health Outcomes Following Firearm-related Injures. Ann Surg 2019;270(4):593–601; https://doi.org/10.1097/SLA.0000000000003473.
[73] American Trauma Society. Trauma Survivors Network. Available at: https://www.traumasurvivorsnetwork.org/pages/home. Accessed September 2, 2021.
[74] Juillard C, Smith R, Anaya N, et al. Saving lives and saving money: hospital-based violence intervention is cost-effective. J Trauma Acute Care Surg 2015;78(2):252–8; https://doi.org/10.1097/TA.0000000000000527.
[75] Loveland-Jones C, Ferrer L, Charles S, et al. A prospective randomized study of the efficacy of "Turning Point," an inpatient violence intervention program. J Trauma Acute Care Surg 2016;81(5):834–42; https://doi.org/10.1097/TA.0000000000001226.
[76] Purtle J, Dicker R, Cooper C, et al. Hospital-based violence intervention programs save lives and money. J Trauma Acute Care Surg 2013;75(2):331–3; https://doi.org/10.1097/TA.0b013e318294f518.
[77] Dicker RA, Gaines BA, Bonne S, et al. Violence intervention pro- grams: a primer for developing a comprehensive program for trauma centers. Bull Am Coll Surg 2017;102(10): 20–9.
[78] The HAVI. The Health Alliance for Violence Intervention. Available at: https://www.thehavi.org/. Accessed November 14, 2021.

Advances in Surgery 56 (2022) 69–78

ADVANCES IN SURGERY

Reducing Complications After Surgery for Benign Anorectal Conditions

Alton Sutter, MD, PhD[a], Vitaliy Poylin, MD[b,*]

[a]Wake Forest Baptist Hospital, Medical Center Boulevard, Winston-Salem, NC 27157, USA; [b]Division of Gastrointestinal and Oncologic Surgery, Feinberg School of Medicine, Northwestern Medical Group, 676 North St. Clair Street, Suite 650, Chicago, IL 60611, USA

Keywords

• Anorectal • Hemorrhoidectomy • Fistula • Abscess • Incontinence

Key points

- Meticulous planning, patient education, and clinical judgment during index procedure can significantly decrease the chance of complications.
- Multimodal pain management can reduce the risk of primary and secondary complications.
- Judicious perioperative fluid management is recommended to reduce the risk of urinary retention.
- Few risk-avoiding strategies in anorectal surgery are supported by rigorous research.

INTRODUCTION

While generally perceived as mundane and low-risk procedures, anorectal surgeries by virtue of their anatomic real-estate–dense with nerves, blood supply, and structures critical to the quality of life–are fraught with the potential for complications. While these complications are generally not life-threatening, their impact on the quality of life can be severe. Furthermore, the sheer volume of anorectal procedures performed each year means that even low complication rates or less severe complications can have a significant economic impact. To this end, we must strive to do everything in our power to reduce the incidence of these complications, as well as to manage them effectively, safely, and economically. While some types of colorectal complications have been studied

*Corresponding author. *E-mail address:* vitaliy.poylin2@nm.org

https://doi.org/10.1016/j.yasu.2022.05.001

extensively (eg, anastomotic leaks), anorectal complications have received a relative smattering of attention over the years. More importantly, there is a relative dearth of evidence on which to base practices on reducing these complications. Nonetheless, we will focus on the available data as it pertains to *modifiable* factors which affect the rate of postoperative complications from anorectal surgery.

While patient modifiable risk factors such as smoking, obesity, and diabetes are loosely associated with complications from anorectal procedures, these linkages are often weak. As with many factors requiring lifestyle modifications (such as smoking), they are often difficult to address effectively perioperatively [1].

COMPLICATIONS

Urinary Retention: Urinary retention is a common complication after anorectal surgery with reported rates of 16.7% [2]. It is related to postoperative pain and use of pain medications especially opioids, perianal blocks, and general manipulation and subsequent inflammation of the area. Higher rates of urinary retention correlate with more extensive anorectal procedures such as hemorrhoidectomy when compared with less extensive ones such as lateral internal sphincterotomy. Urinary retention after anorectal procedures is linked to the modifiable factors of postoperative pain levels and perioperative fluid administration. Urinary retention rates may be halved by restricting perioperative fluids to less than 1 L, while being further reduced by effective analgesia [2]. When spinal anesthetic is used, lower doses of anesthetic are associated with decreased retention rates [3]. Multi-modality pain management and attention to proper preoperative counseling are extremely beneficial in decreasing opioid requirement and subsequently urinary retention. On the other hand, prophylactic alpha-adrenergic blockade does not seem to prevent urinary retention after anorectal surgery [4]. Most of the time, short-term (1–2 day) placement of a catheter is adequate to resolve retention. Patients should be counseled pre and postoperatively about urinary retention. Promptly addressing urinary retention is critical to avoid the possible complication of acute renal injury from postrenal obstruction [5]. Retention can also be an early sign of infection and pelvic sepsis, whereby early intervention can be lifesaving. Patients should be instructed to return to the hospital or proceed to the emergency room promptly if urinary retention is suspected.

Bleeding: While minor bleeding is common and expected after anorectal surgery, significant hemorrhage is encountered in only 1% to 2% of cases. Hemorrhoidectomy is associated with bleeding rates higher than other anorectal procedures [6], around 2%. The definition of bleeding after anorectal surgery is not well defined, but it generally includes the need for blood transfusion, return to the hospital or operating room, or symptoms associated with blood loss anemia. Bleeding is quite distressing for patients and, when combined with the subjective nature of what constitutes significant bleeding, this can create uncertainty especially when not evaluating the patient in person.

Patients should be counseled that bloody and mucus discharge is normal and expected after all anorectal surgery. In the operating room, in addition to meticulous hemostasis, a few measures can be taken to minimize the risk of postoperative bleeding. "Last look" – performing anoscopy at the end of the procedure combined with irrigation can help identify small bleeding vessels before one leaves the operating room. Although electrocautery works well for most bleeding in the area, utilization of absorbable sutures on hemorrhoidal pedicles and areas of concern can improve outcomes. Closing mucosal defects after hemorrhoidectomy may decrease the chances of bleeding, but may come at the price of a slight increase in infectious complications. As there is no quality evidence supporting the use of pharmacologic thromboprophylaxis in patients undergoing ambulatory surgery without additional venous thromboembolism risk factors, ASCRS guidelines recommend an individualized approach in low-risk patients, weighing risk/benefit with bleeding.

Particular care should be taken with hemodialysis patients as they have higher postoperative bleeding rates, up to more than 11% after hemorrhoidectomy [7].

Another frequently encountered issue is the patient on routine anticoagulation. There is no evidence that the use or low or regular dose aspirin increases the chances of bleeding [8]. However, risk of bleeding with other anticoagulants including newer antiplatelet agents can be substantial. This risk can be mitigated by holding anticoagulants pre and postoperatively and should generally be conducted in the coordination with the physician who prescribed it to help assess the risks [8].

If significant bleeding is encountered the patient should be promptly evaluated. Common presenting symptoms include frequent passage of small volume of bright red blood or clots as well as systemic symptoms such as dizziness, tachycardia, and in some cases hypotension. Timely evaluation is key.

Infection: Infection after anorectal surgery is uncommon, for example, a review of 969 patients identified 4 infectious complications yielding a rate of less than 0.5%, or about a tenth of the rate generally observed for surgical procedures [9,10]. Yet, prompt recognition and definitive management (usually with a return to the operating room) are critical to avoid catastrophe. While rates of catastrophic complications such as pelvic sepsis and Fournier's gangrene are exceedingly low, rates of less severe complications, such as abscess formation after hemorrhoidectomy may be as high as 0.5% to 4% [11]. Signs and symptoms of infection include fever, drainage (especially when this changes from serous to purulent), urinary retention, and worsening pain after the initial period of improvement. Some of these can be expected as part of recovery after anorectal surgery, thus there should be a low threshold for evaluating a patient in person.

While rates of surgical site infection in immunosuppressed patients have been debated, retrospective data show them to be similar for patients with HIV undergoing minor anorectal procedures, with or without prophylactic antibiotic administration [12].

Modifications of surgical techniques are common, yet studies have not found infection rates to be decreased by modifying technique (such as open vs closed hemorrhoidectomy) or by perioperative antibiotics [13].

While fistulas are reported as a potential complication after anorectal procedures, the prevention thereof generally lies in careful dissection and attention to other critical structures such as the vaginal wall and urethra as well as careful examination at the end of the case [14]. In addition, higher risk procedures for fistula-in-ano such as Ligation of Intersphincteric Fistula Track (LIFT) or endoanal advancement flap have inherently high risk of failure and recurrence/persistence of symptoms of fistula and abscess. Earlier return for a routine check and preoperative discussion about expectations can be useful in early identification and symptom control.

Incontinence: Incontinence may occur secondary to excessive damage to the sphincter from direct mechanical or thermal trauma during dissection, or subsequent infection. Meticulous surgical technique and clear identification of the sphincter muscle are key to the prevention of these injuries. Some common procedures, however, rely on the division of the sphincter such as fistulotomy and lateral internal sphincterotomy. Adequate preoperative evaluation and patient counseling are extremely important to avoid these problems. The anal canal length, sphincter bulk, tone on the preoperative examination, and preexisting continence must all be taken into account when exercising good clinical judgment before sacrificing sphincter muscle in the course of an operation. Preoperative imaging, such as MRI (fistula protocol) and endoanal ultrasound can aid in delineating the degree of sphincter involvement and the bulk and anatomy of the remaining tissue. The risk of incontinence after lateral internal sphincterotomy can be minimized by performing tailored sphincterotomy and dividing less than 25% of the internal anal sphincter [15]. Postoperative implications and alternatives whereby possible (eg, Botox injection for anal fissure, draining seton for fistula) should be clearly discussed and documented before surgery and communicated to the operating room team. Although LIFT and advancement flap have not been directly implicated in significant worsening of continence, repeated and more extensive anorectal procedures are linked to increased risk of impact on continence. For this reason, a successful first repair or procedure is often the best approach to reduce the risk of incontinence. For instance, recurrent infections are more likely to alter sphincter function than fistulotomy at the index presentation [16]. Debated in the literature for a while, variations in surgical approach do not seem to consistently provide improvement in the rate of continence complications; for instance, it is not reliably shown that there is any difference in incontinence risk between fistulotomy and cutting seton [17]. In the operating room, if doubts are raised about the potential effect on the sphincter complex, one should lean toward the more conservative approach–it is better to return to an operating room for another procedure than to try to deal with the consequences of significant postprocedure fecal incontinence.

Constipation: Constipation after anorectal surgery is common, affecting up to a quarter of patients [18]. Contributing factors include hesitancy/fear of bowel movements, opioids, and immobility. Constipation, beyond its own intrinsic complication, can exacerbate the risks of bleeding, pain, and infection due to the increased trauma of associated bowel movements. The risk of constipation can be addressed by adherence to an adequate bowel regimen, multimodal analgesia limiting narcotic requirements, and addressing lifestyle factors preoperatively [18].

Delayed wound healing: Delayed wound healing can be a concern despite the generally excellent perfusion in the anorectal region, particularly if working in a field that has been subject to chronic infection or radiation. General principles of surgical wound healing apply including management of diabetes, smoking cessation, and nutritional optimization. Extensive packing of anorectal wounds is felt to be associated with delayed healing and the potential for sphincteric injury, probably secondary to nerve injury [19].

Stenosis: While anal stenosis is a potential complication of any procedure causing trauma to the anus, hemorrhoidectomy poses the greatest risk, and rates are reported up to 1.5% [20]. This is thought to be a consequence of overzealous extirpation of anoderm and subsequent scaring; it can be avoided by limiting the dissection and extent of hemorrhoidectomy. Although only supported by expert opinion, at least a 2 cm mucosal bridge should be left between each excised hemorrhoidal column. Additionally, patients undergoing other anorectal procedures may suffer from stenosis secondary to injury to the underlying sphincter muscle. As mild strictures can often be treated with dietary modification and fiber supplements, utilizing the consistent passage of formed stool to provide some intrinsic dilation, it is reasonable to assume this may also be an effective preventative strategy.

Pain: Anorectal procedures are frequently associated with somewhat painful recovery due to the dense sensory innervation of the anatomy. While opioid medications have long been a mainstay in postoperative analgesia of anorectal surgery patients, there has been interesting over the years in decreasing or at least controlling this given not only the abuse potential of opioids but also to control their side effects which further exacerbate recovery after anorectal surgery and potentially increase the risks of other complications (constipation). Multimodal pain control has become standard at many centers given its ability to reduce opioid requirements. These include the addition of nonsteroidal anti-inflammatory medications such as celecoxib given preoperatively, ketorolac at the conclusion of the procedure, and scheduled ibuprofen and acetaminophen at discharge. Gabapentin has been used both as premedication and a postoperative adjunct, although data on its effects are mixed [21–23]. Topical anesthetics, suppositories, metronidazole, and intrathecal injections have all been studied; however, these studies have frequently been plagued by small size and limited scope. For instance, the PROSPECT group reported in 2010 that while numerous publications (>100 meeting inclusion criteria) had addressed analgesia after hemorrhoidectomy, these studies were of heterogeneous design and frequently questionable methodologic quality, limiting their interpretation as a whole [24]. The PROSPECT group did in a 2017 update recommend local anesthetic with a combination of analgesics and other adjuncts postoperatively including NSAIDs, opioids, topical lidocaine, laxatives, but noted that their recommendations are largely based on single intervention studies, not multimodal trials [25]. The use of longer acting liposomal bupivacaine seems like an attractive solution as it should provide pain control for up to 72 hours, yet studies showed only minimal improvement when compared with shorter acting medications. Combined with high-cost, adoption of this medication has been limited. Recently, multimodal strategies involving patient and provider education (all levels including nurses, anesthesia, house staff, and surgeons), as well as the medications previously mentioned, have been shown to drastically reduce both narcotic prescribed and narcotic used while still effectively managing postoperative pain [26]. Clearly, managing patient expectations and educating all stakeholders is critical. Overall, varying approaches to anesthesia (propofol intravenous sedation, spinal anesthesia, and general anesthesia) have met with equivalent outcomes in anorectal surgery [27]. Multiple studies have failed to provide data to support the use of sitz baths or related adjuncts, either on wound healing or symptom management [28].

Several procedures warrant addressing specifically due to their prevalence and potential for complications.

Hemorrhoidectomy: Hemorrhoidectomy is associated with significant postoperative pain, associated narcotic requirements, and convalescence. It also carries the risks of anal stenosis from over-exuberant excision of anoderm, urinary retention, bleeding, chronic pain, incontinence, and pelvic sepsis. Strictures may occur in up to 5% of hemorrhoidectomy patients [29]. An approach to limit the risks associated with hemorrhoidectomy is to limit the initial resection to 1 or 2 columns rather than performing the traditional 3-column procedure. Ectropion can be avoided by avoiding the introduction of rectal mucosa external to the anal canal. While a number of adjuncts including glyceryl-trinitrate and metronidazole have been used in attempts to improve wound healing and reduce postoperative pain, studies have not shown reliable benefits [30,31]. Antibiotic prophylaxis is not indicated for hemorrhoidectomy and does not seem to reduce the incidence of postoperative infection [32]. In addition to surgical bleeding that happens shortly after surgery, delayed bleeding, likely related to medications (NSAIDs) and falling off of the clot from the pedicle can be seen and can happen as late as 2 weeks postoperatively and is associated with infection or trauma (eg, from straining) [33–35].

While the use of circular staplers for the management of hemorrhoids, first begun in the late 1990s, showed initial promise of more favorable bleeding rates and postoperative pain, many have shied away from their use due to high recurrence rates as well as some unsettling complications such as instances of rectovaginal and rectourethral fistula formation.

Other, less invasive, techniques for the management of hemorrhoids may have lower complication rates (such as lower bleeding rates reported for

Doppler-guided hemorrhoidal dearterialization). However, this must be balanced with the likelihood of achieving definitive management [36]. Rubber band ligation of hemorrhoids is overall very safe and can be performed in the office, but is associated with a less durable long-term response. Main potential complications include bleeding (some minor delayed bleeding is expected) and pain if the band is placed in the anatomically incorrect position (below the dentate line or in the anal transitional zone whereby somatic enervation is dense). This can be easily avoided by taking care to ensure adequate visualization of the anatomy before placement, as well as keeping the patient for a short period of time (around 15 minutes) in the clinic to assess for the development of symptoms as the band can be removed if this occurs (with a small vein hook or other devices). While therapeutic anticoagulation is considered a contraindication to banding, a retrospective study that identified significant bleeding in less than 3% of patients found this also linked to ASA and NSAID use [37]. Other investigators suggest bleeding is more related to untreated hemorrhoids than the banding itself and failure of the procedure is also linked to more extensive hemorrhoidal disease. Finally, while exceedingly rare, infectious complications including necrotizing pelvic sepsis and liver and retroperitoneal abscesses have been reported–antibiotics are not felt to be indicated for periprocedural prophylaxis [32,38].

Transanal Excision: Transanal excision of polyps and masses is associated with all the potential complications listed above. In some cases, full-thickness excision may be needed and caries higher risk of perforation into the peritoneal cavity (eg, resection of anterior lesion in thin woman) or damage to surrounding organs such as the vagina and urethra. Adequate counseling and planning for good exit strategies are key in safely moving patients through this procedure. The use of large operating scopes used in Transanal Endoscopic Microsurgery (TEM) and Transanal endoscopic minimally invasive surgery (TAMIS) can be associated with damage to the sphincter. Utilization of local anesthetic and gentle dilation before placing the operating scope can minimize these complications. Recurrence is a potential complication; studies have demonstrated similar outcomes to total mesorectal excision when patients are appropriately selected [39].

ANAL FISTULA

The management of fistulas can be particularly taxing due to their high recurrence rate and potential for associated complications such as incontinence and infection. LIFT and advancement flap have become workhorses for the management of transsphincteric fistulas. The procedure is less likely to be successful in patients with Crohn's disease or prior fistula surgery. The most common complication is dehiscence of the perineal wound and infection which may be precluded by leaving it open [40]. Trials comparing the LIFT procedure with other approaches such as mucosal advancement flap have generally favored LIFT with trends toward lower complication rates and decreased postoperative pain [41,42].

Anal fissure: Lateral internal sphincterotomy is the gold standard for the treatment of anal fissure. It has a very high success rate, but is associated with up to 5% chance of incontinence to stool and 8% chance of incontinence of gas, although these can be minimal when present. Tailored sphincterotomy as described above and alternatives such as the injection of Botox should be considered.

Anal condyloma and dysplasia: Treatment of anal condyloma and dysplasia generally involves the eradication of superficial disease, and is considered very safe. However, some patients, especially from higher risk groups such as immunosuppressed patients, will require multiple procedures over their lifetime, which can result in decreased sensitivity and incontinence as well as strictures related to the damage of anal mucosa. Careful treatment of only involved tissues is important to avoid these complications long term.

References

[1] Mei Z, Wang Q, Zhang Y, et al. Risk Factors for Recurrence after anal fistula surgery: A meta-analysis. Int J Surg 2019;69:153–64.

[2] Toyonaga T, Matsushima M, Sogawa N, et al. Postoperative urinary retention after surgery for benign anorectal disease: potential risk factors and strategy for prevention. Int J Colorectal Dis 2006;21(7):676–82.

[3] Haleem S, Ozair A, Singh A, et al. Postoperative urinary retention: A controlled trial of fixed-dose spinal anesthesia using bupivacaine versus ropivacaine. J Anaesthesiol Clin Pharmacol 2020;36(1):94–9.

[4] Cataldo PA, Senagore AJ. Does alpha sympathetic blockade prevent urinary retention following anorectal surgery? Dis Colon Rectum 1991;34(12):1113–6.

[5] Zaheer S, Reilly WT, Pemberton JH, et al. Urinary retention after operations for benign anorectal diseases. Dis Colon Rectum 1998;41(6):696–704.

[6] MacRae HM, McLeod RS. Comparison of hemorrhoidal treatment modalities. A meta-analysis. Dis Colon Rectum 1995;38(7):687–94.

[7] Sheikh F, Khubchandani IT, Rosen L, et al. Is anorectal surgery on chronic dialysis patients risky? Dis Colon Rectum 1992;35(1):56–8.

[8] Nelson RS, Ewing BM, Ternent C, et al. Risk of late bleeding following hemorrhoidal banding in patients on antithrombotic prophylaxis. Am J Surg 2008;196(6):994–9 [discussion: 9].

[9] Hubner M, Diana M, Zanetti G, et al. Surgical site infections in colon surgery: the patient, the procedure, the hospital, and the surgeon. Arch Surg 2011;146(11):1240–5.

[10] Hyman NH, Cataldo PA, Trevisani GT, et al. Tracking outcomes of anorectal surgery: the need for a disease-specific quality assessment tool. Dis Colon Rectum 2008;51(8):1221–4 [discussion: 4].

[11] Kunitake H, Poylin V. Complications Following Anorectal Surgery. Clin Colon Rectal Surg 2016;29(1):14–21.

[12] Patel SA, Kucejko RJ, Fazendin EA, et al. Are Prophylactic Antibiotic Agents Indicated in Anorectal Surgery for Patients with Human Immunodeficiency Virus? Surg Infect (Larchmt) 2017;18(8):924–8.

[13] Sözener U, Gedik E, Kessaf Aslar A, et al. Does Adjuvant Antibiotic Treatment After Drainage of Anorectal Abscess Prevent Development of Anal Fistulas? A Randomized, Placebo-Controlled, Double-Blind, Multicenter Study. Dis Colon Rectum 2011;54(8):923–9.

[14] Nisar PJ, Acheson AG, Neal KR, et al. Stapled hemorrhoidopexy compared with conventional hemorrhoidectomy: systematic review of randomized, controlled trials. Dis Colon Rectum 2004;47(11):1837–45.

[15] Murad-Regadas SM, Fernandes GO, Regadas FS, et al. How much of the internal sphincter may be divided during lateral sphincterotomy for chronic anal fissure in women? Morphologic and functional evaluation after sphincterotomy. Dis Colon Rectum 2013;56(5): 645–51.
[16] Knoefel WT, Hosch SB, Hoyer B, et al. The initial approach to anorectal abscesses: fistulotomy is safe and reduces the chance of recurrences. Dig Surg 2000;17(3):274–8.
[17] Ritchie RD, Sackier JM, Hodde JP. Incontinence rates after cutting seton treatment for anal fistula. Colorectal Dis 2009;11(6):564–71.
[18] Crain N, Aboulian A. Unplanned Returns to Care within Seven Days after Anorectal Surgery: Can they be Avoided? Am Surg 2019;85(1):92–7.
[19] Kyle S, Isbister WH. Management of anorectal abscesses: comparison between traditional incision and packing and de Pezzer catheter drainage. Aust N Z J Surg 1990;60(2): 129–31.
[20] Liberman H, Thorson AG. Anal stenosis. Am J Surg 2000;179(4):325–9.
[21] Kumar AH, Habib AS. The role of gabapentinoids in acute and chronic pain after surgery. Curr Opin Anaesthesiol 2019;32(5):629–34.
[22] Van Backer JT, Jordan MR, Leahy DT, et al. Preemptive Analgesia Decreases Pain Following Anorectal Surgery: A Prospective, Randomized, Double-Blinded, Placebo-Controlled Trial. Dis Colon Rectum 2018;61(7):824–9.
[23] Poylin V, Quinn J, Messer K, et al. Gabapentin significantly decreases posthemorrhoidectomy pain: a prospective study. Int J Colorectal Dis 2014;29(12):1565–9.
[24] Joshi GP, Neugebauer EA, Collaboration P. Evidence-based management of pain after haemorrhoidectomy surgery. Br J Surg 2010;97(8):1155–68.
[25] Sammour T, Barazanchi AW, Hill AG, et al. Evidence-Based Management of Pain After Excisional Haemorrhoidectomy Surgery: A PROSPECT Review Update. World J Surg 2017;41(2):603–14.
[26] Hartford LB, Murphy PB, Gray DK, et al. The Standardization of Outpatient Procedure (STOP) Narcotics after anorectal surgery: a prospective non-inferiority study to reduce opioid use. Tech Coloproctol 2020;24(6):563–71.
[27] Li S, Coloma M, White PF, et al. Comparison of the costs and recovery profiles of three anesthetic techniques for ambulatory anorectal surgery. Anesthesiology 2000;93(5):1225–30.
[28] Gupta P. Randomized, controlled study comparing sitz-bath and no-sitz-bath treatments in patients with acute anal fissures. ANZ J Surg 2006;76(8):718–21.
[29] Wang JY, Lu CY, Tsai HL, et al. Randomized controlled trial of LigaSure with submucosal dissection versus Ferguson hemorrhoidectomy for prolapsed hemorrhoids. World J Surg 2006;30(3):462–6.
[30] Wesarachawit W, Pattana-arun J. Antibiotics and early post operative complications of closed hemorrhoidectomy: a retrospective matched pair study. J Med Assoc Thai 2007;90(9):1828–32.
[31] Elton C, Sen P, Montgomery AC. Initial study to assess the effects of topical glyceryl trinitrate for pain after haemorrhoidectomy. Int J Surg Investig 2001;2(5):353–7.
[32] Nelson DW, Champagne BJ, Rivadeneira DE, et al. Prophylactic antibiotics for hemorrhoidectomy: are they really needed? Dis Colon Rectum 2014;57(3):365–9.
[33] Jeong HY, Hwang DY, Cho DH, et al. Analysis of risk factors for delayed bleeding after semi-closed hemorrhoidectomy. Int J Colorectal Dis 2021;36(4):857–64.
[34] Lee KC, Liu CC, Hu WH, et al. Risk of delayed bleeding after hemorrhoidectomy. Int J Colorectal Dis 2019;34(2):247–53.
[35] Chen HH, Wang JY, Changchien CR, et al. Effective management of posthemorrhoidectomy secondary hemorrhage using rectal irrigation. Dis Colon Rectum 2002;45(2):234–8.
[36] Giordano P, Overton J, Madeddu F, et al. Transanal hemorrhoidal dearterialization: a systematic review. Dis Colon Rectum 2009;52(9):1665–71.
[37] Iyer VS, Shrier I, Gordon PH. Long-term outcome of rubber band ligation for symptomatic primary and recurrent internal hemorrhoids. Dis Colon Rectum 2004;47(8):1364–70.

[38] Khan KI, Akmal M, Waqas A, et al. Role of prophylactic antibiotics in Milligan Morgan hemorrhoidectomy - a randomized control trial. Int J Surg 2014;12(8):868–71.
[39] Hakiman H, Pendola M, Fleshman JW. Replacing Transanal Excision with Transanal Endoscopic Microsurgery and/or Transanal Minimally Invasive Surgery for Early Rectal Cancer. Clin Colon Rectal Surg 2015;28(1):38–42.
[40] Emile SH, Khan SM, Adejumo A, et al. Ligation of intersphincteric fistula tract (LIFT) in treatment of anal fistula: An updated systematic review, meta-analysis, and meta-regression of the predictors of failure. Surgery 2020;167(2):484–92.
[41] Madbouly KM, El Shazly W, Abbas KS, et al. Ligation of intersphincteric fistula tract versus mucosal advancement flap in patients with high transsphincteric fistula-in-ano: a prospective randomized trial. Dis Colon Rectum 2014;57(10):1202–8.
[42] Mushaya C, Bartlett L, Schulze B, et al. Ligation of intersphincteric fistula tract compared with advancement flap for complex anorectal fistulas requiring initial seton drainage. Am J Surg 2012;204(3):283–9.

Advances in Surgery 56 (2022) 79–87

ADVANCES IN SURGERY

ELSEVIER
MOSBY

Private Equity and Its Increasing Role in US Healthcare

Kristen M. Beyer, MBA, Lyudmyla Demyan, MD, Matthew J. Weiss, MD, MBA*

Northwell Health Cancer Institute, Zucker School of Medicine at Hofstra Univeristy, 1111 Marcus Avenue, Lake Success, NY 11042, USA

Keywords

- Health care • Surgical care • Private equity investment in health care
- Private equity investment in surgical care
- Advantages of private equity investment in health care
- Drawbacks of private equity investment • Value-based care
- Fragmented health care market

Key points

- Private equity investments in health care and surgery are rising exponentially.
- Private equity investment in health care has the potential to be beneficial if done under the right parameters.
- Private equity firms should be diligent about finding solutions that deliver the best quality health care while maximizing the greatest return on investment.
- In health care, mission drives margin and having a keen focus on financial incentives that combat the traditional health care silos can theoretically produce high-quality products.

INTRODUCTION

Private equity (PE) investments have been rapidly expanding over the last decade. Most recently, the health care field has been a spotlight for PE investment. PE firms consist of individual fund managers often referred to as "General Partners" and outside investors called "Limited Partners" that infuse capital directly into a private, nonpublicly traded company or fund [1]. Investors in private firms are paid in distributions through the life of their investment rather

Funding/Support: This research did not receive any support from funding agencies in the public, commercial, or not-for-profit sector.

*Corresponding author. *E-mail address:* MWeiss8@northwell.edu

https://doi.org/10.1016/j.yasu.2022.02.003
0065-3411/22/

than stock accumulations. PE firms closely resemble venture capital firms in the sense that they invest directly into private companies or purchase them with the intent of optimizing and streamlining their operations to create value greater than the initial purchase price. However, Venture capitalists tend to invest in more start-up companies, which results in taking on more aggressive risks. PE firms generally are attracted to companies with longer turnaround or larger consolidation opportunities leading to potentially lucrative returns on investment.

PE firms approach their investments with a keen focus to enhance value and growth. Like hedge funds, PE companies require a large balance per investor. However, the investor has a greater lock-up period where their funds cannot be withdrawn until the period has elapsed. Compared with Hedge Funds with a lock-up period varying months to a year, PE firms can have lock-up periods for up to 10 years, which allows the opportunity to turn a company's financial health and operations around over a longer investment period [2]. PE firms frequently use subject matter experts in the fields that they invest in to run the operations and finances. The last decade has seen a remarkable increase in PE investment in health care and the field of surgery.

HEALTH CARE AND PE FIRMS

A recent study found that health care has become the second largest sector of PE investment. From 2010 to 2020, PE deals in health care have increased more than 250% (Fig. 1) [3,4]. Health care is appealing to PE firms because consumer demand remains stable throughout volatile economic periods. In addition, the health care industry remains fragmented, which provides opportunities for optimizing and potentially consolidating care across large markets with broad patient populations [5]. Most recently, PE firms have shifted their interest from buying out large hospitals and health systems to acquiring independent practices and physicians with the goal of consolidating, improving economies of scale, and negotiating enhanced reimbursements from payors.

Currently, surgical services account for 51% of all Medicare spending [4]. According to researchers at the University of Michigan, PE firms have increasingly purchased more surgical practices over the last 20 years, specifically Ambulatory Surgery Centers (ASCs). ASCs typically have a more efficient operational flow due to minimal interruptions from emergencies. The streamlined operations at ASCs are both appealing and convenient to providers and patients. In addition, ASCs offer lower costs than inpatient settings and Centers for Medicare and Medicaid Services (CMS) recently expanded the number of procedures that are covered under ASCs including 13 coronary intervention procedures [6]. All these factors are appealing to PE firms as they may protect from potential economic downturns. This is particularly true during the COVID pandemic where independently run ASCs have fewer restrictions and potential staff repurposing.

During the rise of PE investments in health care, particularly in surgical care, there has been limited research on the influence of PE deals on both the delivery and quality of patient care (Table 1). There are vastly conflicting opinions

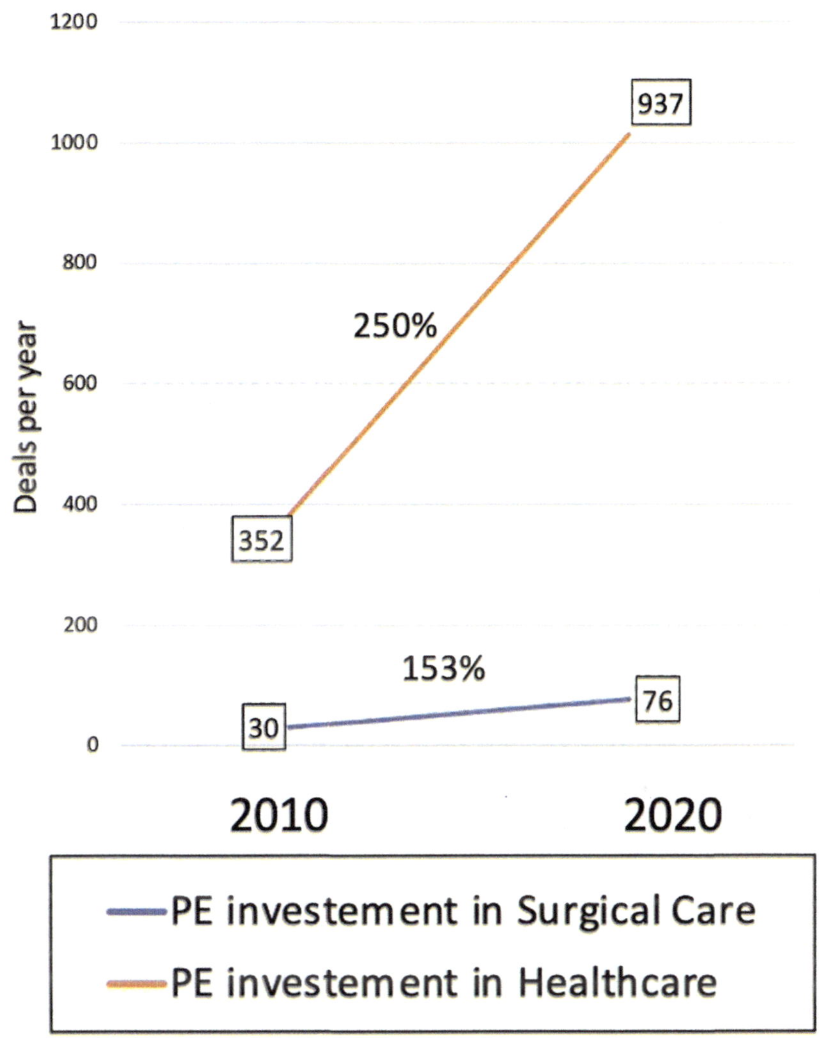

Fig. 1. PE investment in health care and surgical care between 2010 and 2020 [3,5].

on the benefits and shortfalls of PE investment into health care, making this a vigorously debated topic.

POTENTIAL DRAWBACKS OF PE INVESTMENTS IN HEALTH CARE

For years, it has been debated whether health care should be run as a for-profit business. Historically, it has been shown that nonprofit hospitals have lower cost of care, lower mortality rates, and better outcomes than for-profit hospitals [7]. These aspects are attributed to the quality of clinical staff caring for the

Table 1
Potential advantages and drawbacks of PE investment in health care in relation to stakeholders of care delivery: patients, health care providers, and health care systems

Stakeholders	Pros	Cons
Patients	• Streamline care delivery • Improve management for complex diseases • Enhance value-based care • Improve patient outcomes	• Increase out of pocket cost • Decrease quality of care • Reduce access to care • Lack of patient-centered model
Health care providers	• Access to innovative technology/science • Enhance reimbursement • Ensure streamlined operations	• Loss of autonomy • Liquidation of small practice • Disincentivize delivery of care to low-income patients • Conflict of interest
Health care systems	• Provide cost-effective care • Improve patient care outcomes • Liquidate fragmented health care • Eliminate insufficiencies/ eliminate waste	• Threat to public health • Concern for access to care for vulnerable communities • Unsustainable PE business practices

patients and the proper organizational protocols and processes put into place. This known fact combined with the notion that the goal of PE firms is consolidation and quick revenue generation, leads to the perception that PE companies will solely focus on their bottom line by cutting labor costs and using unsustainable business practices to quickly achieve profit.

PE in health care is also a contributor to the surprise billing epidemic. As a lightly regulated entity, PE-supported medical groups have the jurisdiction to charge higher prices for the services they render. For example, a patient may receive a disproportionally high bill from an out-of-network provider while receiving care at an in-network hospital [8,9]. A recent study from Stanford University found that 43% of patients received surprise bills from emergency room or inpatients services in 2016, which is considerably higher compared with 2010 [10]. Surprise billing may also occur for other health care–related services such as ambulance or airlift transportation, given that two-thirds of medical helicopters belong to for-profit providers [11]. As a recent example, an intubated coronavirus patient who was airlifted from one in-network hospital to another by a PE-owned air ambulance service was charged over $52k [12]. The 2020 legislation efforts to solve the surprise billing problem, unfortunately, left loopholes for companies to continue charging high prices.

The laser-focus of PE investors on profit may undermine the autonomy of health care practice owners. Once the acquisition occurs and a rapid period of process improvement initiatives are completed, the PE firm may ultimately sell to produce a high rate of return [2]. Most firms sell within 7 to 10 years, but the timing can be unpredictable. Although this tactic is the primary reason PE firms can be so lucrative, it may leave many health care owners wary of ultimately losing autonomy and strategic agility once the firm sells again. To mitigate this risk, before finalizing a relationship, health care owners should develop a solid exit plan that includes fulfilling active roles on the board and obtaining voting rights to ensure their voice and opinions remain represented. This can be accomplished through personally investing in the company or practice itself, sitting on the Board of Directors, or even through a contractual agreement.

Furthermore, the effects of PE investment in surgical care are not well understood. PE funding could lead to improved technology and advancement of surgical science; however, such advances usually come with a high price tag [5]. This also has the potential to affect the availability of certain surgical procedures and patient outcomes [4]. Further research is needed to understand the implications of PE funding in surgical care and surgical outcomes.

Besides potentially increasing costs and reducing the quality of care, PE investment in health care may also compromise access to care. Merger and acquisition of health care market drives small independent practices out of business, further decreasing physician practice choices and access to care [13]. Once acquired by PE investors, physicians might also be discouraged from providing care to low-income patients. This is critical because Bruch and colleagues [14] showed that hospitals in rural and low-income areas are more likely to be PE-owned compared to urban hospitals, further jeopardizing quality and access to care for an already vulnerable population.

An example of significant harm to patients related to PE investment was the closure of Hahnemann University Hospital in Philadelphia, which was previously owned by Tenet Healthcare Corporation until it was sold to Paladin Healthcare Capital. Economists predicted the Hahnemann University Hospital was bought based solely on their valuable real estate holdings located near the burgeoning arts district of Philadelphia and not on its mission to provide health care to low-income communities. Once the acquisition occurred, no steps were taken by management to enhance revenue streams by placing medical practices and services in wealthier communities, instead the hospital went into more debt over the next 18 months until ultimately filing for bankruptcy [15].

Health care is a unique industry that is government regulated and highly sensitive to consumer sentiment. Private investor-backed companies that use strategies such as inflating prices to maximize short-term profits without delivering any true health care benefits become quickly unsustainable and may lead to consumer outrage. This can quickly invoke government intervention and further regulation that risks derailing the PE strategy and profitability [9]. There is a potential need for a regulatory system to monitor health care economics and quality metrics of PE-acquired medical entities to ensure patient-centered care delivery.

POTENTIAL ADVANTAGES OF PE INVESTMENT IN HEALTH CARE

PE involvement in health care can be beneficial and can potentially solve some of today's most complex health care issues. The first is health care spending. Currently, health care represents approximately 20% of gross domestic product (GDP). It is anticipated that by the year 2030, as more of the population enter their seventies and eighties, health care spending will be approximately 16 trillion per year in the United States, or 32% of the GDP [16]. One reason for increased health care spending may be attributed to poor productivity and inefficiencies in the health care industry [17].

In addition, health care consumers are becoming increasingly educated on health care quality and value-based care. Aside from medical emergencies, patients increasingly seek out their own health care services and research which institutions provide best in class care [18]. These factors can influence PE firms to streamline health care inefficiencies and ensure both quality and cost-effective care to dominate the health care market. The reality is that hospitals and health systems have been slow to address these issues on their own. Providing high-quality services at affordable prices to patients while eliminating waste may increase market share and decrease overall health care spending.

The health care payer market is volatile and ever-changing. The payer shift to value-based care may create the opportunity for better alignment with other specialty groups, whereas fee-for-service models have long incentivized financial performance and fee-for-service over quality and comprehensive care. This new value-based care payment model holds physicians and health care systems more financially accountable on the total cost of the patient's treatment and recovery [19]. A PE firm that invests in a health care company under this payment model would focus on investments and operational changes that support better outcomes and lower costs regardless if they act purely out of financial self-interest [20]. PE firms also could provide the opportunity to negotiate better enhanced rates for commercial payers especially if they consolidate a company and eliminate waste.

There are numerous examples of PE investments improving the quality of care delivered. According to a case study on CareMore Health acquired by PE firm CCMP Capital in 2006, CareMore increased from 4 to 27 care centers and 22,000 to 55,000 patients over a 5-year period. Data support that the quality of care improved under the PE ownership. Colorectal screening increased from 56% to 74% surpassing the national average of 58% in 2011. Hemoglobin A1C and blood pressure control improved from 10% to 20% above the national average [21]. Another case study on Oak Street Health, a primary care group that serves older adults, found that their PE acquisition led to fewer hospital admissions, fewer 30-day readmissions, and emergency department visits after expanding to 54 clinics across 8 states. In either case study, no adverse outcomes were reported [20].

Consolidation of fragmented health care market may improve care delivery for diseases that require complex management. Bundled payments for cancer diagnoses emphasize the most effective clinical and efficient treatments, which can further accentuate the need to build comprehensive models [22]. This is now a health care culture shift occurring that requires breaking down the current silos in the health care market. PE investment may provide access to innovative technology, which is imperative to ensure streamlined operations and fluid provider communication. As cancer care has evolved into multidisciplinary approaches, the relative value of treatments such as chemotherapy, immunotherapy, surgery, and radiation has now led payors to consider the cost of such treatments with respect to life-years gained. Bundling payments for a specific cancer diagnosis are already pushing systems to develop treatment regimens that are both clinically and cost-effective [23]. PE firms have the potential to address such complicated clinical and financial decisions if engaged properly.

According to a John's Hopkins study, the third leading cause of death in the United States is medical errors [24]. We are antiquated in providing the most efficient quality care possible to our patients. Such inefficiencies that contribute to poor patient care and outcomes may be solved with improved technology infrastructure. PE firms may provide health care businesses access to funds that allow investments in innovative technology and data integration platforms [25]. These platforms have the potential to make the patient experience more seamless and collect the best quality data for a complex system. The access to key quality data may help to address the deficiencies and shortfalls of the operations, which directly affect quality of care. Furthermore, advances in technology can produce quicker access to information for patients and providers and the ability to capture key data in an organized and seamless fashion to measure quality and growth. In addition, technology can help administrators better understand coding opportunities to enhance revenue and other areas of improvement.

SUMMARY

PE investments in health care are on the rise and as leaders, we need to understand how PE can fit into the current health care environment. Finding ways to use the vast resources and capital of PE has the potential to improve patient care. Although PE does focus on a high operating margin, that does not mean the quality of care necessarily has to be compromised. Changes in health care delivery and the management of PE has the potential to address some of the difficult challenges and inefficiencies that we have failed to address for decades.

Disclosure

The authors have nothing to disclose.

References

[1] The enduring appeal of private equity. WMS. 2019. Available at: https://www.wms-partners.com/insights/the-enduring-appeal-of-private-equity. Accessed October, 2021.

[2] Ivashina V. Pay now or pay later?: the economics within the private equity partnership. Journal of Financial Economics (JFE), Forthcoming 2016;51.
[3] Scheffler RM. Soaring Private Equiry Investment in the healthcare sector: consolidation accelerated, competition undermined, and patients at risk. 2021. Available at:https://publichealth.berkeley.edu/wp-content/uploads/2021/05/Private-Equity-I-Healthcare-Report-FINAL.pdf. . Accessed October, 2021.
[4] Billig JI, Kotsis SV, Chung KC. Trends in funding and acquisition of surgical practices by private equity firms in the US From 2000 to 2020. JAMA Surg 2021;156(11): 1066–8.
[5] Bruch JD, Gondi S, Song Z. Changes in hospital income, use, and quality associated with private equity acquisition. JAMA Intern Med 2020;180(11):1428–35.
[6] Private Equity Transactions for Ambulatory Surgery Centers (ASCs). Answers to the what? why? and who? questions. Available at: https://www.garfunkelwild.com/wp-content/ASC/ASC%202020/11-10-2020%20Reibolt,%20Goettling%20-%207th%20Annual%20ASC%20-%20Post-COVID%20Keys%20To%20Private%20Equity%20Transactions.pdf 2020. Accessed November 1, 2020.
[7] Himmelstein DU, Woolhandler S, Hellander I, et al. Quality of care in investor-owned vs not-for-profit HMOs. JAMA 1999;282(2):159–63.
[8] Meindl JaWS. Healthcare M&A report. Chicago (IL): VMG Health: American Medical Association (AMA); 2019.
[9] Lovisa Gustafsson SS, Blumenthal David. The Role of Private Equity in Driving Up Health Care Prices. In. Harward Business Review. Available at: https://hbr.org/2019/10/the-role-of-private-equity-in-driving-up-health-care-prices 2019. Accessed October 1, 2019.
[10] Sun EC, Mello MM, Moshfegh J, et al. Assessment of out-of-network billing for privately insured patients receiving care in in-network hospitals. JAMA Intern Med 2019;179(11): 1543–50.
[11] Tozzi J. Air Ambulances Are Flying More Patients Than Ever, and Leaving Massive Bills Behind. Bloomberg 2018.
[12] Kliff S. A $52,112 Air Ambulance Ride: Coronavirus Patients Battle Surprise Bills. The New York Times2020.
[13] Reinhardt UE. The rise and fall of the physician practice management industry. Health Aff (Millwood) 2000;19(1):42–55.
[14] Characteristics of private equity–owned hospitals in 2018. Ann Intern Med 2021;174(2): 277–9.
[15] Pomorski C. The death of hahnemann hospital. In. The New Yorker 2021.
[16] Burner ST, Waldo DR, McKusick DR. National health expenditures projections through 2030. Health Care Financ Rev 1992;14(1):1–29.
[17] David Champagne AD, J Littlejohns, D Podpolny. Private equity opportunities in healthcare tech. 2019. Accessed October 2021.
[18] Weil AR. Patients as consumers. Health Affairs; 2019.
[19] What is value-based healthcare? USA; NEJM Catalyst 2019.
[20] Powers BWS, William H, Navathe AS. Private equity and health care delivery: value-based payment as a guardrail? JAMA 2021;326(10):907–8.
[21] Huckman RS, Powers BW. CareMore health system. Harvard Business School. 2017. Available at: https://www.hbs.edu/faculty/Pages/item.aspx?num=52933. Accessed December 18, 2021.
[22] Oncology care model. Available at: https://innovation.cms.gov/innovation-models/oncology-care. Accessed December, 2021.
[23] Kline RM, Muldoon LD, Schumacher HK, et al. Design challenges of an episode-based payment model in oncology: the centers for medicare & medicaid services oncology care model. J Oncol Pract 2017;13(7):e632–45.

[24] Study Suggests Medical Errors Now Third Leading Cause of Death in the U.S. 2016. Available at: https://www.hopkinsmedicine.org/news/media/releases/study_suggests_medical_errors_now_third_leading_cause_of_death_in_the_us. Accessed November 2021.
[25] Anaeze C. Offodile II MC, Mohini Bindal, Jose Alejandro Rauh-Hain, and Vivian Ho. Private Equity Investments In Health Care: An Overview Of Hospital And Health System Leveraged Buyouts, 2003–17. Health Aff 2021;40(5):719–26.

Advances in Surgery 56 (2022) 89–109
ADVANCES IN SURGERY

Facts and Fallacy of Benchmark Performance Indicators

James P. Byrne, MD, PhD, FRCSC*, Elliott R. Haut, MD, PhD
Division of Acute Care Surgery, Department of Surgery, Johns Hopkins Hospital, Sheikh Zayed 6107 1800 Orleans Street, Baltimore, MD 21287, USA

Keywords

• Surgery • Performance improvement • Benchmarking • Quality • Risk-adjustment • Performance indicator

Key points

- Quality improvement in health care in the United States has evolved over time, with the Donabedian model of structure, process, and outcome at the center of the current framework.
- Although performance benchmarking arose in industry, it is now ubiquitous across surgical disciplines with the goal of using risk-adjusted outcomes to improve surgeon and hospital performance.
- Performance benchmarking initiatives are not without their challenges, including the definition of certain outcomes as quality measures, the potential for unmeasured confounding, and the potential for participants to prioritize measured performance over optimal patient care.

BACKGROUND

The case of need to improve quality in health care

It is an expectation of the American public that when they fall ill, they will receive health care that both meets their needs and is based on best scientific knowledge [1]. The care received should meet this standard irrespective of the geographic location at which the illness or injury occurs, or the facility or medical team treating the patient. Simply stated, patients should receive the right treatment, at the right place, at the right time to achieve the best possible outcome. Unfortunately, this is often not realized. An illustrative case occurred in 1976 when an orthopedic surgeon piloting

*Corresponding author. Division of Trauma and Acute Care Surgery, Department of Surgery, Johns Hopkins Hospital, Sheikh Zayed 6107E 1800 Orleans Street, Baltimore, MD 21287, USA *E-mail address:* Jbyrne13@jh.edu
Twitter: @dctrjbyrne (J.P.B.); @elliotthaut (E.R.H.)

https://doi.org/10.1016/j.yasu.2022.03.002

a plane crashed in rural Nebraska. Reflecting on the inadequate and disorganized care he and his family received, he stated: "When I can provide better care in the field with limited resources than what my children and I received at the primary care facility, there is something wrong with the system, and the system has to be changed" [2] prompting creation of the American College of Surgeons Advanced Trauma Life Support (ATLS) course. The discordance between expectation and actual care persists. Although two-thirds of the United States public believe that they would receive "the best medical care" should they be seriously injured [3], Minei and colleagues found that case fatality rates after severe injury ranged from 14% to 51% between nine North American geographic regions [4]. The risk of mortality varies further between specialized trauma centers [5]–the centers designed to house the optimal resources for care of injured patients [6]. More broadly, this has been similarly true between hospitals for patients undergoing general surgical, vascular, thoracic, urologic, orthopedic, and neurosurgical procedures [7]. This concern applies to both elective and emergency surgical conditions. Therefore, the quality of medical treatment a patient receives continues to depend on the location at which illness occurs and the facility in which it is treated. It is the recognition of this challenge, which continues to the present day, that has driven the need to define and evaluate the quality of care.

Defining quality in modern health care: structure, process, and outcome

The Institute of Medicine has defined quality in health care as "the degree to which health services for individuals and populations increase the likelihood of desired health outcomes and are consistent with current professional knowledge" [8]. Avedis Donabedian, a physician and epidemiologist whose work was foundational to the conceptualization of quality in medicine [9], provided the framework to measure quality in three key domains: structure, process, and outcomes [10,11]. Structures of care relate to the material attributes and resources of the environment in which health care is delivered (ie, hospital buildings, operating rooms). Processes of care describe the sequence of events that take place during the delivery of care (ie, timing of antibiotic administration), reflect physician decision-making, and the interaction between clinician and patients. Outcomes describe the effect of care on the health status of patients (ie, mortality, complications), a reflection of both structures and processes. As variation in structures and processes of care influence outcomes, all three dimensions provide valuable information with which to evaluate quality [1]. The comparison of structures or processes to determine which factors result in more favorable outcomes is central to quality improvement.

Evolution of benchmarking: from private industry to health care

Evaluation of quality requires that there be comparators. The word 'benchmark', defined as "a point of reference from which measurements may be made" [12], was first implemented as a verb ('benchmarking') and business practice at Xerox in 1979 [13,14] in response to deteriorating market share. By evaluating the best practices of their direct competitors (competitive benchmarking) as well as the efficiencies of companies in different industries (process benchmarking), Xerox improved the quality of their processes to the degree that it was awarded a Presidential award for performance in manufacturing by the National Institute of Standards and Technology in 1989 [15]. Performance benchmarking has since become a ubiquitous practice in business and finance.

Contemporaneous with the advent of benchmarking in business and finance, the practice of collecting data for the purpose of evaluating performance improvement arose in health care. However, the concept was not new. Ernest Codman was a surgeon in Boston in the early 1900s and is credited with developing the concept of the "end result idea" suggesting that outcomes should be measured for surgical patients. At the time, his ideas were not embraced, and he was shunned from standard medical practice. Only now, nearly a century after his death, do we realize how important his insights were. One of the earliest examples of benchmarking in health care in the modern era was the study and public reporting of outcomes after coronary artery bypass grafting beginning in the late 1980s. This example has improved the overall care of patients with cardiovascular disease by specifically improving patient outcomes when comparing both individual surgeons [16] and institutions [17]. The application of risk-adjusted outcomes to improve the quality of care for patients undergoing elective surgical procedures arose in the Veterans Health Administration in the 1990s [18] and more broadly into the private sector in the early 2000s via the National Surgical Quality Improvement Program (NSQIP) [19]. Benchmarking of trauma care began with the major trauma outcomes study (MTOS) in the 1980s [20]. This concept of collecting data and outcomes in trauma evolved into the American College of Surgeons (ACS) National Trauma Data Bank (NTDB). The study of trauma center outcomes is now well accepted to improve performance in the care of injured patients by the ACS via the ACS Committee on Trauma (ACS COT), and the Trauma Quality Improvement Program (TQIP) [5,21]. Similar quality improvement initiatives in other surgical specialties have been successfully implemented.

QUALITY MEASUREMENT AND PERFORMANCE IMPROVEMENT

A national framework for evaluating and improving quality in health care

The Agency for Healthcare Research and Quality (AHRQ), the lead federal agency charged with improving quality, safety, efficiency, and effectiveness in health care in the United States [22], has sought to provide a common language with which to approach the quality improvement process (Table 1). The Institute of Medicine has provided the framework that quality health care achieves the following six aims: safe, effective, patient centered, timely, efficient, and equitable [1,23]. Within these six aims, quality measures can be classified under the three domains of the Donabedian model as relating to structure, process, or outcomes [24].

The data sources from which quality measures are derived and studied must be carefully considered. These range in scope of the patient population captured, the granularity of clinical detail, and nature of information available

Table 1
Framework for measuring and evaluating quality in health care

Aims of the health care system: six domains of quality	
Safe	Avoiding harm
Effective	Providing evidence-based care that benefits patients
Patient-centered	Providing care that is respectful and responsive to patient preferences
Timely	Minimizing harmful delays in care
Efficient	Avoiding waste and unnecessary cost
Equitable	Providing quality care irrespective of patient characteristics
Types of Health Care Quality Measures	
Structural Measures	Features of the system that affect its capacity to provide high-quality care
Process Measures	Reflect physician decision-making and treatments delivered
Outcome Measures	Reflect the impact of structures and processes on the patient health status
Data Sources for Health Care Quality Measurement	
Administrative Data	• Often population-based, linked to payments or health encounters • Benefits: Broad evaluations of health care processes • Drawbacks: Lack granular clinical data for patient-level risk adjustment • Example: Healthcare Cost and Utilization Project (HCUP) databases
Standardized Clinical Data	• Data collected from facilities by trained abstractors • Benefits: Granular clinical data useable for evaluations of patient-level processes of care • Drawbacks: Not collected for purpose of secondary analyses • Examples: NSQIP, TQIP, STS
Quality Measures	
Standardization	Standardized at the national level
Comparability	Risk-adjusted to allow for true measurement of performance
Availability	Available across all relevant health institutions
Timeliness	Available at points in time that fit needs of the participating institutions
Relevance	Reflects the outcome of concern
Validity	Tested for accuracy and reliability
Experience	Institutions have experience with the measure so that data errors are unlikely
Stability	Will remain in use over time
Evaluability	Clearly reflects an outcome that is good or bad
Distinguishable	Can be used to demonstrate significant differences between institutions
Credibility	Has been demonstrated to represent the true outcome through audit

This framework is derived from the Agency for Healthcare Research and Quality [1].

[25]. Administrative databases are often linked to the payment claims or patient encounters within health systems. These allow for broad, population-based evaluations of the administration of health care but often lack granular clinical details necessary for the risk adjustment at the patient level. Examples of administrative databases include the Healthcare Cost and Utilization Project databases that aim to track health care utilization and access in the United States [26]. These datasets can be used for benchmarking but also are routinely used for other types of health services, outcomes, and comparative effectiveness research [27]. Conversely, there are also databases or registries that capture granular clinical information at the patient level from hospitals in a standardized fashion. Such datasets allow for the evaluation of associations between processes of care and outcomes. Examples include the NSQIP[28] database, the Metabolic and Bariatric Surgery Accreditation and Quality Improvement Program (MBSAQIP), and the National Trauma Databank [29] maintained under the Quality Programs of the ACS. Other major surgical societies also maintain well-respected and validated registries. The Society for Thoracic Surgeons registry may be one of the largest of its type including both cardiac and thoracic procedures.

Finally, quality measures selected for evaluation must be carefully considered. Measures should be available and standardizable across institutions, relevant to the end user, and validated to accurately reflect the clinical process or outcome of concern [30]. Although the relevant quality measures will vary by medical or surgical discipline and patient population, the National Quality Forum provides an objective and standardized assessment of measures against a list of desired properties [31].

The performance improvement process

The ultimate goal of measuring the quality of care is to provide new insights into how performance can be improved. In other words, what changes can be made to existing structures or processes that will result in improved patient outcomes? The implementation of evidence-based changes tends to follow a process common to performance improvement endeavors. These have been formalized in approaches to quality improvement such as the Plan-Do-Study-Act Worksheet [32], Lean Six Sigma [33], and others. The Translating Evidence Into Practice model [34] is an implementation science framework for implementing evidence-based changes for the purpose of quality improvement [35] and has been used as a backbone by many process improvement initiatives [36]. One model for the performance improvement process is shown in Fig. 1.

The performance improvement process is rooted in high-quality standardized data collected in a manner commensurate with the framework described above. Analysis of data is undertaken following the correct methodology to evaluate the relationship of interest. In the case of benchmarking in surgery, the relationship evaluated is often the association between the individual surgeon (or institution) and the likelihood (or risk) of favorable (or unfavorable) outcome. Careful risk adjustment must be performed in analyses to account

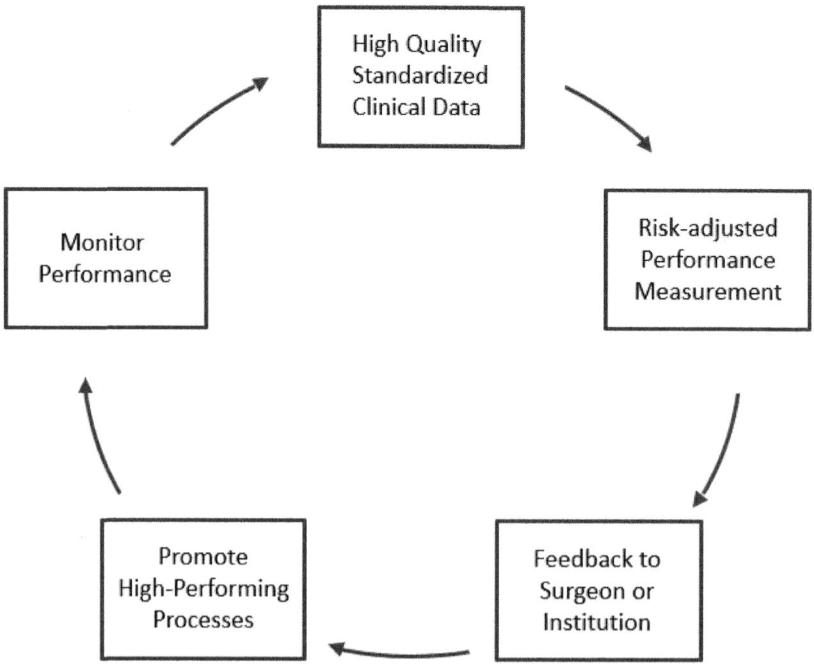

Fig. 1. The cycle of performance improvement.

for confounding factors (ie, differences in patient demographics, comorbidities, presenting characteristics) with the goal of estimating the true causal relationship within margins of error. Once risk-adjusted analysis has yielded estimates of performance, feedback is delivered to the individual surgeon (or institution) in a format that can be easily interpreted and acted upon.

This information is used to promote structures and processes of care that are found to be associated with high performance. For example, among a group of surgeons, those identified to have worse-than-expected rates of a poor outcome might benefit from learning what techniques or approaches are used by surgeons with better performance. Recent data have shown the benefit of coaching by high-performing surgeons of individual lower-performing surgeons [37]. Statewide collaboratives have shown improvement of participant hospital performance as the result of data-driven benchmarking of peer centers [38]. For example, hospitals with higher-than-expected rates of urinary tract infections after elective colorectal surgery might benefit from implementing the catheterization best practices used by hospitals with lower rates of this complication. After implementation of changes, performance is monitored, new data are collected, and the performance improvement cycle repeats. The net result of this iterative process is that all participants move closer to an average state of higher overall performance–the embodiment of the aphorism "a rising tide lifts all boats".

METHODOLOGIES FOR PERFORMANCE BENCHMARKING IN SURGERY

Data collection and management

The need to collect high-quality data is common to all performance benchmarking initiatives. This process is made more complicated by the nature of the data often being collected from multiple hospitals with registries maintained by different groups. Quality of the data collected can be ensured through multiple mechanisms [28,39,40]. Data abstractors should receive dedicated training. Data reliability audits should be performed to ensure the coding accuracy of the variables collected. Many performance benchmarking initiatives require that institutions achieve a minimum standard of data reliability, and that data input is up to date. If the underlying data are not reliable, the inferences made from the data will be flawed. For example, in early iterations of the NTDB, complication reporting was optional. As a result, centers that chose not to report complications might appear as high performers in benchmarking reports. Only by identifying these omissions and excluding such centers could reliable inferences be made [41].

Missing data are a common problem among health care registries [42,43]. The easiest approach to managing missing data is to exclude patients with missing variables from analysis. However, if these data are not missing at random, exclusion of these cases introduces bias into adjusted results [42]. Therefore, the current best practice is to use multiple imputation methodology to deal with missing variables [43,44]. Specifically, a multiple imputation algorithm is used to estimate the missing values based on nonmissing variables, and the final imputed value is the average of multiple estimates. An even better approach is to use software enhancements to require that all fields be completed.

Data are cleaned and cohorts of interest are defined. For example, in the case of the ACS NSQIP patients undergoing targeted procedures (eg, colorectal, pancreas, ventral hernia, appendectomy) are evaluated with additional data elements important to evaluating processes and outcomes specific to those operations. Similarly, ACS TQIP patients with blunt multiple system injuries or hemorrhagic shock might be considered in distinct analyses. In this way, patients with similar characteristics can be compared between hospitals to provide meaningful results.

Estimating risk-adjusted performance: O/E ratios and hierarchical models

Because the characteristics of patients often differ between hospitals, risk adjustment to account for these differences in patient case mix is of utmost importance. To accomplish this, hospital performance was initially reported in the form of risk-adjusted observed-to-expected (O/E) ratios. Logistic regression analysis, adjusted for each patient's unique baseline characteristics, is used to predict the probability of death or complication. Within specific patient cohorts or specific surgical procedures, the probabilities are summed for each hospital to provide the expected number of adverse events. The O/E ratios for each hospital with 95% confidence intervals are then calculated. Hospitals with O/E ratios that are significantly higher or lower than average are identified. This information is fed back to institutions for the purpose of promoting local quality improvement, in keeping with the cycle of performance improvement [19,40].

In recent years, surgical performance improvement initiatives have adopted the use of hierarchical or multilevel models. These models are logistic regression models that both adjust for patient characteristics and account for the clustering of patients within hospitals. The advantage of such hierarchical models is the ability to model the outcome probability for each hospital [45]. In doing so, each hospital's unique odds ratio with a 95% confidence interval for the outcome, adjusted for patient characteristics, is estimated. Hospitals with lower limits of the 95% confidence intervals that are greater than 1 are identified as high outliers–those where the odds of the outcome are significantly higher than average. Conversely, hospitals with upper limits of the 95% confidence intervals that are lower than 1 are identified as low outliers–those where the odds of the outcome are significantly lower than average. By plotting each hospital's odds ratio for mortality with a 95% confidence interval on the same graph, a caterpillar plot is obtained (Fig. 2). Caterpillar plots provide a visual representation of each hospital's performance compared with other hospitals (or individual surgeons compared with peers). In this way, benchmarking reports provide participating hospitals with an objective measure of their performance relative to peers.

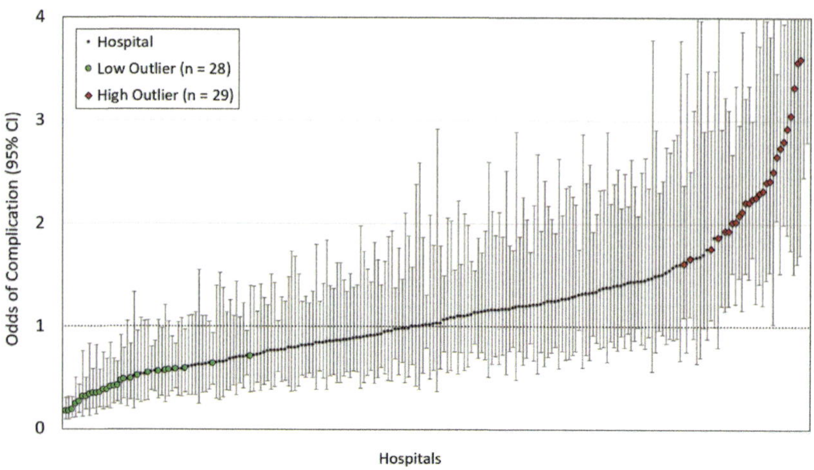

Fig. 2. Caterpillar plot, showing each hospital's unique odds ratio and 95% confidence interval (CI) for the complication under study. Hospitals with the upper limit of the 95% CI less than 1 are low outliers (better than expected—shown in *green*) with significantly lower-than-average odds of complication. Hospitals with the lower limit of the 95% CI greater than 1 are high outliers (worse than expected—shown in *red*) with significantly higher-than-average odds of complication.

SUCCESSFUL PERFORMANCE BENCHMARKING INITIATIVES IN SURGERY

Cardiac surgery

Several performance benchmarking initiatives aimed at improving the care of surgical patients have arisen and matured over the past three decades. Perhaps one of the earliest and longest-standing examples has been in cardiac surgery. Beginning in 1987, a regional intervention study was performed among 23 cardiothoracic surgeons practicing in the states of Maine, New Hampshire, and Vermont [16]. Data were collected for more than 15,000 patients undergoing coronary artery bypass graft surgery (CABG) over a 6-year period. Halfway through the study period, interventions were implemented whereby surgeons were provided feedback on outcomes, training in quality improvement practices, and site visits to other hospitals. In the postintervention period, a statistically significant 24% reduction in mortality was observed to be associated with the implementation of the interventions.

Along a similar timeline, the New York State Department of Health began collecting, analyzing, and disseminating data regarding risk factors, complications, and mortality following CABG in 1989 [46]. These data were used to stimulate quality improvement activities at hospitals across the state. An evaluation of the impact of this initiative at all 30 hospitals in the state performing CABG demonstrated that risk-adjusted patient mortality after surgery decreased by 41%, from 4.2% to 2.5% over the 3-year study period [17]. In another study using similar data, hospitals were grouped into three tertiles based on performance at the beginning of the study. There were significant differences in risk-adjusted mortality between the three groups at baseline. However, by the end of the study period, risk-adjusted mortality was comparable [47]. As these landmark reports, the New York State Cardiac Reporting System has expanded to report outcomes for CABG, percutaneous coronary intervention, and valvular operations [46,48]. The risk-adjusted mortality for each individual cardiothoracic surgeon is also publicly disclosed. National benchmarking of cardiac surgery is now available through the Society of Thoracic Surgeons databases.

Elective non-cardiac surgery

In 1985, a US government mandate sought to solve the problem of high observed rates of complications and mortality after surgery at Veteran's Administration (VA) hospitals [49]. This initiative was hampered by the lack of reliable data for the comparison of outcomes. For this reason, the legislative act specified that improved data collection and use of risk-adjusted outcomes would allow for accurate comparisons between hospitals to allow for quality improvement. In this setting, Khuri and Daley embarked on the implementation of a program to evaluate 30-day mortality and morbidity for patients undergoing elective noncardiac major surgery at Veterans Affairs Medical Centers (VAMCs). Between 1991 and 1993, the National VA Surgical Risk Study demonstrated the feasibility and set the parameters for the risk adjustment using data collected at 44 VAMCs [18,50]. In 1994, the VA-NSQIP was established, providing a means for the comparison of risk-adjusted morbidity and mortality across 10 surgical subspecialties at all 133 VAMCs. In 2002, a report found that since the inception of VA NSQIP, risk-adjusted postoperative mortality among patients undergoing major surgery had decreased by 27% and morbidity had decreased by 45% [50].

The success of VA NSQIP led to the evaluation of the concept outside the VA in a pilot study at a small number of academic and private hospitals [19]. In 2004, NSQIP was implemented at the national level by the ACS. The program provides benchmarking reports that contain caterpillar plots that describe each participating hospital's risk-adjusted performance relative to peers in the domains of 30-day postoperative mortality and complications. Today, approximately 700 participating hospitals submit data to ACS NSQIP and receive benchmarking reports.

NSQIP has grown in scope and number of participating centers. Initially, data collected were the same for all types of surgical procedures. Recently, more granular data are collected for targeted procedures with specific outcomes of interest particular to those procedures. For example, specialty-specific information and outcomes unique to colorectal surgery have been captured (ie, anastomotic leak). Similar initiatives are underway for hepatobiliary, urologic, hernia, and appendectomy.

Trauma

Performance improvement has long been central to the community of surgeons that care for injured patients. Trauma as a specialty was the first to develop regionalized systems of care by establishing dedicated trauma centers [51]. Since its inception in 1979, the ACS COT has promoted a 'systems approach' to improving the quality of care, based on the principles of the Donabedian model [11]. The COT first published its resource document entitled "Optimal Resources for Care of the Injured Patient" [6] 40 years ago. This document outlines the complement of structures and processes of care that should be available to provide high-quality care to trauma patients. At the core is a performance improvement process in which quality of care is monitored and systematically reviewed. The emphasis on the organization of structures and processes within hospitals for optimal patient care led to the establishment of the trauma center verification process in 1987 [52]. The underlying objective of the verification process is to standardize structures and processes of care and to minimize variation in the quality of care.

Despite this emphasis on standardization of care, variation in practices and patient outcomes persisted. In 2006, the COT created TQIP [53] under the mandate to design, test, and validate the measurement of risk-adjusted outcomes for improving trauma care. The COT had already created the National Trauma Databank [29] that captured standardized clinical data for trauma patients treated at trauma centers in the United States. However, the differences in patient case mix between trauma centers were not considered in the National

Trauma Databank initiative. In its landmark report in 2009, the TQIP group reported significant variation in risk-adjusted trauma patient mortality between trauma centers [5]. This finding was notable in the context of the efforts of the COT to standardize care at trauma centers. Following methodology like that implemented by NSQIP, the feasibility of TQIP to provide risk-adjusted trauma center performance for the purpose of benchmarking was demonstrated [54]. The emphasis by TQIP on best practices in data collection, standardization, and validation [5] provides a roadmap for other benchmarking quality improvement initiatives. Today, TQIP provides benchmarking reports to more than 875 level 1, 2, and 3 trauma centers across the United States [53], and participation in TQIP has become a requirement for trauma center verification by the ACS COT.

Other surgical disciplines

In the current era of surgical safety and quality assurance, risk-adjusted performance benchmarking of hospital outcomes has become common across many surgical disciplines. Table 2 provides a list of benchmarking programs run by a variety of national professional organizations. In many cases, these programs

Table 2
Representative benchmarking initiatives across surgical disciplines

Initiative	Website
American College of Surgeons (ACS)	
National Surgical Quality Improvement Program (NSQIP)	https://www.facs.org/quality-programs/acs-nsqip
Trauma Quality Improvement Program (TQIP)	https://www.facs.org/quality-programs/trauma/tqp/center-programs/tqip
Metabolic and Bariatric Surgery Accreditation and Quality Improvement Program (MBSAQIP)	https://www.facs.org/quality-programs/mbsaqip
Society of Thoracic Surgeons (STS)	
Adult Cardiac Surgery Database	https://publicreporting.sts.org/search/acsd
Congenital Heart Surgery Database	https://publicreporting.sts.org/chsd-exp
General Thoracic Surgery Database	https://publicreporting.sts.org/gtsd-about
American Association of Endocrine Surgery (AAES)	
Collaborative Endocrine Surgery Quality Improvement Program (CESQIP)	https://cesqip.org/
Society for Vascular Surgery (SVS)	
Vascular Quality Initiative (VQI)	https://www.vqi.org/quality-improvement/qi-projects/
Americas Hernia Society	
Abdominal Core Health Quality Collaborative	https://www.achqc.org/
United Network for Organ Sharing (UNOS)	
Transplant Center Benchmarking Reports	https://unos.org/data/data-collection/

provide feedback to hospitals (or individual surgeons) via benchmarking reports. Many also allow for their standardized clinical data to be used by participating institutions for research evaluating associations between processes of care and outcomes.

FALLACIES IN PERFORMANCE BENCHMARKING: PITFALLS AND MISPERCEPTIONS

As performance benchmarking has become ubiquitous across surgical disciplines, the implications of comparing performance between peers have been met with skepticism and scrutiny. In disciplines where participation in benchmarking initiatives has become mandatory, the validity of the results of risk-adjusted benchmarking methodology is of utmost importance. Some participants have raised concern about the methodology, whether the comparisons made between hospitals are fair, and whether the results are accurate. Another concern is the possibility of bias is introduced by selecting specific outcomes as measures of performance and quality of care. At a time when performance reporting and quality measurement have become central to medical institutions nationwide, negative outcomes might become attributed to poor quality of care, even if the occurrence of these outcomes are not always preventable. Finally, the measurement and reporting of performance may have inadvertent consequences on decision-making and patient care. Here we describe these potential pitfalls and misperceptions in greater detail. The examples highlight the importance of continued progress of benchmarking initiatives to strive for improved methodologies, open communication with centers that participate in them, and judicious introspection with regards to their impact on patient care.

Never events

The evolving culture of medical safety and quality assurance has been positive for the reasons previously highlighted in this paper. Standardized measurement and reporting of outcomes have decreased practice variation and improved patient care. However, emphasis on patient outcomes as synonymous with quality and performance has the potential to be detrimental to institutions in a manner not justified by medical evidence. An example of where such fallacies might occur is in the concept of 'never events'.

The term 'never event' was first coined by the National Quality Forum [31] to refer to serious medical errors that should never occur (eg, wrong-site surgery, unintentionally retained foreign objects) [55]. Over time, however, the term's use has become more widespread to refer to measured adverse events that might be preventable. Consequently, emphasis on patient safety in the national conversation on health care has led to declaring preventable adverse outcomes as 'never events'. In 2009, the President's Fiscal Year Budget outlined this approach [56,57]. Outcomes such as catheter-associated urinary tract infections, venous thromboembolism, and hospital-acquired or ventilator-associated pneumonia were among labeled 'never events'. The impact of this policy was financial. Medicare would withhold payment for subsequent care related to these outcomes. Mandatory reporting of these events was required. The theoretic positive effects of this policy would be that these outcomes are taken seriously and adherence to practices that minimize their occurrence are promoted. However, the negative effect of the policies lies in the adoption of a punitive approach to enforcing quality of care, rather than rewarding high-quality care. Hospitals may become disincentivized to proactively test for these complications [58,59]. A culture of blame might be fostered for outcomes that might not be completely preventable despite optimal practice.

Venus thromboembolism (VTE), composed of pulmonary embolism (PE) and deep vein thrombosis (DVT), is an important measure that has been widely examined as a performance indicator. Although processes directed at reducing the risk of venous thrombosis such as pharmacologic and mechanical prophylaxis are effective, evidence is clear that even with optimal prophylaxis VTE will occur [59–61]. The measurement of these events might reflect widespread variation in rates of diagnostic testing rather than high-quality care to prevent them–a classic example of surveillance bias. For example, in trauma, the practice of surveillance for DVT with duplex ultrasound for asymptomatic patients varies widely by patient criteria and by institution [61–65]. Centers that actively select high-risk patients for surveillance, with the goal of identifying and treating DVT early, report higher rates of DVT [61,62,65]. Therefore, although there is evidence that screening of high-risk trauma patients for DVT is beneficial in terms of outcomes and costs [66], it may result in erroneously attributing higher DVT rates to worse performance. This biased benchmarking may penalize trauma centers with financial consequences or publicly reported outcomes [60]. This occurs in Maryland where the Maryland Hospital Acquired Complications program financially penalizes hospitals for VTE events even when prophylaxis guidelines have been adhered to [67]. Other outcomes selected for reporting as 'never events' are fraught with similar concerns. Despite optimal practices, evidence shows that catheter-associated urinary tract infections, hospital-acquired and ventilator-associated pneumonia are not always preventable even with strict adherence to best practices in a large part due to patient risk profiles [68–71].

Taken together, caution must be taken in applying broad policies with the goal of promoting quality of care. The use of 'never events' runs the risk of promoting a culture of blame for imperfect outcomes where perfection is rarely attainable, even with optimal structures and processes. A balanced approach that rewards high-quality practices while minimizing punitive policies is preferable. The quote attributed to American football coach Vince Lombardi encapsulates a philosophy apropos to performance improvement: "Perfection is not attainable, but if we chase perfection we can catch excellence".

Apples to oranges?

Another important cause for scrutiny of benchmarking initiatives has been the validity of their comparisons of risk-adjusted hospital performance. As the reporting of a hospital's performance relative to peers has important implications, there has been concern that despite the methodologic rigor underlying these reports, their results might not account for all factors that influence measured outcomes, leaving the potential for residual or unmeasured confounding. Risk-adjustment models used to generate benchmarking reports might not fully account for differences in patient characteristics between hospitals, resulting in possible 'apples to oranges' comparisons.

One such example lies in the heterogeneity of the trauma patient population. Some trauma centers frequently treat patients with gunshot wounds, whereas others rarely do. Patients with gunshot wounds are significantly more likely to suffer injuries that are highly time sensitive and associated with high mortality [72]. Furthermore, urban hospitals that frequently treat such injuries also often receive these patients quickly from the field, with short emergency medical service prehospital times. As a result, there has been concern that hospitals that treat high volumes of gunshot wounds will be unfairly penalized in benchmarking of trauma center performance, as they disproportionately receive patients at high risk of early death [73]. To answer this concern, TQIP evaluated the impact on performance benchmarking of patients that are likely unsalvageable based on presenting characteristics [74]. The exclusion of such patients had a tangible impact on trauma center risk-adjusted mortality among subgroups of patients with penetrating injury and shock. TQIP methodology now routinely excludes these patients meeting the unsalvageable criteria. Similarly, an evaluation of the impact of short prehospital times on trauma center performance found that although hospitals with short prehospital times are more likely to receive patients in extremis and at high risk of emergency department death, this effect did not affect overall risk-adjusted mortality. Therefore, the concern for short prehospital times being a source for meaningful confounding in benchmarking of trauma center performance has been diminished.

These examples serve as important instances in which the methodologic approach and validity of performance benchmarking can be called into question. It is integral for these benchmarking initiatives to continue to adjust their methodology and to build trust with participating centers by answering concerns with evidence-based answers.

Public reporting of outcomes and risk aversion

Performance benchmarking has been shown to promote improved outcomes among surgeons [16] and hospitals [17,47] that participate in them. However, one unintended consequence of public reporting of surgeon outcomes is that surgeons may alter their practice to avoid risk for fear of being identified as low performers [75]. The New York Cardiac Reporting System has publicly reported outcomes for individual surgeons since its inception. A survey of cardiothoracic surgeons in New York State found that 62% reported refusing to perform coronary artery bypass surgery on high-risk patients in the year of the survey, primarily because of the public reporting system [75]. A study of patients with acute myocardial infarction found that patients in New York State may undergo bypass surgery or percutaneous intervention later owing to a reluctance in the state to perform early revascularization in the highest-risk patient groups [76].

There has been further concern that public reporting of outcomes might lead some surgeons and institutions to prioritize their reported performance over the best interests of patients. Two cases reported in the media have raised such concerns. In one example, a 94-year-old patient who "never wanted to go to a nursing home" underwent heart valve replacement surgery complicated by postoperative cardiac arrest. The surgical team told the family they were "optimistic she would recover" for several weeks. Eventually, the patient was transitioned to palliative care and died on postoperative day 31, just after the mortality benchmarking window for 30-day outcomes passed [77]. In a different example, an article titled "Hospital Kept Vegetative Patient on Life Support to Boost Survival Rates" reported the story of a patient who experienced numerous complications after a heart transplant. The authors reported that "recordings show that the transplant team was fixated on keeping him alive, rather than his quality of life or his family's wishes, because of worries about the transplant program's survival rate" (https://www.propublica.org/article/audio-shows-hospital-kept-vegetative-patient-on-life-support-to-boost-survival-rates).

Potential adverse consequences to patient care such as this should be evaluated and weighed where public reporting of outcomes is used. Many performance benchmarking initiatives provide hospital-specific benchmarking reports anonymously, with the purpose that local quality improvement efforts can take place without external scrutiny or influence.

EVOLVING USES OF BIG DATA

The collection of standardized clinical data for the purpose of measuring and comparing quality has led to large repositories of patient information with multiple potential uses beyond the measurement of risk-adjusted hospital outcomes. Among these are research and data-driven risk prediction.

Research

It is worth emphasizing the enormous impact that research using datasets captured for the purpose of benchmarking has had on patient care. Randomized clinical trials evaluating treatment modalities in surgery are often not feasible. Therefore, high-quality observational studies fill an important role in the study of structures and processes of care for patients with surgical diseases [78,79]. Many benchmarking initiatives make de-identified clinical datasets available to participating centers in the form of 'participant use files'. Examples of research performed using TQIP data to evaluate processes of care in trauma have found that utilization of intracranial monitoring in severe traumatic brain injury is associated with lower mortality [80], low molecular weight compared with unfractionated heparin is more effective at preventing PE [81], and experimental endovascular interventions for hemorrhage control are associated with adverse events [82]. Such studies evaluating processes of care using data for millions of patients at hundreds of hospitals would never have been feasible without the high-quality data collection practices made possible through benchmarking programs.

Data-driven outcome prediction

Based on the high-quality data within these standardized clinical datasets, risk calculators have been built for the purpose of informing both physicians and patients about the predicted risks associated with surgery. The ACS developed the Surgical Risk Calculator in 2013 based on risk-adjusted outcomes data for more than 1.4 million patients undergoing surgery captured in NSQIP [83]. As NSQIP has grown, so has the data upon which the risk calculator estimates probabilities. The current risk calculator [84] is based on more than 5 million operations at more than 800 hospitals. Surgeons, or patients, can use the free, web-based, online calculator to estimate risk-adjusted outcome probabilities, based on the planned surgery, comorbidities, and other patient characteristics (https://riskcalculator.facs.org/RiskCalculator/).

Other examples of risk-adjusted outcome prediction derived from clinical datasets are in the form of computer and phone-based applications. The CeDAR app (Carolinas Equation for Determining Associated Risks) for ventral hernia surgery risk prediction is designed to allow providers and patients determine the risk of adverse outcomes after ventral hernia repair [85,86]. The app allows the users to examine how changes in specific risk factors, such as body mass index or smoking, impact risk. The Predictive OpTimal Trees in Emergency Surgery Risk (POTTER) calculator is another example of a downloadable app to use in real time for predicting outcomes after emergency general surgery [87].

SUMMARY

Efforts to ensure the quality of health care for all citizens in the United States have driven the evolution of nationwide quality improvement efforts based on the Donabedian model of process, structure, and outcome. Performance benchmarking, using high-quality data to measure risk-adjusted surgeon and hospital outcomes, has become a ubiquitous and oftentimes mandatory part of the health care landscape. Although this approach has demonstrated its effectiveness across surgical disciplines, it is not without its challenges and potential pitfalls.

CLINICS CARE POINTS

- Performance benchmarking, based on measurement and comparison of the risk-adjusted surgeon or hospital outcomes, has become the gold standard approach for quality improvement initiatives in surgery.
- Many benchmarking programs exist, supported either through the ACS or specialty-specific organizations. Participation in these programs has been shown to be an effective means for improving patient outcomes.

- Essential to the measurement of risk-adjusted outcomes for the purpose of benchmarking is the collection of reliable, standardized clinical data by trained abstractors.
- When selecting quality measures to be captured in data collection, consideration should be given to the three domains in which quality can be measured in health care, described by Avedis Donabedian: structures, processes, and outcomes.
- Potential pitfalls of performance benchmarking include punitive enforcement of quality measures, surgeon or institution skepticism toward methodology, or incentivizing participants to 'game the system'.
- In any performance benchmarking or quality improvement program, a continuous process of re-evaluation and communication with participating surgeons or hospitals is mandatory to foster a culture of transparency and trust.

Disclosure

The authors have nothing to disclose.

References

[1] Institute of Medicine Committee on Quality of Health Care in A. Crossing the quality chasm: a new health system for the 21st century. Washington (DC): National Academies Press (US); 2001.

[2] American College of Surgeons Committee on Trauma. Advanced trauma life support student course manual. 10th edition. Chicago, IL: American College of Surgeons; 2018.

[3] Champion HR, Mabee MS, Meredith JW. The state of US trauma systems: public perceptions versus reality–implications for US response to terrorism and mass casualty events. J Am Coll Surg 2006;203(6):951–61.

[4] Minei JP, Schmicker RH, Kerby JD, et al. Severe traumatic injury: regional variation in incidence and outcome. Ann Surg 2010;252(1):149–57.

[5] Shafi S, Nathens AB, Cryer HG, et al. The trauma quality improvement program of the american college of surgeons committee on trauma. J Am Coll Surg 2009;209(4):521–30.

[6] American College of Surgeons Committee on Trauma. Resources for Optimal care of the injured patient. 2014. Available at. https://www.facs.org/quality%20programs/trauma/vrc/resources. Accessed: Nov 1, 2021.

[7] Khuri SF, Daley J, Henderson W, et al. The department of veterans affairs' national surgical quality improvement program: the first national, validated, outcome-based, risk-adjusted, and peer-controlled program for the measurement and enhancement of the quality of surgical care. Ann Surg 1998;228(4):491–507.

[8] Institute of Medicine (US). Committee to design a strategy for quality review and assurance in medicare. In: Lohr KN, editor. Medicare: a strategy for quality assurance. Washington (DC): National Academies Press (US); 1990.

[9] Best M, Neuhauser D. Avedis donabedian: father of quality assurance and poet. Qual Saf Health Care 2004;13(6):472–3.

[10] Donabedian A. The quality of medical care. Science 1978;200(4344):856–64.

[11] Donabedian A. The quality of care. how can it be assessed? JAMA 1988;260(12):1743–8.

[12] Merriam-Webster.com. Benchmarking. 2021. Available at. https://www.merriam-webster.com/dictionary/benchmark. Accessed: Nov 1, 2021.

[13] Camp RC. Benchmarking: the search for industry best practices that lead to superior performance. Milwaukee, WI: ASQC Quality Press; 1989.

[14] Cross Ral A. The rank xerox experience: benchmarking ten years on benchmarking — theory and practice. Milwaukee, WI: Springer Science and Business Media; 1995.
[15] National Institute of Standards and Technology. Baldrige award recipients listing. 2021. Available at. https://www.nist.gov/baldrige/award-recipients. Accessed: Nov 1, 2021.
[16] O'Connor GT, Plume SK, Olmstead EM, et al. A regional intervention to improve the hospital mortality associated with coronary artery bypass graft surgery. the northern new england cardiovascular disease study group. JAMA 1996;275(11):841–6.
[17] Hannan EL, Kilburn H Jr, Racz M, et al. Improving the outcomes of coronary artery bypass surgery in New York State. JAMA 1994;271(10):761–6.
[18] Khuri SF, Daley J, Henderson W, et al. The national veterans administration surgical risk study: risk adjustment for the comparative assessment of the quality of surgical care. J Am Coll Surg 1995;180(5):519–31.
[19] Fink AS, Campbell DA Jr, Mentzer RM Jr, et al. The national surgical quality improvement program in non-veterans administration hospitals: initial demonstration of feasibility. Ann Surg 2002;236(3):344–53.
[20] Champion HR, Copes WS, Sacco WJ, et al. The major trauma outcome study: establishing national norms for trauma care. J Trauma 1990;30(11):1356–65.
[21] Shafi S, Nathens AB, Parks J, et al. Trauma quality improvement using risk-adjusted outcomes. J Trauma 2008;64(3):599–604.
[22] Department of Health and Human Services. Agency for healthcare research and quality. 2021. Available at. https://www.ahrq.gov/. Accessed: Nov 1, 2021.
[23] Agency for Healthcare Quality and Research. Six domains of healthcare quality. 2021. Available at. https://www.ahrq.gov/talkingquality/measures/six-domains.html. Accessed: Nov 1, 2021.
[24] Agency for Healthcare Quality and Research. Types of healthcare quality measures. 2021. Available at. https://www.ahrq.gov/talkingquality/measures/types.html. Accessed: Nov 1, 2021.
[25] Agency for Healthcare Quality and Research. Datasources for healtcare quality measures. 2021. Available at. https://www.ahrq.gov/talkingquality/measures/understand/index.html. Accessed: Nov 1, 2021.
[26] Agency for Healthcare Quality and Research. Healthcare cost and utilization project. 2021. Available at. https://www.hcup-us.ahrq.gov/databases.jsp. Accessed: Nov 1, 2021.
[27] Stulberg JJ, Haut ER. Practical guide to surgical data sets: healthcare cost and utilization project national inpatient sample (NIS). JAMA Surg 2018;153(6):586–7.
[28] American College of Surgeons. National surgical quality improvement program. 2021. Available at. https://www.facs.org/quality-programs/acs-nsqip. Accessed: Nov 1, 2021.
[29] American College of Surgeons. ACS national trauma databank 2021. Available at. https://www.facs.org/quality-programs/trauma/tqp/center-programs/ntdb. Accessed: Nov 1, 2021.
[30] Agency for Healthcare Quality and Research. Key questions when choosing health care quality measures. 2021. Available at. https://www.ahrq.gov/talkingquality/measures/measure-questions.html. Accessed: Nov 1, 2021.
[31] National Quality Forum. Maintenance of NQF-endorsed performance measures. 2021. Available at. https://www.qualityforum.org/Measuring_Performance/Endorsed_Performance_Measures_Maintenance.aspx. Accessed: Nov 1, 2021.
[32] Institute for Healthcare Improvement. Plan-do-study-Act (PDSA) worksheet 2021. Available at: http://www.ihi.org/resources/Pages/Tools/PlanDoStudyActWorksheet.aspx. Accessed: November 1, 2021.
[33] American Society for Quality. What is six sigma? 2021. Available at: https://asq.org/quality-resources/six-sigma#Lean%20Six%20Sigma. Accessed November 1, 2021.
[34] Pronovost PJ, Berenholtz SM, Needham DM. Translating evidence into practice: a model for large scale knowledge translation. BMJ 2008;337:a1714.

[35] Neuman HB, Kaji AH, Haut ER. Practical guide to implementation science. JAMA Surg 2020;155(5):434–5.
[36] Streiff MB, Carolan HT, Hobson DB, et al. Lessons from the Johns Hopkins multi-disciplinary venous thromboembolism (VTE) prevention collaborative. BMJ 2012;344:e3935.
[37] Greenberg CC, Byrnes ME, Engler TA, et al. Association of a statewide surgical coaching program with clinical outcomes and surgeon perceptions. Ann Surg 2021;273(6):1034–9.
[38] Hemmila MR, Cain-Nielsen AH, Jakubus JL, et al. Association of hospital participation in a regional trauma quality improvement collaborative with patient outcomes. JAMA Surg 2018;153(8):747–56.
[39] Newgard CD, Fildes JJ, Wu L, et al. Methodology and analytic rationale for the American college of surgeons trauma quality improvement program. J Am Coll Surg 2013;216(1): 147–57.
[40] Khuri SF, Daley J, Henderson W, et al. Risk adjustment of the postoperative mortality rate for the comparative assessment of the quality of surgical care: results of the national veterans affairs surgical risk study. J Am Coll Surg 1997;185(4):315–27.
[41] Kardooni S, Haut ER, Chang DC, et al. Hazards of benchmarking complications with the national trauma data bank: numerators in search of denominators. J Trauma 2008;64(2): 273–7, ; discussion 7-9.
[42] Haukoos JS, Newgard CD. Advanced statistics: missing data in clinical research–part 1: an introduction and conceptual framework. Acad Emerg Med 2007;14(7):662–8.
[43] Newgard CD, Haukoos JS. Advanced statistics: missing data in clinical research–part 2: multiple imputation. Acad Emerg Med 2007;14(7):669–78.
[44] Sterne JA, White IR, Carlin JB, et al. Multiple imputation for missing data in epidemiological and clinical research: potential and pitfalls. BMJ (Clinical research ed) 2009;338:b2393.
[45] Merlo J, Chaix B, Ohlsson H, et al. A brief conceptual tutorial of multilevel analysis in social epidemiology: using measures of clustering in multilevel logistic regression to investigate contextual phenomena. J Epidemiol Community Health 2006;60(4):290–7.
[46] New York State Department of Health. Cardiac reporting system overview. 2013. Available at. https://health.data.ny.gov/api/assets/9327BAEB-8F27-4382-BCBF-6173944447A3?download=true. Accessed: Nov 1, 2021.
[47] Hannan EL, Kumar D, Racz M, et al. New York State's Cardiac Surgery Reporting System: four years later. Ann Thorac Surg 1994;58(6):1852–7.
[48] New York State Department of Health. Adult Cardiac Surgery in New York State 2015-2017. 2020. Available at. https://www.health.ny.gov/statistics/diseases/cardiovascular/heart_disease/docs/2015-2017_adult_cardiac_surgery.pdf. Accessed: Nov 1, 2021.
[49] Veterans' Administration Health-Care Amendments of 1985, Pub L No 99–166, 99 Stat 941. Dec 3, 1985. Title II: Health-Care Administration, Sec. 201– 4.
[50] Khuri SF, Daley J, Henderson WG. The comparative assessment and improvement of quality of surgical care in the Department of Veterans Affairs. Arch Surg 2002;137(1):20–7.
[51] Maier RV. Trauma: the paradigm for medical care in the 21st century. J Trauma 2003;54(5): 803–13.
[52] American College of Surgeons Committee on Trauma. About the verification, review and consultation program. 2021. Available at. https://www.facs.org/quality-programs/trauma/tqp/center-programs/vrc/about. Accessed: Nov 1, 2021.
[53] American College of Surgeons Committee on Trauma. Trauma quality improvement program (TQIP). 2021 Available from. https://www.facs.org/quality-programs/trauma/tqp/center-programs/tqip. Accessed: Nov 1, 2021.
[54] Hemmila MR, Nathens AB, Shafi S, et al. The Trauma Quality Improvement Program: pilot study and initial demonstration of feasibility. J Trauma 2010;68(2):253–62.
[55] Agency for Healthcare Quality and Research. Never events. 2019. Available at. https://psnet.ahrq.gov/primer/never-events. Accessed: Nov 1, 2021.

[56] Sutedjo JL, Ng RK, Piazza G, et al. Medicare's new regulations for deep vein thrombosis as a "never event": wise or worrisome? Am J Med 2009;122(11):975–6.
[57] Centers for Medicare and Medicaid Services, HHS. Medicare program: Changes to the hospital inpatient prospective payment systems and fiscal year 2009 rates; payments for graduate medical education in certain emergency situations; changes to disclosure of physician ownership in hospitals and physician self-referral rules; updates to the long-term care prospective payment system; updates to certain IPPS excluded hospitals; and collection of information regarding financial relationships between hospitals. Fed Regist 2008;73: 48433–9084.
[58] Pronovost PJ, Goeschel CA, Wachter RM. The wisdom and justice of not paying for "preventable complications. JAMA 2008;299(18):2197–9.
[59] Streiff MB, Haut ER. The CMS ruling on venous thromboembolism after total knee or hip arthroplasty: weighing risks and benefits. JAMA 2009;301(10):1063–5.
[60] Thorson CM, Ryan ML, Van Haren RM, et al. Venous thromboembolism after trauma: a never event? Crit Care Med 2012;40(11):2967–73.
[61] Shackford SR, Cipolle MD, Badiee J, et al. Determining the magnitude of surveillance bias in the assessment of lower extremity deep venous thrombosis: A prospective observational study of two centers. J Trauma Acute Care Surg 2016;80(5):734–9.
[62] Haut ER, Chang DC, Pierce CA, et al. Predictors of posttraumatic deep vein thrombosis (DVT): hospital practice versus patient factors-an analysis of the National Trauma Data Bank (NTDB). J Trauma 2009;66(4):994–9.
[63] Haut ER, Noll K, Efron DT, et al. Can increased incidence of deep vein thrombosis (DVT) be used as a marker of quality of care in the absence of standardized screening? The potential effect of surveillance bias on reported DVT rates after trauma. J Trauma 2007;63(5): 1132–5.
[64] Haut ER, Pronovost PJ. Surveillance bias in outcomes reporting. JAMA 2011;305(23): 2462–3.
[65] Bilimoria KY, Chung J, Ju MH, et al. Evaluation of surveillance bias and the validity of the venous thromboembolism quality measure. JAMA 2013;310(14):1482–9.
[66] Malhotra AK, Goldberg SR, McLay L, et al. DVT surveillance program in the ICU: analysis of cost-effectiveness. PLoS One 2014;9(9):e106793.
[67] Haut ER, Lau BD, Kraus PS, et al. Preventability of Hospital-Acquired Venous Thromboembolism. JAMA Surg 2015;150(9):912–5.
[68] Croce MA, Brasel KJ, Coimbra R, et al. National Trauma Institute prospective evaluation of the ventilator bundle in trauma patients: does it really work? J Trauma Acute Care Surg 2013;74(2):354–60.
[69] Guo WA. Pneumonia after trauma: a "never event. J Surg Res 2013;185(2):539–40.
[70] Kuy S, Gupta R, Roy C, et al. Incidence of Catheter-Associated Urinary Tract Infections With Compliance With Preventive Guidelines. JAMA Surg 2020;155(7):661–2.
[71] Wahl WL, Zalewski C, Hemmila MR. Pneumonia in the surgical intensive care unit: is every one preventable? Surgery 2011;150(4):665–72.
[72] Acosta JA, Yang JC, Winchell RJ, et al. Lethal injuries and time to death in a level I trauma center. J Am Coll Surg 1998;186(5):528–33.
[73] Heaney JB, Guidry C, Simms E, et al. To TQIP or not to TQIP? that is the question. Am Surg 2014;80(4):386–90.
[74] Byrne JP, Xiong W, Gomez D, et al. Redefining "dead on arrival": Identifying the unsalvageable patient for the purpose of performance improvement. J Trauma Acute Care Surg 2015;79(5):850–7.
[75] Burack JH, Impellizzeri P, Homel P, et al. Public reporting of surgical mortality: a survey of New York State cardiothoracic surgeons. Ann Thorac Surg 1999;68(4):1195–200.
[76] Apolito RA, Greenberg MA, Menegus MA, et al. Impact of the New York state cardiac surgery and percutaneous coronary intervention reporting system on the management of

patients with acute myocardial infarction complicated by cardiogenic shock. Am Heart J 2008;155(2):267–73.

[77] Span P. A surgery standard under fire: New York times. 2015. Available at. https://www.nytimes.com/2015/03/03/health/a-30-day-surgical-standard-is-under-scrutiny.html. Accessed: Nov 1, 2021.

[78] Haut ER, Kalish BT, Cotton BA, et al. Prehospital intravenous fluid administration is associated with higher mortality in trauma patients: a National Trauma Data Bank analysis. Ann Surg 2011;253(2):371–7.

[79] Byrne JP, Witiw CD, Schuster JM, et al. Association of venous thromboembolism prophylaxis after neurosurgical intervention for traumatic brain injury with thromboembolic complications, repeated neurosurgery, and mortality. JAMA Surg 2021;157(3):e215794.

[80] Alali AS, Fowler RA, Mainprize TG, et al. Intracranial pressure monitoring in severe traumatic brain injury: results from the American College of Surgeons Trauma Quality Improvement Program. J Neurotrauma 2013;30(20):1737–46.

[81] Byrne JP, Geerts W, Mason SA, et al. Effectiveness of low-molecular-weight heparin versus unfractionated heparin to prevent pulmonary embolism following major trauma: a propensity-matched analysis. J Trauma Acute Care Surg 2017;82(2):252–62.

[82] Joseph B, Zeeshan M, Sakran JV, et al. Nationwide analysis of resuscitative endovascular balloon occlusion of the aorta in civilian trauma. JAMA Surg 2019;154(6):500–8.

[83] Bilimoria KY, Liu Y, Paruch JL, et al. Development and evaluation of the universal ACS NSQIP surgical risk calculator: a decision aid and informed consent tool for patients and surgeons. J Am Coll Surg 2013;217(5):833–42.

[84] American College of Surgeons National Surgical Quality Improvement Program. Surgical risk calculator. 2021. Available at. https://riskcalculator.facs.org/RiskCalculator/PatientInfo.jsp. Accessed: Nov 1, 2021.

[85] Augenstein V, Colavita P, Wormer B, et al. CeDAR: Carolinas equation for determining associated risks. J Am Coll Surg 2015;221(4):S65–6.

[86] Center PSH. CeDAR app is a free resource for hernia patients 2021. Available at: https://www.premierherniacenter.com/03/cedar-app-is-a-free-resource-for-hernia-patients/. Accessed November 1, 2021.

[87] Bertsimas D, Dunn J, Velmahos GC, et al. Surgical risk is not linear: derivation and validation of a novel, user-friendly, and machine-learning-based predictive optimal trees in emergency surgery risk (POTTER) calculator. Ann Surg 2018;268(4):574–83.

Advances in Surgery 56 (2022) 111–127

ADVANCES IN SURGERY

Transcarotid Artery Revascularization: Is It Better than Carotid Endarterectomy?

Patric Liang, MD, Marc L. Schermerhorn, MD*

Beth Israel Deaconess Medical Center, Division of Vascular and Endovascular Surgery, Harvard Medical School, 110 Francis Street, Suite 5B, Boston, MA 02215, USA

Keywords

• Carotid • Endarterectomy • Stenting • Transcarotid • Revascularization • Stroke

Key points

- Transcarotid artery revascularization (TCAR) is a novel carotid stenting approach that is associated with a lower perioperative stroke or death risk compared with transfemoral carotid stenting.
- TCAR is associated with a similar risk of perioperative stroke or death risk compared with carotid endarterectomy.
- Compared with carotid endarterectomy, TCAR is associated with a lower risk of myocardial infarction, cranial nerve injuries, and shorter operative times.
- TCAR is associated with a higher risk of bleeding complications compared with transfemoral carotid artery stenting; however, this bleeding risk can be mitigated by the use of protamine for heparin reversal.
- Inadequate clavicle to carotid bifurcation distance is the most common anatomic limitation for patients being considered for TCAR with flow reversal neuroprotection.

INTRODUCTION

Carotid endarterectomy for the treatment of symptomatic and asymptomatic extracranial carotid artery disease has been one of the most studied procedures in vascular surgery, to be only further scrutinized over the past 2 decades by the introduction of transfemoral carotid artery stenting as a minimally invasive alternative to open carotid surgery. However, transfemoral carotid artery stenting never gained universal acceptance among vascular surgeons due to an

*Corresponding author. *E-mail address:* mscherm@bidmc.harvard.edu

https://doi.org/10.1016/j.yasu.2022.02.004
0065-3411/22/

increased risk of periprocedural stroke compared with traditional endarterectomy. Transcarotid artery revascularization (TCAR), a novel carotid stenting method that uses a transcervical approach and a unique flow reversal neuroprotection system, was developed to mitigate the high-risk stroke maneuvers associated with the transfemoral carotid stenting approach. TCAR has been found to have perioperative stroke risks comparable with carotid endarterectomy and has led to a recent resurgence in carotid artery stenting in the United States. As TCAR use continues to grow and its treatment indications broaden, it is imperative to evaluate its role in the current landscape of carotid artery revascularization and assess whether it has the potential to supplant endarterectomy as the standard-of-care for carotid revascularization.

THE HISTORY AND LIMITATIONS OF CAROTID ENDARTERECTOMY

The first successful carotid revascularization procedure was performed by Carrera, Molins, and Murphy in 1951 for a male patient suffering from a stroke, and they published this case report in 1955 [1]. DeBakey performed a carotid endarterectomy procedure in 1953, but did not publish his case report until after the patient died 19 years later from coronary artery disease complications [2]. The first published report of a carotid revascularization procedure was by Eastcott, Pickering, and Rob in 1954 for the treatment of a patient suffering from recurrent transient ischemic attacks secondary to high-grade carotid stenosis [3]. These seminal carotid revascularization procedures used to treat symptomatic carotid lesions were performed using varying surgical approaches. Carrera and his colleagues performed an end-to-end external carotid artery to internal carotid artery anastomosis after resecting the stenosed internal carotid lesion, DeBakey performed an endarterectomy of the carotid lesion followed by primary arterial closure, and Eastcott and colleagues created an end-to-end common carotid to internal carotid artery anastomosis after excising the internal carotid lesion. These procedures ultimately spurred a global carotid revascularization movement that would expand over the next few decades and define the surgical treatment of carotid artery disease.

The carotid endarterectomy procedure is currently an accepted and well-established procedure, but in its early stages, there was a wide range of surgical techniques and outcomes. The Joint Study of Extracranial Arterial Occlusion study group, consisting of 24 institutions, published a report of 2400 carotid endarterectomy procedures performed between 1961 and 1968 and found an overall surgical mortality rate of 4.5%, ranging widely from less than 2% to 36% among the institutions [4]. Lower mortality rates were found in institutions performing higher volume of cases, whereas higher mortality rates were found in institutions performing lower volume of cases, suggesting a significant learning curve to the procedure as well as a lack of standardization in technique. For example, thromboendarterectomy closure using a patch was not widely adopted at the time and primary closure was most often performed. Data from several studies have since shown that the use of patch closure is more likely to result in lower risk of perioperative stroke and of recurrent stenosis compared with primary closure alone [5,6]. Through advancements in preoperative medical optimization, developments in intraprocedural management strategies, including carotid shunting and or neuromonitoring, and standardization of surgical technique and postoperative care management, carotid endarterectomy has now become a routine procedure for vascular surgeons with excellent results in standard-risk patients.

Several pivotal trials have shown the benefit of carotid endarterectomy compared with best medical management to prevent stroke in symptomatic and asymptomatic patients [7,8,9,10]. However, carotid endarterectomy is only beneficial if the risks of stroke or death from the procedure itself are low. The importance of maintaining a low periprocedural risk with endarterectomy is of particular concern in high surgical-risk patients who have multiple baseline comorbidities. Consensus guidelines have advised that the perioperative stroke or death rate for carotid endarterectomy be less than 3% in asymptomatic patients and less than 6% for symptomatic patients [11,12]. An analysis of the 2011 to 2017 data from the American College of Surgeons National Surgical Quality Improvement Program (ACS-NSQIP) registry showed an acceptable 1.5% rate of 30-day stroke or death in asymptomatic standard-risk patients undergoing carotid endarterectomy in the United States, but found that high medical-risk patients undergoing carotid endarterectomy for asymptomatic carotid disease had an unacceptably high, 4.7% rate of perioperative stroke or death [13]. These findings suggest the need for an alternative, more minimally invasive option for the treatment of medically complex patients.

In addition to baseline medical comorbidities, certain anatomic characteristics can make carotid endarterectomy surgery more challenging and increase the risk of adverse events. Compared with standard-risk patients, high anatomic-risk patients undergoing carotid endarterectomy have been found to have a significantly higher risk of 30-day stroke or death in the ACS-NSQIP, and these differences were evident in both the treatment of asymptomatic (2.6% vs 1.5%) and symptomatic patients (4.8% vs 3.4%) [13]. Anatomic characteristics that can make carotid endarterectomy more challenging include redo carotid surgery for carotid restenosis following prior endarterectomy, prior radical neck dissection, neck radiation, and high internal carotid lesions. Although redo endarterectomy for carotid restenosis has been found to have an acceptable 30-day stroke rate in selected patients with both asymptomatic and symptomatic disease, redo surgery is associated with a 2.8-fold increase in the risk of stroke and 2.2-fold increase in death compared with the treatment of primary carotid lesions [14]. In addition, carotid endarterectomy for high internal carotid lesions results in the need for adjunct maneuvers to achieve high carotid exposure, which can increase the risk of cranial nerve injuries and perioperative morbidity. Surgical treatment of high carotid lesions has been found to be an independent risk factor for perioperative stroke [15]. Therefore, a safe, alternative approach to carotid endarterectomy for patients with challenging anatomy is needed.

THE SHORTCOMINGS OF TRANSFEMORAL CAROTID ARTERY STENTING

Transfemoral carotid stenting was developed as an alternative treatment option for carotid stenosis and theoretically addresses the medical and anatomic risks of open carotid surgery by eliminating the need for surgical exposure of the carotid artery. The history of percutaneous intraluminal carotid artery interventions dates back to 1977 when Mathias published the first report detailing the treatment of a stenotic carotid lesion using balloon angioplasty [16]. However, it was not until the 1990s that carotid stenting was popularized and studied for the treatment of carotid stenosis [17]. Several multi-institutional randomized trials have since been performed over the past 2 decades to compare transfemoral carotid stenting with carotid endarterectomy, but unfortunately, none have shown a clear advantage of carotid stenting over endarterectomy despite its minimally invasive approach [18,19,20,21,22].

The recurring theme found in these clinical trials is an increased risk of stroke from carotid stenting compared with endarterectomy for the treatment of higher risk symptomatic and elderly patients, and a statistically equivalent risk of stroke for the treatment of lower risk, asymptomatic patients. In randomized clinical trials evaluating treatment of only symptomatic patients, the perioperative 30-day risk of stroke or death has been found to be significantly higher for transfemoral carotid stenting compared with endarterectomy; the EVA-3S trial reported a 9.6% 30-day stroke death rate following carotid stenting compared with a 3.9% event rate for endarterectomy, and the ICSS trial reported a 7.4% rate for endarterectomy compared with 3.4% for endarterectomy. In contrast, the ACT-1 trial evaluated low-risk, asymptomatic patients younger than 80 years of age and found that carotid artery stenting was statistically noninferior to endarterectomy, albeit with a nearly 2-fold increased risk of stroke or death in the stenting arm (stenting 2.9% vs endarterectomy 1.7%) [22].

The CREST trial, regarded as the largest and most rigorously designed trial comparing carotid stenting and endarterectomy, evaluated a study population of both asymptomatic and symptomatic patients. The study found a significantly higher risk of stroke or death for those undergoing stenting, but a higher risk of myocardial infarction for those undergoing carotid endarterectomy [18]. A health-related quality of life study using the CREST data showed that perioperative stroke following revascularization had a greater and more sustained impact on quality of life compared with postprocedural myocardial infarction [23]. A subanalysis of the CREST trial further highlighted that age was a significant treatment effect modifier and the risk of stroke increased with age, placing elderly patients at higher risk of adverse events following carotid artery stenting [24].

The role of a minimally invasive alternative carotid revascularization procedure should be heralded by its ability to decrease the perioperative risk of its more invasive counterpart and provide a safer option for the treatment of high-risk patients. In this sense, transfemoral carotid stenting fails at its intended design, placing higher risk, symptomatic patients at a higher risk of perioperative stroke and death. Despite these findings, carotid stenting is only reimbursed by the Centers for Medicare and Medicaid Services (CMS) for the treatment of medically and anatomically high surgical-risk, symptomatic patients (or asymptomatic high-risk patients enrolled in an approved clinical trial) and CMS has outlined several medical and anatomic risk factors to determine which patients are high-risk for carotid endarterectomy (Table 1). The listed CMS medical high-risk factors are unsurprisingly related to patients suffering from significant cardiac or pulmonary disease, whereas the anatomic criteria are specific factors that make carotid endarterectomy challenging.

Despite these proposed CMS high-risk guidelines, there is little to no evidence that transfemoral carotid artery stenting reduces the risk of adverse events in CMS-defined high-risk patients, compared with endarterectomy. Using the Vascular Quality Initiative (VQI) registries to identify and evaluate CMS high-risk patients undergoing carotid endarterectomy and carotid stenting, transfemoral carotid artery stenting was found to be associated with a significantly higher perioperative stroke risk compared with carotid endarterectomy in this patient population [25]. In addition, only a few of the CMS-defined risk factors have actually been found to be independently associated with 30-day stroke or death following carotid endarterectomy. These risk factors included congestive heart failure class III or IV, left ventricular ejection fraction less than 30%, unstable angina, contralateral occlusion, and high internal carotid artery lesion [15]. Notably, age greater or equal to 80 and redo carotid endarterectomy for restenosis have not been found to be independently associated with 30-day stroke or death.

The shortcomings of the transfemoral carotid artery stenting are likely secondary to its approach in accessing the carotid vessel and a failure of intraprocedural neuroprotection. In transfemoral carotid artery stenting, percutaneous access is first obtained via the common femoral artery and a wire and catheter are navigated through a patient's aortic arch to cannulate the carotid artery, followed by the advancement of a sheath for intervention. Patients with advanced atherosclerotic carotid disease are likely to have concomitant disease in the aortic arch, so the manipulation of a diseased aortic arch during these steps

Table 1
CMS medical and anatomic risk factors for carotid endarterectomy

Medical high-risk criteria	Anatomic high-risk criteria
• Congestive heart failure class III/IV • Left ventricular ejection fraction <30% • Unstable angina	• Contralateral carotid occlusion • Recent myocardial infarction • Previous carotid endarterectomy with recurrent stenosis • Prior radiation treatment to the neck

The Centers for Medicare and Medicaid Services also accept the use of any other conditions that were used to determine patients at high risk for carotid endarterectomy in prior carotid artery stenting trials and studies, such as ARCHER, CABERNET, SAPPHIRE, BEACH, and MAVERIC II.

of the stenting procedure can lead to inadvertent plaque embolization to the brain. The right carotid artery can also be particularly difficult to cannulate in patients with type III aortic arches, leading to the need for additional arch manipulation. After cannulating the proximal common carotid artery, the carotid lesion is then crossed using a wire to then deploy a distal filter and initiate neuroprotection. Therefore, the wire and catheter maneuvers used to cannulate the carotid artery and cross the carotid lesion are all performed without a neuroprotection device in place, placing the patient at risk for iatrogenic strokes from the aortic arch or carotid plaque. In addition, distal embolic filter devices can also allow the passage of small embolic particles through the filter pores and or around the filter, especially if the filter is undersized or inadequately opposed to the arterial wall [26,27].

The inability to initiate early neuroprotection with distal embolic filter devices led to the development of alternative transfemoral embolic protection systems that can initiate neuroprotection before crossing the internal carotid artery lesion. These embolic protection systems work on the basis for flow-arrest or flow-reversal. The first carotid stenting procedure performed using flow reversal neuroprotection through a transcervical approach was by Parodi 1998 [28]. Parodi had first observed flow reversal in the middle cerebral artery on transcranial Doppler when inserting a shunt into the distal internal carotid artery during carotid endarterectomy and found that patients tolerated flow reversal in the internal carotid artery quite well. Translating this concept for flow reversal to prevent antegrade iatrogenic embolization during carotid stenting, Parodi was able to create flow-arrest by external carotid artery balloon occlusion and surgical clamping of the common carotid artery through an open transcervical approach. Flow reversal was then established passively by opening the side port of the carotid sheath via exsanguination and by active aspiration of blood and debris. Stenting of the internal carotid lesion was then performed after flow-stasis or flow-reversal neuroprotection was established. Later, an extracorporeal circuit from the carotid arterial to the venous system was devised to allow for continuous flow reversal and reduce blood loss during neuroprotection. This neuroprotection system was soon developed for the transfemoral approach, and this device was termed the Parody AntiEmoblic System (PAES).

The concept of flow-stasis and reversal for neuroprotection during carotid stenting was first commercially adapted in the United States for the transfemoral approach. Medtronic (Dublin, Ireland) developed a transfemoral Mo.Ma neuroprotection system that can initiate flow-stasis by occlusion of the external and common carotid artery, followed by the manual aspiration of blood and any debris through its sheath after carotid angioplasty and stenting. W.L. Gore and Associates (Flagstaff, AZ) later adopted and commercialized the PAES which included an extracorporal arteriovenous shunt system for continuous flow-reversal. While the Mo.Ma device is still on the market today, the Gore device has since been discontinued due to poor sale projections.

Unfortunately, the use of these transfemoral flow arrest devices has not translated to improved perioperative stroke outcomes for the transfemoral carotid artery stenting approach. In a study evaluating all transfemoral carotid stenting procedures performed using transfemoral flow-arrest/reversal neuroprotection systems in the VQI from 2005 to 2019, use of transfemoral flow-arrest/reversal for neuroprotection did not confer a significantly decreased risk of perioperative in-hospital stroke or death compared with the use of distal embolic filter devices (flow-arrest 3.2% vs distal filter 3.7%) [29]. The benefits of the transfemoral flow-arrest system in initiating neuroprotection before crossing a carotid lesion may be negated by the need to advance its large, 8 or 9Fr, sheath system through the aortic arch and a small flow reversal channel that may be suboptimal for cerebral protection. These findings implicate the need for an alternative approach for carotid artery stenting that can avoid aortic arch manipulation and use robust flow reversal before engaging the lesion.

DEVELOPMENT OF TRANSCAROTID ARTERY REVASCULARIZATION AND THE RESURGENCE OF CAROTID ARTERY STENTING

The TCAR procedure uses an open surgical common carotid access approach for carotid stenting in conjunction with a flow reversal neuroprotection system that is specifically designed for the transcervical approach (Silk Road Medical, Sunnyvale, CA). TCAR avoids the need for aortic arch manipulation and can initiate neuroprotection before crossing a carotid lesion. These theoretic benefits have translated to findings of low periprocedural stroke rates in an initial single-arm clinical trial [30]. Furthermore, comparative studies using prospectively collected data of TCAR procedures performed in the United States and Canada have found significantly lower risks of stroke or death compared with the transfemoral carotid stenting approach and equivalent stroke or death rates compared with endarterectomy [31,32].

The TCAR procedure is performed through a small 2 to 4 cm transverse or longitudinal incision just above the clavicle, between the 2 heads of the sternocleidomastoid muscle [33]. The common carotid artery is exposed through this incision and circumferentially controlled. A purse string or U-stitch is placed using a 5-0 prolene suture at the desired common carotid puncture location. A micropuncture needle is then used to puncture the artery between the prolene stitch in antegrade fashion followed by the advancement of a microwire. The Silk Road micropuncture needle has a marking to help ensure that the needle is not advanced more than 2 mm into the artery, so that the backwall of the carotid artery is not injured (Fig. 1A). Additionally, the microwire is also marked to help ensure the wire is not advanced more than 4 cm into the common carotid artery to avoid inadvertently manipulating the carotid bifurcation before starting flow reversal (see Fig. 1B). A micropuncture sheath with 1 cm length markings is then advanced over this wire and advanced 3–4 cm into the artery, and an arteriogram is performed (see Fig. 1C). At this point, the microwire and sheath can

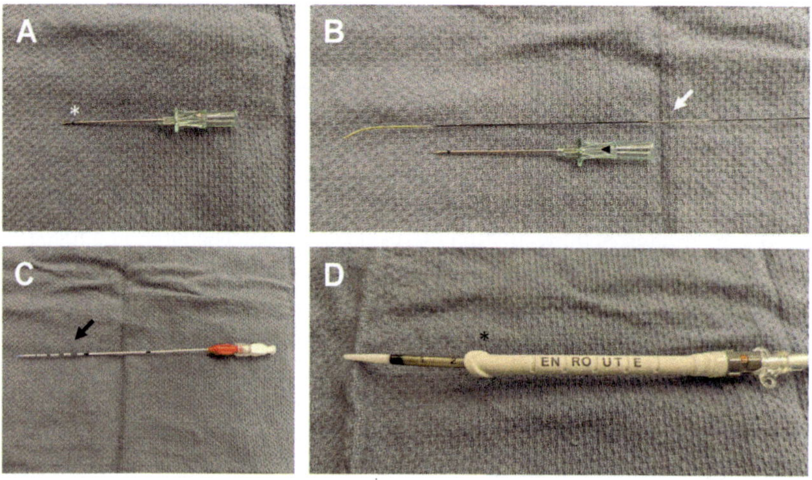

Fig. 1. (*A*) Micropuncture introducer needle with black marking (white star) to indicate 2 mm distance from the tip of the needle. (*B*) Microwire with silver marking (*white arrow*) to indicate a safe distance to insert the wire through the introducer needle. (*C*) Microsheath with 1 cm markings (*black arrow*) to indicate distance from the tip of sheath. (*D*) Flow reversal arterial sheath with adjustable bumper (black star) to control distance of sheath insertion.

be advanced into the external carotid artery to exchange out for a stiffer .035 wire for the insertion of the arterial flow-reversal sheath. The arterial flow reversal sheath has a bumper that prevents the arterial sheath from being inserted too far (see Fig. 1D). If the external carotid artery is diseased or not easily accessible with a stiff wire, and there is adequate common carotid artery distance to the carotid bifurcation, the stiff wire can be advanced just short of the carotid bifurcation, and the arterial flow-reversal sheath inserted.

Femoral vein access is obtained percutaneously through ultrasound guidance and a venous return sheath is placed. “Passive” flow reversal can then be initiated by connecting the arterial and venous sheaths. A flow switch system with an embedded filter connects the arterial and venous sheaths to allow capture of debris and control of the amount of flow reversal, that is, low-flow versus high-flow. Due to the pressure gradient difference between the arterial and venous systems, blood flow is preferentially directed away from the carotid arterial system and to the venous system. However, antegrade common carotid blood flow around the arterial carotid sheath prevents complete flow-reversal in the carotid artery from occurring despite this pressure difference. Therefore, to initiate true flow reversal in the carotid artery, the common carotid artery proximal to the arterial sheath is clamped using a vascular clamp or a Rummel tourniquet. Once flow reversal is established and blood flow is directed away from the carotid artery, the carotid lesion is crossed using a 0.14-inch wire, predilated using a balloon, and a stent is deployed. Following carotid stent placement, 2 additional minutes of flow reversal is allowed to retrieve any additional debris resulting from the intervention. A completion angiogram is performed, and postdilation may be performed as needed. Once the procedure is completed, blood in the flow reversal system is returned to the patient through the venous sheath, the arterial sheath is removed, and hemostasis is achieved by tying the previously placed prolene suture.

The TCAR technique combines open and endovascular surgical techniques that are familiar to the modern vascular surgeon. In contrast to the learning curve needed in the 1960s after the introduction of carotid endarterectomy, TCAR has proven to have a short learning curve and is performed with low rates of stroke or death complications even in the early stages of the surgeon's experience [34]. This has resulted in rapid and widespread adoption of the TCAR procedure across the United States for the treatment of high surgical-risk patients (Fig. 2), with TCAR supplanting transfemoral carotid artery stenting in 2019 among institutions participating in the VQI. To evaluate and monitor the outcomes of this novel stenting procedure, the VQI TCAR Surveillance Project was launched in 2016 through a collaborative effort among the Society for Vascular Surgery, the US Food and Drug Administration, and the CMS. This prospective TCAR registry currently captures more than 95% of all TCAR procedures performed in the United States and Canada, and its data have been critical in evaluating the safety and efficacy of this new procedure.

Using a propensity-score matched analysis of patients undergoing TCAR and transfemoral carotid artery stenting in the TCAR Surveillance Project registry and the VQI transfemoral carotid stent registry data, respectively, TCAR was found to be associated with a significantly lower risk of stroke or death at 1-year compared with transfemoral carotid artery stenting (TCAR 5.1% vs transfemoral

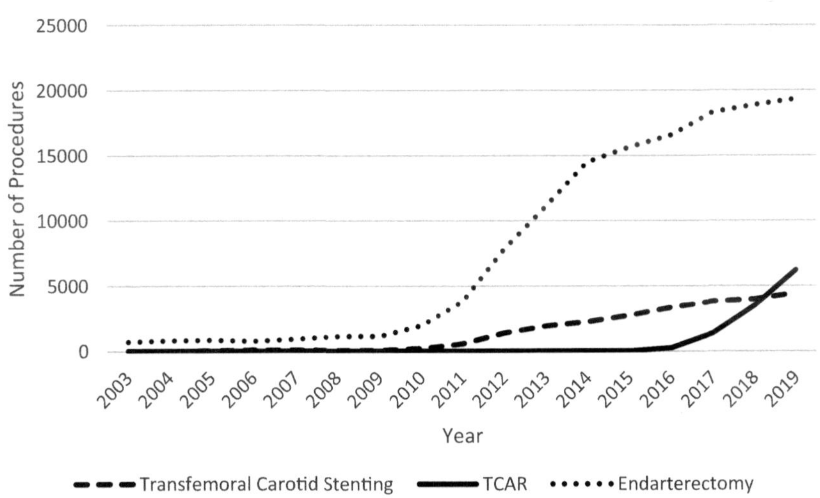

Fig. 2. Trend in carotid artery revascularization procedure utilization in the Vascular Quality Initiative.

carotid stenting 9.6%) [31]. These differences were found to be more pronounced for the treatment of symptomatic lesions. There were no statistically significant differences found in the rates of perioperative myocardial infarction between the 2 cohorts. TCAR was associated with less radiation time and less contrast needed to complete the procedure. However, TCAR was found to be associated with a higher risk of access site complications resulting in reoperation or interventional treatment given the need to make a small cervical incision.

Intraoperative therapeutic heparin anticoagulation is used for both carotid endarterectomy and carotid stenting to reduce the risk of thrombosis during the manipulation of the carotid artery. Bleeding complications following carotid endarterectomy have been shown to be strongly associated with stroke, death, and myocardial infarction, whereas protamine use has been shown to reduce this perioperative bleeding risk without increasing the risk of stroke, MI, or CHF [35]. Given the increased risk of adverse events with bleeding complications, routine use of protamine in carotid endarterectomy has become widely accepted by vascular surgeons. For carotid artery stenting, concerns regarding increased risk of stent thrombosis with protamine use led to the discouragement of protamine use in large carotid stenting studies, including the CREST trials. However, these concerns are unsubstantiated as protamine use has more recently been found to be safe for both transfemoral carotid artery stenting and TCAR, without increasing risk of thromboembolic complications [36,37]. Given the need for a surgical incision to expose the carotid artery for the TCAR procedure as well as dual-antiplatelet therapy use for carotid stenting, routine protamine use is now recommended to mitigate the incidence of access site bleeding complications.

The clinical trial comparing TCAR with carotid endarterectomy in conjunction with the SVS VQI TransCarotid Artery Surveillance Project is currently in an active enrollment phase (NCT02850588). However, an early preliminary analysis evaluating these data found equivalent in-hospital stroke or death outcomes between TCAR and endarterectomy [38]. In addition, TCAR was associated with lower rates of cranial nerve injuries and patients undergoing TCAR were less likely to have a prolong hospital stay. An interim, propensity-matched analysis of this trial, which consisted of more than 6000 patients in each cohort, observed no statistically significant differences between TCAR and CEA in terms of in-hospital stroke or death (TCAR 1.6% vs endarterectomy 1.6%), but TCAR was found to be associated with significant lower rates of in-hospital myocardial infarction (TCAR 0.5% vs endarterectomy 0.9%), highlighting the advantage of the more minimally invasive TCAR approach [32]. The final results from this clinical trial with 1-year follow-up are forthcoming, but because most adverse events occur in the peri-operative period following carotid revascularization, it is unlikely that a difference will be seen at longer-term follow-up. Therefore, based on the currently available data from the VQI TransCarotid Artery Revascularization Surveillance Project trial, TCAR is equivalent to endarterectomy in terms of perioperative stroke or death risk, but has the added advantage of decreased myocardial infarction risk, cranial nerve injuries, hospital length of stay, and overall operative times.

ANATOMIC CONSIDERATIONS FOR TRANSCAROTID ARTERY REVASCULARIZATION

Safe placement and use of the only FDA-approved flow reversal device is dependent on several anatomic factors as listed in the device's instructions for use (IFU) (Box 1). All patients being considered for carotid stenting should undergo preoperative CTA imaging of the carotid vessels to determine anatomic eligibility. A single-institution study found that 72% of carotid arteries being assessed for revascularization met the TCAR IFU anatomic requirements, and the most common reason for not meeting the device's IFU requirements was an insufficient ≥5 cm distance between the clavicle and carotid bifurcation [39]. In addition to the TCAR IFU anatomic restrictions, carotid stenting is not advised for carotid lesions with bulky or circumferential calcification due to the risk of adequate stent expansion (Fig. 3). While circumferential carotid disease with inner calcific plaque is not amenable to stenting, circumferential outer wall calcific lesions with inner uncalcified plaque can be treated with stenting. Balloon lithotripsy and atherectomy could be used to treat calcified lesions to make them amendable for stenting, but these adjuncts have not been proven to be safe or beneficial and should be considered experimental. Up to 7% of carotid arteries are ineligible for carotid stenting due to excessive circumferential calcification burden of the lesion [39].

The depth of the common carotid artery is also an important consideration that is not explicitly listed in the TCAR device's anatomic IFU requirements. Common carotid arteries with extended CCA depth are technically more challenging and can increase the risk of carotid artery injury or dissection given the steeper angle needed to enter the artery. Additionally, access to a deep common carotid artery will result in higher common carotid artery punctures above the clavicle given the angle and trajectory needed for the access, further decreasing the distance to the carotid bifurcation available for arterial sheath placement (Fig. 4). Although insufficient clavicle to carotid bifurcation distance is the most common reason for TCAR ineligibility, a prosthetic Dacron conduit can be sewn onto the common carotid artery to gain the additional carotid length needed to safety insert the arterial sheath. While this modification is technically feasible and would make most patients anatomically eligible for TCAR, it should be used with caution as it is outside the device IFU and there is currently no data to support its long-term safety.

Box 1: Silk road enroute flow reversal device anatomic requirements

Silk Road EnRoute Flow Reversal Anatomic Requirements

- Clavicle to carotid bifurcation distance of >5 cm above the clavicle as measured by duplex ultrasound or computerized axial tomography (CT)
- Common carotid artery reference diameter of >6 mm
- Common carotid artery puncture site free of atherosclerotic disease
- Internal carotid artery diameter >4 mm and <9 mm

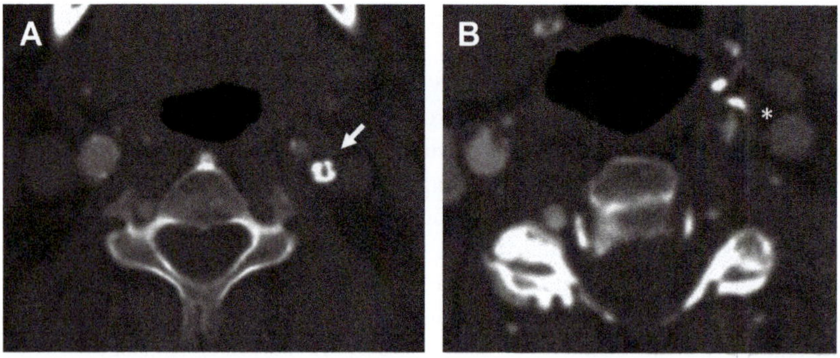

Fig. 3. (*A*) Heavy circumferential calcification of the left internal carotid artery that is not amendable to carotid stenting (*B*) Circumferential calcification of the left internal carotid artery with inner uncalcified plaque that is amendable to stenting. Images obtained with permission on behalf of Silk Road Medical Inc.

TCAR has not proven to be superior to endarterectomy in terms of risk of stroke or death, but TCAR makes the treatment of high carotid bifurcation lesions significantly easier. In turn, vascular surgeons who adopt and use the TCAR option for the treatment of high carotid lesions will be left with standard and low carotid lesions that can be treated with a technically straightforward endarterectomy procedure. In patients with standard and low carotid lesions,

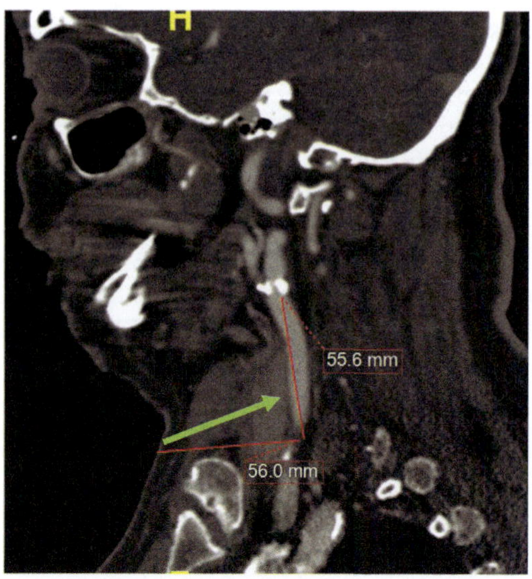

Fig. 4. Clavicle to carotid bifurcation distance measured on the sagittal view of computed tomography angiography images. Given the depth of the common carotid artery, the actual trajectory (green *arrow*) of the sheath will decrease the clavicle to the carotid distance available.

carotid duplex can be used to identify the bifurcation to perform endarterectomy through a small 3–4 cm transverse incision. Centers with vascular surgeons who adopt TCAR have been found to be associated with a 10% decrease in the overall likelihood of stroke, myocardial infarction, or death for all carotid revascularization procedures compared with centers that only perform endarterectomy [40]. However, given its higher procedural costs compared with endarterectomy, TCAR has not been found to be cost-effective as a first-line carotid intervention [41,42]. Therefore, despite the minimally invasive advantages of TCAR, endarterectomy is currently still the preferred procedure for standard-risk patients with normal carotid anatomy.

SUMMARY

TCAR with flow reversal neuroprotection is currently the safest approach for carotid artery stenting and should be preferentially performed over the transfemoral approach for patients who are high risk for carotid endarterectomy and are suitable anatomic TCAR candidates. Based on currently available data, TCAR has a similar risk of major adverse outcomes compared with endarterectomy, but has several advantages including lower myocardial infarction risk, decreased cranial nerve injuries, and shorter operative times. TCAR has been quickly adopted by vascular surgeons based on these outcomes and its overall ease-of-use. For patients with anatomic risk factors that make carotid endarterectomy challenging, such as those with high carotid lesions, restenosis following carotid surgery, and prior neck radiation, TCAR provides a much easier and safer approach. Long-term follow-up outcomes comparing TCAR and CEA are forthcoming, but several randomized trials have shown no difference in stroke or death occurring beyond the perioperative period between transfemoral carotid stenting and endarterectomy [43,44]. It is, therefore, unlikely that long-term results would be different for carotid stents placed from the transcervical approach. TCAR is also currently only approved for patients with CMS-defined high-risk criteria but TCAR may be expanded to standard-risk patients in the future given its low procedural risk profile. If TCAR reimbursement is expanded to standard-risk patients and if the procedural costs of TCAR can be reduced, it would not be surprising if TCAR becomes the predominant method for the treatment of carotid artery stenosis.

CLINICS CARE POINTS

- Transfemoral carotid artery stenting has a higher periprocedural stroke risk compared with carotid endarterectomy, particularly in patients with symptomatic carotid disease and those who are elderly.
- TCAR is associated with a lower risk of stroke or death compared with transfemoral carotid artery stenting, and an equivalent risk of stroke or death compared with endarterectomy.

- Compared with endarterectomy, TCAR is associated with a lower risk of myocardial infarction, cranial nerve injuries, hospital length of stay, and overall operative times.
- Protamine should be used following TCAR to reverse the effects of heparin and reduce periprocedural bleeding complications.
- Computed tomography imaging of the head and neck is necessary to determine if a patient is anatomically suitable for the TCAR device.

DISCLOSURE

The authors have nothing to disclose.

References

[1] Carrea R, Molins M, Murphy G. [Surgery of spontaneous thrombosis of the internal carotid in the neck; carotido-carotid anastomosis; case report and analysis of the literature on surgical cases]. Medicina (B Aires) 1955;15(1):20–9, Tratamiento quirurgico de la trombosis espontanea de la carotida interna en el cuello; anastomosis carotido-carotidea; relato de un caso y analisis de la literatura sobre casos operados.

[2] DeBakey ME. Successful carotid endarterectomy for cerebrovascular insufficiency. Nineteen-year follow-up. JAMA 1975;233(10):1083–5.

[3] Eastcott HH, Pickering GW, Rob CG. Reconstruction of internal carotid artery in a patient with intermittent attacks of hemiplegia. Lancet 1954;267(6846):994–6; https://doi.org/10.1016/s0140-6736(54)90544-9.

[4] Blaisdell WF, Clauss RH, Galbraith JG, et al. Joint study of extracranial arterial occlusion. IV. A review of surgical considerations. *JAMA* Sep 22 1969;209(12):1889–95.

[5] AbuRahma AF, Robinson PA, Saiedy S, et al. Prospective randomized trial of carotid endarterectomy with primary closure and patch angioplasty with saphenous vein, jugular vein, and polytetrafluoroethylene: long-term follow-up. J Vasc Surg 1998;27(2):222–32.

[6] Bond R, Rerkasem K, Naylor AR, et al. Systematic review of randomized controlled trials of patch angioplasty versus primary closure and different types of patch materials during carotid endarterectomy. J Vasc Surg 2004;40(6):1126–35; https://doi.org/10.1016/j.jvs.2004.08.048.

[7] Endarterectomy for asymptomatic carotid artery stenosis. Executive Committee for the Asymptomatic Carotid Atherosclerosis Study. JAMA 1995;273(18):1421–8.

[8] Halliday A, Mansfield A, Marro J, et al. Prevention of disabling and fatal strokes by successful carotid endarterectomy in patients without recent neurological symptoms: randomised controlled trial. Lancet 2004;363(9420):1491–502; https://doi.org/10.1016/S0140-6736(04)16146-1.

[9] North American Symptomatic Carotid Endarterectomy Trial C, Barnett HJM, Taylor DW, et al. Beneficial effect of carotid endarterectomy in symptomatic patients with high-grade carotid stenosis. N Engl J Med 1991;325(7):445–53; https://doi.org/10.1056/NEJM199108153250701.

[10] Randomised trial of endarterectomy for recently symptomatic carotid stenosis: final results of the MRC European Carotid Surgery Trial (ECST). Lancet 1998;351(9113):1379–87.

[11] Ricotta JJ, Aburahma A, Ascher E, et al. Updated Society for Vascular Surgery guidelines for management of extracranial carotid disease: executive summary. J Vasc Surg 2011;54(3):832–6; https://doi.org/10.1016/j.jvs.2011.07.004.

[12] Brott TG, Halperin JL, Abbara S, et al. 2011 ASA/ACCF/AHA/AANN/AANS/ACR/ASNR/CNS/SAIP/SCAI/SIR/SNIS/SVM/SVS guideline on the management of patients with extracranial carotid and vertebral artery disease: executive summary: a report of the

American College of Cardiology Foundation/American Heart Association Task Force on Practice Guidelines, and the American Stroke Association, American Association of Neuroscience Nurses, American Association of Neurological Surgeons, American College of Radiology, American Society of Neuroradiology, Congress of Neurological Surgeons, Society of Atherosclerosis Imaging and Prevention, Society for Cardiovascular Angiography and Interventions, Society of Interventional Radiology, Society of NeuroInterventional Surgery, Society for Vascular Medicine, and Society for Vascular Surgery. Developed in collaboration with the American Academy of Neurology and Society of Cardiovascular Computed Tomography. Catheter Cardiovasc Interv 2013;81(1):E76–123; https://doi.org/10.1002/ccd.22983.

[13] Rao V, Liang P, Swerdlow N, et al. Contemporary outcomes after carotid endarterectomy in high-risk anatomic and physiologic patients. J Vasc Surg 2020;71(1):104–10; https://doi.org/10.1016/j.jvs.2019.05.041.

[14] Arhuidese IJ, Faateh M, Nejim BJ, et al. Risks Associated With Primary and Redo Carotid Endarterectomy in the Endovascular Era. JAMA Surg 2018;153(3):252–9; https://doi.org/10.1001/jamasurg.2017.4477.

[15] Schermerhorn ML, Fokkema M, Goodney P, et al. The impact of Centers for Medicare and Medicaid Services high-risk criteria on outcome after carotid endarterectomy and carotid artery stenting in the SVS Vascular Registry. J Vasc Surg 2013;57(5):1318–24; https://doi.org/10.1016/j.jvs.2012.10.107.

[16] Mathias K. [A new catheter system for percutaneous transluminal angioplasty (PTA) of carotid artery stenoses]. Fortschr Med 1977;95(15):1007–11, Ein neuartiges Katheter-System zur perkutanen transluminalen Angioplastie von Karotisstenosen.

[17] Diethrich EB, Ndiaye M, Reid DB. Stenting in the carotid artery: initial experience in 110 patients. J Endovasc Surg 1996;3(1):42–62; https://doi.org/10.1583/1074-6218(1996)003<0042:SITCAI>2.0.CO.

[18] Brott TG, Hobson RW 2nd, Howard G, et al. Stenting versus endarterectomy for treatment of carotid-artery stenosis. N Engl J Med 2010;363(1):11–23; https://doi.org/10.1056/NEJMoa0912321.

[19] Mas JL, Chatellier G, Beyssen B, et al. Endarterectomy versus stenting in patients with symptomatic severe carotid stenosis. N Engl J Med 2006;355(16):1660–71; https://doi.org/10.1056/NEJMoa061752.

[20] International Carotid Stenting Study i, Ederle J, Dobson J, et al. Carotid artery stenting compared with endarterectomy in patients with symptomatic carotid stenosis (International Carotid Stenting Study): an interim analysis of a randomised controlled trial. Lancet 2010;375(9719):985–97; https://doi.org/10.1016/S0140-6736(10)60239-5.

[21] Yadav JS, Wholey MH, Kuntz RE, et al. Protected carotid-artery stenting versus endarterectomy in high-risk patients. N Engl J Med 2004;351(15):1493–501; https://doi.org/10.1056/NEJMoa040127.

[22] Rosenfield K, Matsumura JS, Chaturvedi S, et al. Randomized Trial of Stent versus Surgery for Asymptomatic Carotid Stenosis. N Engl J Med 2016;374(11):1011–20; https://doi.org/10.1056/NEJMoa1515706.

[23] Cohen DJ, Stolker JM, Wang K, et al. Health-related quality of life after carotid stenting versus carotid endarterectomy: results from CREST (Carotid Revascularization Endarterectomy Versus Stenting Trial). J Am Coll Cardiol 2011;58(15):1557–65; https://doi.org/10.1016/j.jacc.2011.05.054.

[24] Voeks JH, Howard G, Roubin GS, et al. Age and outcomes after carotid stenting and endarterectomy: the carotid revascularization endarterectomy versus stenting trial. Stroke 2011;42(12):3484–90; https://doi.org/10.1161/STROKEAHA.111.624155.

[25] Hicks CW, Nejim B, Locham S, et al. Association between Medicare high-risk criteria and outcomes after carotid revascularization procedures. J Vasc Surg 2018;67(6):1752–1761 e2; https://doi.org/10.1016/j.jvs.2017.10.066.

[26] Muller-Hulsbeck S, Jahnke T, Liess C, et al. In vitro comparison of four cerebral protection filters for preventing human plaque embolization during carotid interventions. J Endovasc Ther 2002;9(6):793–802; https://doi.org/10.1177/152660280200900612.
[27] Vos JA, van den Berg JC, Ernst SM, et al. Carotid angioplasty and stent placement: comparison of transcranial Doppler US data and clinical outcome with and without filtering cerebral protection devices in 509 patients. Radiology 2005;234(2):493–9; https://doi.org/10.1148/radiol.2342040119.
[28] Parodi J, Bates MC, Ohki T, et al. The history of proximal carotid protection and flow reversal to prevent stent angioplasty embolization. Semin Vasc Surg 2018;31(1):9–14; https://doi.org/10.1053/j.semvascsurg.2018.03.002.
[29] Liang P, Soden P, Wyers MC, et al. The role of transfemoral carotid artery stenting with proximal balloon occlusion embolic protection in the contemporary endovascular management of carotid artery stenosis. J Vasc Surg 2020;72(5):1701–10; https://doi.org/10.1016/j.jvs.2020.02.036.
[30] Kwolek CJ, Jaff MR, Leal JI, et al. Results of the ROADSTER multicenter trial of transcarotid stenting with dynamic flow reversal. J Vasc Surg 2015;62(5):1227–34; https://doi.org/10.1016/j.jvs.2015.04.460.
[31] Schermerhorn ML, Liang P, Eldrup-Jorgensen J, et al. Association of Transcarotid Artery Revascularization vs Transfemoral Carotid Artery Stenting With Stroke or Death Among Patients With Carotid Artery Stenosis. JAMA 2019;322(23):2313–22; https://doi.org/10.1001/jama.2019.18441.
[32] Malas MB, Dakour-Aridi H, Kashyap VS, et al. TransCarotid Revascularization with Dynamic Flow reversal versus Carotid Endarterectomy in the Vascular Quality Initiative Surveillance Project. Ann Surg 2020; https://doi.org/10.1097/SLA.0000000000004496.
[33] Malas MB, Leal J, Kashyap V, et al. Technical aspects of transcarotid artery revascularization using the ENROUTE transcarotid neuroprotection and stent system. J Vasc Surg 2017;65(3):916–20; https://doi.org/10.1016/j.jvs.2016.11.042.
[34] Kashyap VS, King AH, Liang P, et al. Learning Curve for Surgeons Adopting Transcarotid Artery Revascularization Based on the Vascular Quality Initiative-Transcarotid Artery Revascularization Surveillance Project. J Am Coll Surg 2020;230(1):113–20; https://doi.org/10.1016/j.jamcollsurg.2019.09.020.
[35] Stone DH, Giles KA, Kubilis P, et al. Editor's Choice - Protamine Reduces Serious Bleeding Complications Associated with Carotid Endarterectomy in Asymptomatic Patients without Increasing the Risk of Stroke, Myocardial Infarction, or Death in a Large National Analysis. Eur J Vasc Endovasc Surg 2020;60(6):800–7; https://doi.org/10.1016/j.ejvs.2020.08.047.
[36] Liang P, Motaganahalli R, Swerdlow NJ, et al. Protamine use in transfemoral carotid artery stenting is not associated with an increased risk of thromboembolic events. J Vasc Surg 2021;73(1):142–150 e4; https://doi.org/10.1016/j.jvs.2020.04.526.
[37] Liang P, Motaganahalli RL, Malas MB, et al. Protamine use in transcarotid artery revascularization is associated with lower risk of bleeding complications without higher risk of thromboembolic events. J Vasc Surg 2020;72(6):2079–87; https://doi.org/10.1016/j.jvs.2020.02.019.
[38] Schermerhorn ML, Liang P, Dakour-Aridi H, et al. In-hospital outcomes of transcarotid artery revascularization and carotid endarterectomy in the Society for Vascular Surgery Vascular Quality Initiative. J Vasc Surg 2020;71(1):87–95; https://doi.org/10.1016/j.jvs.2018.11.029.
[39] Wu WW, Liang P, O'Donnell TFX, et al. Anatomic eligibility for transcarotid artery revascularization and transfemoral carotid artery stenting. *J Vasc Surg* May 2019;69(5):1452–60; https://doi.org/10.1016/j.jvs.2018.11.051.
[40] Columbo JA, Martinez-Camblor P, O'Malley AJ, et al. Association of Adoption of Transcarotid Artery Revascularization With Center-Level Perioperative Outcomes. JAMA Netw

Open 2021;4(2):e2037885; https://doi.org/10.1001/jamanetworkopen.2020.37885.

[41] Cui C, Ramakrishnan G, Murphy J, et al. Cost-effectiveness of transcarotid artery revascularization versus carotid endarterectomy. *J Vasc Surg* Dec 2021;74(6):1910–1918 e3; https://doi.org/10.1016/j.jvs.2021.05.051.

[42] Sridharan ND, Chaer RA, Smith K, et al. Carotid Endarterectomy remains cost-effective for the surgical management of carotid stenosis. J Vasc Surg 2021; https://doi.org/10.1016/j.jvs.2021.09.039.

[43] Brott TG, Howard G, Roubin GS, et al. Long-Term Results of Stenting versus Endarterectomy for Carotid-Artery Stenosis. N Engl J Med 2016;374(11):1021–31; https://doi.org/10.1056/NEJMoa1505215.

[44] Bonati LH, Dobson J, Featherstone RL, et al. Long-term outcomes after stenting versus endarterectomy for treatment of symptomatic carotid stenosis: the International Carotid Stenting Study (ICSS) randomised trial. *Lancet* Feb 7 2015;385(9967):529–38; https://doi.org/10.1016/S0140-6736(14)61184-3.

Advances in Surgery 56 (2022) 129–150

ADVANCES IN SURGERY

Endovascular Repair of Descending Thoracic Aortic Aneurysms

Michol A. Cooper, MD, PhD[a,*], Zain Shahid, MD[a], Gilbert R. Upchurch, Jr, MD[b]

[a]University of Florida College of Medicine, Division of Vascular Surgery and Endovascular Therapy, 1600 SW Archer Road, Room NG-45, Gainesville, FL 32610-0128 USA; [b]University of Florida College of Medicine, Department of Surgery, 1600 SW Archer Road, Room 6174, Gainesville, FL 32610-0286 USA

Keywords

• Thoracic aortic aneurysm • Penetrating aortic ulcer • TEVAR
• Spinal cord protection

Key points

- Descending thoracic aortic aneurysms (DTAAs) have an incidence of up to 10 cases per 100,000 individuals/y, affect men and women equally and have a significant genetic component.
- DTAAs should be repaired at 5.5 cm in low-risk patients with a higher threshold in patients with higher anatomic or physiologic risk. Thoracic endovascular aortic repair (TEVAR) is the preferred approach for repair.
- There are multiple procedural adjuncts, both open and endovascular, which can expand the indications for and use of TEVAR.
- Spinal cord injury (SCI) is one of the most devastating complications after DTAA repair, occurring in up to 4% of patients. It is imperative to use a multimodal approach with defined protocols to mitigate this risk.

INTRODUCTION

Descending thoracic aortic aneurysms (DTAAs) are an important cause of morbidity and mortality in the elderly with an incidence of up to 10 cases per 100,000 individuals/y [1]. Unlike abdominal aortic aneurysms (AAAs),

*Corresponding author: University of Florida College of Medicine Division of Vascular Surgery and Endovascular Therapy 1600 SW Archer Road, Room NG-45 Gainesville, FL 32610-0128 USA, *E-mail address:* Michol.cooper@surgery.ufl.edu

https://doi.org/10.1016/j.yasu.2022.02.005

they affect men and women equally and have a significant genetic component with 20% of affected family members having a first-degree relative affected by aneurysm disease [2–4]. Risk factors for progression include hypertension, smoking, COPD, and aortic dissection [5–9]. For aneurysm repair, although more sophisticated criteria are needed, aneurysm diameter is the most commonly used indication for repair as it most reliably predicts rupture. Maximum aneurysm diameter greater than 6 cm for DTAAs is associated with rupture and rupture-associated complications. Aneurysm repair is recommended at 5.5 cm in normal risk patients and higher diameters if the patient is high risk medically or anatomically [10,11]. Repair can be performed either in a traditional open fashion or with a thoracic endovascular aortic repair (TEVAR). There are no randomized control trials comparing TEVAR to open repair, as there were with EVAR. However, based on the best available data, TEVAR for DTAs is associated with lower morbidity, mortality, and hospital length of stay compared with open repair. The SVS recommends TEVAR as the preferred approach to DTA aneurysms [11,12]. Adjuncts including proximal and distal open and endovascular debranching can be used to extend proximal and distal landing zones and expand indications for TEVAR. One of the most devastating complications after DTA repair with TEVAR is spinal cord injury (SCI), which has an incidence of 1% to 4%, depending on the length of aorta treated and patient risk factors [11]. A multimodal approach with preoperative, intraoperative, and postoperative protocols for SCI prevention, as well as rescue protocols for those with delayed SCI, is imperative [11]. After endovascular repair for DTAAs, initial long-term data suggest excellent outcomes with only 11% of patients requiring re-intervention at 5 years [13]. TEVAR has changed the treatment paradigm for DTAAs. As technology continues to evolve and improve, the indications for endovascular repair of the thoracic aorta will undoubtedly continue to expand.

Epidemiology

Incidence

Aortic disease is one of the top 20 causes of death in the United States [14]. DTAAs are less common than abdominal and ascending aortic aneurysms, but they are a significant cause of morbidity and mortality with an incidence of 6 to 10 cases per 100,000 individuals/y [1]. Aneurysms isolated to the descending thoracic aorta account for about 35% of TAAs; those of the ascending aorta comprise 40%, aortic arch 15%, and thoracoabdominal aorta 10% [15]. The population affected by DTAAs are primarily elderly patients with an average age at diagnosis of 65. Unlike AAA, whereby the incidence in men is 6 times that of women, DTAAs have an equal incidence in men and women [2–4].

Risk factors for disease

The pathogenesis for DTAAs is multifactorial, with many risk factors being similar to those for patients with AAA. Modifiable risk factors inherent to both include hypertension, especially diastolic blood pressure greater than

100 mm Hg, and smoking [16–18]. Additionally, in DTAAs, there is a clear genetic component with more than 20% of patients with DTAA having a first-degree relative affected by aneurysm disease [19]. Finally, while 80% of DTAAs are due to medial degeneration, up to 20% are a result of a chronic aortic dissection [18].

Risk of progression and rupture

Due to isolated DTAAs being not as prevalent as ascending or infrarenal aortic aneurysms, their natural history is not as well known or described in the literature. Furthermore, most of the published DTAA data includes thoracoabdominal aortic aneurysms and aneurysms associated with dissections, which likely have distinct clinical progressions [20]. A 2002 review of 721 patients with TAA, which included ascending, descending and thoracoabdominal aortic aneurysms, found a significantly higher growth rate for DTAAs and TAAAs (0.19 cm/y) compared with ascending TAAs (0.07 cm/y). Dissected aneurysms also grew faster (0.14 cm/y) than nondissected aneurysms (0.09 cm/y). They also found that aneurysm size greater than 6 cm was associated with higher rates of rupture and dissection-associated complications [10]. Other smaller natural history studies of TAAs and TAAAs have demonstrated that COPD, larger aortic diameter, pain, older age, and chronic renal failure were associated with aneurysm growth, dissection, and rupture [5–9].

Anatomy

Aortic zones

The thoracic aorta contains the aortic root, ascending aorta, aortic arch, and descending aorta down to the level of the diaphragm. In normal aortas, the size of the thoracic aorta increases in size as it goes distally from the root to the diaphragm, with an average size of 2 to 3 cm. Of note, the TAA is approximately 10% smaller in women [15]. To better classify the anatomy of the aorta for treatment planning and reporting, the Society for Vascular Surgery (SVS) published guidelines dividing the aorta into 11 zones (Fig. 1) [21]. These zones aid in the description of how much of the aorta is affected by both aneurysmal and other diseases (including penetrating aortic ulcers (PAUs), intramural hematoma (IMH), dissection), which branches will be covered and the extent of coverage needed for treatment [21].

Another important consideration, particularly in the era of endovascular repair, is the angulation of the arch due to difficulty with navigating a device into the appropriate position as well as for the likelihood of seal. Type I arches are the easiest arches to treat and navigate, while type III are the most difficult (Fig. 2). [22].

Common anatomic variants

There are many common anatomic aortic arch variants, which can impact the ease and ability to treat DTAAs. The most common anatomic variant is the bovine arch in which one or more of the great vessels arise from a common trunk. The most common bovine arch variant is a common origin of the left

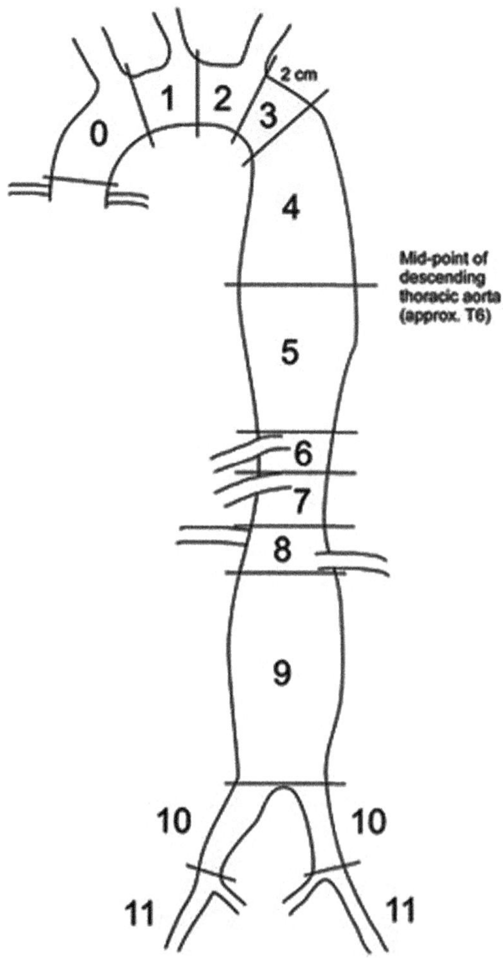

Fig. 1. Zones of aorta as defined by the Society for Vascular Surgery. (From [Fillinger MF, Greenberg RK, McKinsey JF, Chaikof EL, Society for Vascular Surgery Ad Hoc Committee on TEVAR Reporting Standards. Reporting standards for thoracic endovascular aortic repair (TEVAR). J Vasc Surg. 2010;52(4):1022–1033]; with permission).

common carotid artery and brachiocephalic artery at the aortic arch. Another common variant is a vertebral artery coming directly off of the aortic arch, either proximal or distal to the left subclavian. A third common variant is an aberrant right subclavian arising distal to the left subclavian artery off of the descending thoracic aorta. In this variant, the subclavian crosses through the posterior mediastinum posterior to the esophagus toward the right upper extremity (Fig. 3) [23]. Due to its course, it can cause a vascular ring around the trachea and esophagus and can cause dysphagia and palsy of the recurrent laryngeal nerve due to anatomic position. Additionally, these variants are often

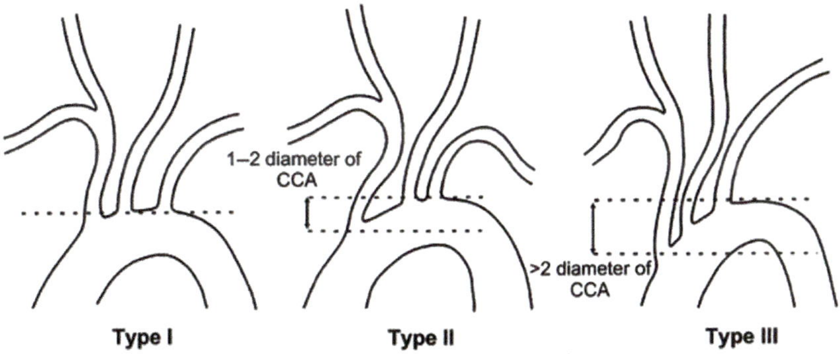

Fig. 2. Classification of the aortic arch based on type I, II, and III based on the cranial-caudal distance of the innominate from the left subclavian. CCA, Common carotid artery. (From [Marrocco-Trischitta MM, Rylski B, Schofer F, et al. Prevalence of type III arch configuration in patients with type B aortic dissection. Eur J Cardiothorac Surg. 2019;56(6):1075–1080]; with permission).

associated with a Kommerell diverticulum, or aneurysm, of the origin of the subclavian artery (Fig. 4) [24,25].

Spinal cord perfusion

There are multiple vessels that supply blood flow to the spinal cord that are at risk both during open and endovascular repair. These include the dorsal branches from the intercostal arteries, the lumbar arteries, and the artery of Adamkiewicz [26–28]. Many of the branches are either excluded during open repair or covered during TEVAR. For this reason, it is important that

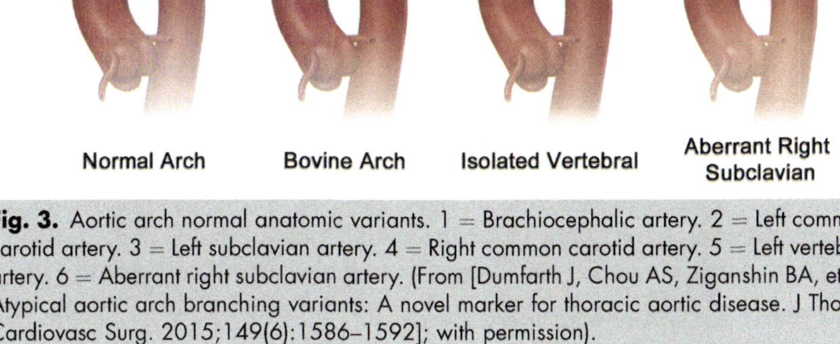

Fig. 3. Aortic arch normal anatomic variants. 1 = Brachiocephalic artery. 2 = Left common carotid artery. 3 = Left subclavian artery. 4 = Right common carotid artery. 5 = Left vertebral artery. 6 = Aberrant right subclavian artery. (From [Dumfarth J, Chou AS, Ziganshin BA, et al. Atypical aortic arch branching variants: A novel marker for thoracic aortic disease. J Thorac Cardiovasc Surg. 2015;149(6):1586–1592]; with permission).

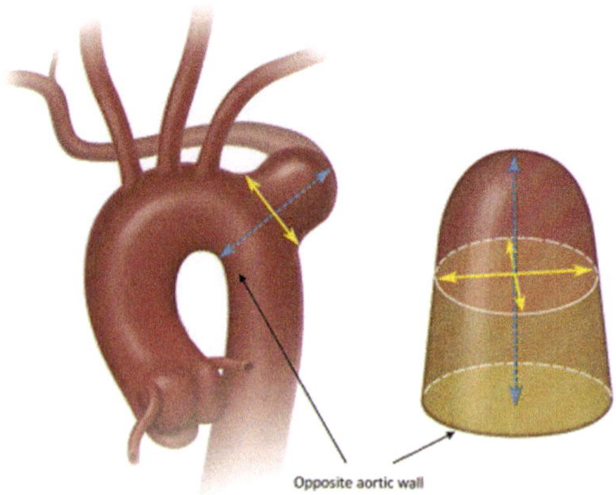

Fig. 4. Diagrammatic representation of a Kommerell diverticulum (KD) with a replaced right subclavian artery. This includes a representation of the usual measurements to record growth on the KD including KD diameter (yellow *arrow*) and the distance to the opposite aortic wall (DAW; blue dashed *arrow*). (From [Erben Y, Brownstein AJ, Velasquez CA, et al. Natural history and management of Kommerell's diverticulum in a single tertiary referral center. J Vasc Surg. 2020;71(6):2004–2011]; with permission).

neuroprotective strategies be applied, both with maintaining as much of the collateral flow as possible and with spinal drain placement as well as other adjuncts discussed later in the article. Collateral flow is provided by the subclavian and vertebral arteries, as well as the iliolumbar branches of the hypogastric arteries. It is imperative to maintain flow to these if possible (Fig. 5)[26,27,28].

Diagnosis and preoperative surveillance

Thoracic aortic aneurysms are mostly asymptomatic and found incidentally on imaging performed for other indications [11]. Due to higher numbers of imaging studies being performed, higher image quality, increased patient and physician awareness and an aging population, the incidence of TAA disease is higher than previously reported and has been steadily increasing over time [11,29]. However, unlike the low-cost, low-risk ultrasound screening for AAAs, there is no low-cost modality that can be used to image the descending thoracic aorta [11,30]. Thus, screening for TAA disease is based largely on patient and family history, including genetic testing as well as patient comorbidities.

Once a DTAA has been diagnosed, aneurysms can be followed with either CTA or MRA, depending on what is most readily available at the institution whereby they are being followed [11]. Ideally, serial studies should be performed using the same imaging modality/protocol in the same center for best image comparison over time. Once an aneurysm has been detected, for patients without connective tissue disorders, a reasonable surveillance protocol is:

- 3 to 4 cm: CTA or MRA every 2 years
- 4 to 4.9 cm: CTA or MRA yearly

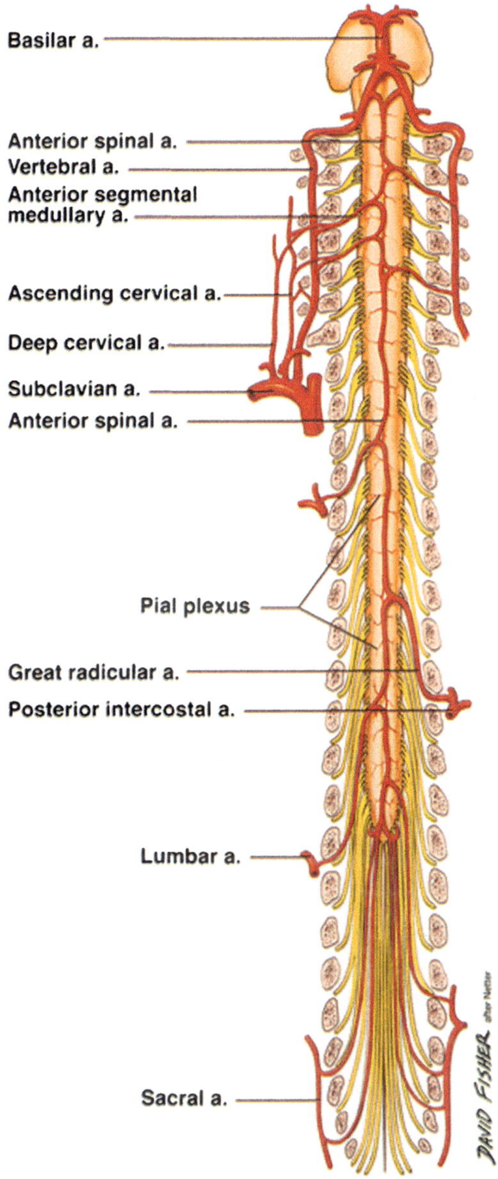

Fig. 5. Spinal cord perfusion and collaterals. (From [Taterra D, Skinningsrud B, Pękala PA, et al. Artery of Adamkiewicz: a meta-analysis of anatomical characteristics. Neuroradiology. 2019;61(8):869–880]; with permission).

- 5 to 6 cm: CTA or MRA every 6 months

For patients with connective tissue disorders, surveillance should be performed every 6 months of the entire aorta [31].

Indications for repair

Size

Although more sophisticated criteria are needed, maximum aneurysm diameter is the most commonly used indication for repair as it most reliably predicts rupture. In a 2002 study of 721 patients with TAAs, an aneurysm of $\geq$ 6 cm was associated with a nearly 4-fold increase in the incidence of rupture [10]. In another study of 57 patients with DTA not considered operative candidates, aneurysm size greater than 5 cm was independently associated with rupture [5]. Due to the rarer incidence of DTA compared with AAA, data for treatment thresholds are not as clear. Based on the best available evidence, the SVS [11] recommends TEVAR in:

- Asymptomatic, low-risk patients at maximum diameter $\geq$ 5.5 cm
- Higher diameter for patients deemed high risk of death, renal failure, or paraplegia

Additionally, for patients with connective tissue disorder, a lower threshold can be considered.

Special considerations

Penetrating aortic ulcers. A PAU can form when an atherosclerotic plaque becomes ulcerated and penetrates the internal elastic lamina, resulting in a hematoma formation within the media [11]. PAUs are typically not aneurysmal, but can occur within an aneurysm. The natural history of PAUs is not well defined, but the presence of symptoms, associated IMH, or pleural effusion are risk factors for complications [32,33]. Additionally PAU depth greater than 10 mm and diameter greater than 20 mm are risks for disease progression [33]. Based on this, treatment of PAUs with TEVAR is recommended in asymptomatic patients who have at-risk characteristics for growth and rupture. Additionally, it is recommended in patients who have persistent symptoms or progression despite optimal blood pressure control [11].

Intramural hematoma and aortic dissection. Aortic IMH is likely a variant of aortic dissection without a clear entry tear, intimal flap, or flow in the false lumen. IMH is believed to be secondary to the rupture of the vasa vasorum into the aortic wall. This disease can progress and rupture into the intima, leading to progression to a dissection [11,34]. In a systematic review of 925 patients with IMH, predictors for progression and complications included persistent pain, IMH thickness greater than 10 mm, aortic diameter greater than 45 mm, hemodynamic instability, pleural effusion, or hemomediastinum or periaortic hemorrhage [35]. For patients with asymptomatic IMH, optimal medical therapy with blood pressure control and follow-up imaging is recommended. For patients with persistent symptoms despite optimal medical control or those with the progression of disease on follow-up imaging, treatment with TEVAR is recommended [11].

Kommerell diverticulum. As described above, a Kommerell diverticulum is an outpouching of the aorta typically associated with an aberrant subclavian artery.

The risk of dissection or rupture associated with these aneurysms is highly variable in the literature, ranging from 19% to 53% in different case series, likely due to cystic medial necrosis in the diverticulum wall [11,24]. Because of the high rates of rupture and dissection, surgical intervention should be considered with the maximum diameter of the diverticulum is > 30 mm or when the adjacent aorta is ≥ 50 mm [36].

Mycotic aneurysms. Mycotic, or infected, aneurysms can be secondary to seeding from bacteremia, extension from an infection in adjacent tissue, or iatrogenic introduction during an intra-arterial procedure. Pre-existing atherosclerotic plaque, aneurysm, or aortic wall trauma can predispose a patient to mycotic aneurysm formation [11]. These are life-threatening infections that often progress rapidly and should be treated when diagnosed if the patient will tolerate it. Of note, any saccular TAA should be worked up for an infectious etiology as greater than 90% of mycotic aneurysms are saccular in appearance [37].

Repair types

Thoracic endovascular aortic repair versus open repair

Traditional open repair of DTAAs remains one of the most technically and physiologically demanding procedures with a nationwide mortality of 22% for elective cases [38]. In highly specialized centers, the mortality for elective cases drops significantly to 4.8%, but remains high at 26% for ruptured TAA [39,40]. In contrast, TEVAR for isolated DTAAs is associated with significantly lower morbidity, mortality, and hospital length of stay, although we are still lacking long-term data on the need for open conversion, endoleak, and late mortality [12]. There are no randomized control trials comparing TEVAR to open repair, as there were with EVAR. Thus, most of the current data on TEVAR is from industry-sponsored, nonrandomized comparisons to open repair as well as single-center experiences and registry data that combine different pathologies and indications. However, based on the current best available data, the SVS recommends TEVAR as the preferred approach for DTAAs [11].

Special populations

One population whereby we have very little data for open versus endovascular repair is in patients with connective tissue disease. There has been increasing use of TEVARs in this patient population with good short-term results [41]. However, the long-term outcomes remain to be seen and TEVAR in this patient population should be performed with caution in high volume centers with experienced vascular and cardiovascular surgeons. Another population where TEVARs have had some increasing use is in patients with mycotic aneurysms. It is often used as a good temporizing measure in patients too sick for open repair, but data demonstrating long-term benefits are lacking[11].

Thoracic endovascular aortic repair

Dake and colleagues reported the first thoracic aortic endovascular repair in 1994 [42]. These grafts were constructed from self-expanding stainless steel stents covered with woven Dacron and were custom-designed for each patient. The first commercially available endograft, the GORE TAG device, was then released almost 20 years later in 2005. TEVAR graft development has lagged behind the pace of EVAR due to lower incidence of DTAA, need for larger devices, and more challenging hemodynamics. Despite this, there are now 4 commercially available device platforms available in the United States (Table 1)[11].

Approach

Due to the large access needed for the introduction of TEVAR devices, TEVARs were originally performed through open femoral access. However, there are now closure devices that permit a percutaneous approach with minimal morbidity and mortality. In a meta-analysis including 469 percutaneous TEVARs, the overall technical success rate was 94% for percutaneous access with only 1.6% of patients requiring open repair of the groin [43]. Factors associated with successful percutaneous access include ultrasound guidance, sheath size less than 20 Fr, greater than 1 cm segment of common femoral artery without anterior calcification, abscess of severe scarring in the groin, native arterial access, and access diameter greater than 5 mm [43–45].

In patients in which femoral and/or iliac artery size or disease precludes the introduction of a TEVAR device, the following adjuncts can be used.

- Serial angioplasty and dilators
- Direct common iliac or infrarenal aortic access with primary closure
  - Most commonly performed during debranching or other procedure
- Iliac conduit
  - Open: retroperitoneal exposure of the common iliac artery (CIA) or distal infernal aorta and the left or right femoral artery is performed, depending on patient anatomy. A 10 mm prosthetic (Dacron or PTFE) bypass is then performed to the CIA or aorta to the CFA. This can then be used not only for the DTA treatment but also for future interventions if needed.
  - Endovascular: 10 mm or 12 mm stent grafts are placed through the length of the diseased/small iliac vessel and the vessel is then angioplastied, often with intentional rupture of the vessel to expand it to the needed diameter for graft introduction.
- Carotid/axillary access
  - Can be used in selected patients with iliac/distal aortic occlusions
  - The stent graft will be deployed in an inverted fashion
  - This approach can also be used to facilitate the introduction of the graft from femoral access in tortuous iliac and/or aortic anatomy. In this approach, a wire is introduced from the left or right brachial or axillary artery into the aorta and the wire is snared from below. A stiff (usually Lunderquist) wire is then placed from the femoral access out through the axillary/brachial access to facilitate graft delivery by straightening the aorta and allowing for a push–pull technique [11].

Thoracic endovascular aortic repair adjuncts

For most devices, a landing zone of 2 to 3 cm is adequate, although a longer seal zone may be preferable to improve seal and decrease the occurrence of

Table 1
Currently commercially available TEVAR devices for the treatment of thoracic aortic aneurysms. Graft oversizing is based on the diameter of the graft compared with the diameter of healthy aorta in the proximal and distal landing zones.

Manufacturer	Device name	Graft material	Minimum access size needed (mm)	Aortic diameter	Graft diameter oversizing (%)	Minimum proximal landing zone (mm)	Minimum distal landing zone (mm)
W.L. Gore & Associates	Conformable Thoracic Aortic Graft with Active Control	Expanded PTFE[a] reinforced with an ePTFE film with external self-expanding nitinol stent	4–8.7	16–42	8–32	20	20
Medtronic	Valiant Captivia	Monofilament polyester graft with external self-expanding nitinol stents	7.3–8.3	18–42	10–20	20	20
Cook Medical	Zenith Alpha	Dacron with external self-expanding stainless steel Z stents	6–7.7	20–42	10–25	20	20
Bolton Medical	RelayPro	Woven polyester with external self-expanding Duralloy stents	6.3–7.6	19–42	9–20	15–30	25–30

[a]PTFE is polytetrafluoroethylene.

(Adapted from [Upchurch Jr GR, Escobar GA, Azizzadeh A, et al. Society for Vascular Surgery clinical practice guidelines of thoracic endovascular aortic repair for descending thoracic aortic aneurysms. J Vasc Surg. 2021;73(1S):55S-83S]; with permission).

late endoleaks. Where there is more angulation in the aorta, typically in zones 2 and 3, apposition of the TEVAR device against the aortic wall can be hindered. Due to this, the landing zone should be determined based on the length of the seal along the inner curve. To increase the seal proximally and distally, there are multiple adjunctive procedures that can be performed.

Open hybrid repairs

Proximal debranching.

- Left carotid-subclavian bypass (Fig. 6): Up to 40% of patients with DTAs may need left subclavian coverage to obtain adequate proximal seal for a TEVAR [46]. This maintains not only flow to the left arm but also posterior circulation flow through the left vertebral artery and collateral spinal cord flow through the left vertebral artery, LIMA, subscapular artery, and lateral thoracic artery [46]. Additionally, in patients with prior CABG and LIMA grafts, it is imperative to maintain left subclavian artery flow. In emergencies, such as unstable ruptures, the left subclavian artery can be covered without revascularization. However, this is associated with a combined stroke, paraplegia, and death rate of up to 28% [47].
- Right to left carotid-carotid bypass or right to left axillo-axillary artery bypass: these can be performed in combination with a left carotid-subclavian bypass in aneurysms whereby the graft needs to land in zone 1 (Fig. 7).
- Bilateral carotid-subclavian bypass: this is most often performed with an aberrant right subclavian artery and a Kommerell Diverticulum as the right carotid-subclavian alone most often does not leave enough of a proximal landing zone.
- Debranching off of the ascending aorta: debranching of the innominate and left common carotid can be performed through a sternotomy with a side biting

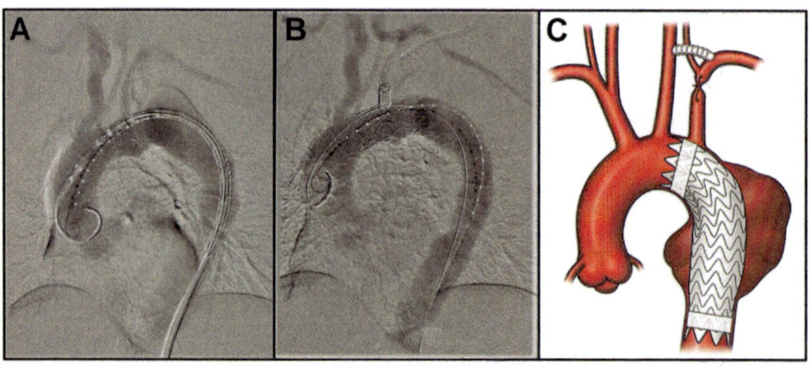

Fig. 6. Debranching with a left carotid-subclavian bypass and TEVAR. (*A*) The TEVAR graft was introduced and placed into zone 2 to cover the left subclavian artery. (*B*) The TEVAR graft was deployed and the left subclavian was coil embolized with excellent exclusion of the aneurysm. The left carotid-subclavian bypass can also be seen providing flow to the left subclavian artery. (*C*) A schematic demonstrating left subclavian artery debranching with left carotid-subclavian bypass and TEVAR with open ligation of the proximal left subclavian proximal to the vertebral artery (Adapted from [Riesenman PJ, Farber MA, Mendes RR, Marston WA, Fulton JJ, Keagy BA. Coverage of the left subclavian artery during thoracic endovascular aortic repair. J Vasc Surg. 2007;45(1):90–94; discussion 94]; with permission).

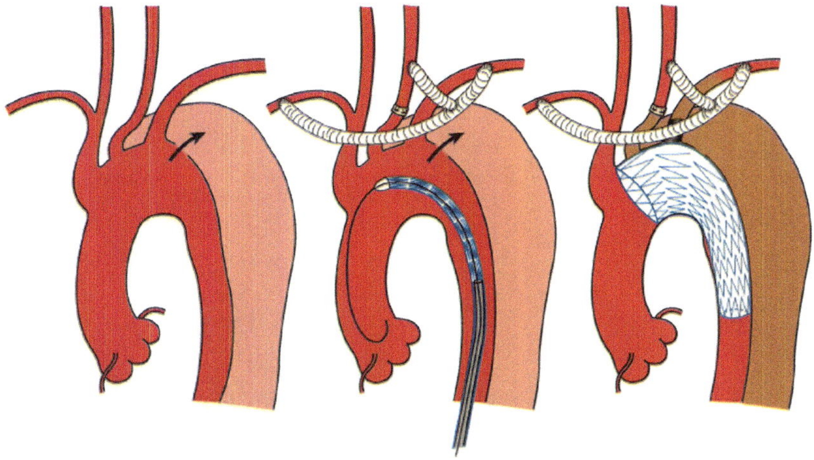

Fig. 7. A thoracic aortic aneurysm extending into Zone 2 with the need for coverage into Zone 1. An axillary–axillary artery bypass with left carotid-subclavian bypass was performed for debranching before TEVAR placement. (From [atani T. Best surgical option for arch extension of type B dissection: the endovascular approach. Ann Cardiothorac Surg. 2014;3(3):292–299]; with permission).

proximal aortic clamp without the need for cardiopulmonary bypass. A left carotid-subclavian is then performed through a supraclavicular approach followed by TEVAR and subclavian artery embolization for TAA exclusion (Fig. 8).

Distal debranching.

- Celiac artery coverage can add between 1 and 2.5 cm of additional distal seal for a TEVAR and is necessary for treatment in about 4% to 6% of DTAAs [11,48]. There is generally extensive collateralization between the celiac and SMA, but this is not reliably determined by preoperative CTA or intraoperative angiogram [48]. Complications including foregut ischemia, paraplegia, and death are more common in patients who do not undergo celiac artery revascularization [48]. However, this has to be weighed against the mortality of celiac artery revascularization for each patient. Distal debranching of the celiac artery can be performed through multiple techniques including hepatorenal bypass, splenorenal bypass, and retrograde ilio-celiac bypass.
- For patients with associated thoracoabdominal aortic aneurysms that need to be treated, visceral-renal debranching can be performed using bifurcated or trifurcated grafts off of the right or left iliac arteries, and then TEVAR can be placed across the affected segment (Fig. 9). This approach has decreased early morbidity and similar late survival to traditional open repair [49,50].

Endovascular techniques

Chimney and periscope grafts: patients considered too high risk for open debranching can also undergo parallel graft placement with chimney and

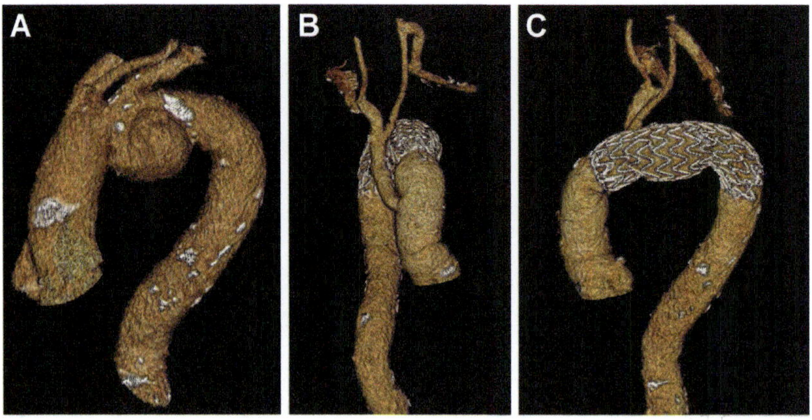

Fig. 8. Debranching and TEVAR for Zone 2 aneurysm. (*A*) The aneurysm before repair with the proximal aneurysm extending into Zone 1. (*B*) Anterior view of the aorta after debranching of the innominate and left common carotid off of the ascending thoracic aorta and a left carotid-subclavian bypass followed by aneurysm exclusion with a TEVAR (*C*) Lateral view post debranching and TEVAR placement demonstrating excellent aneurysm exclusion.

periscope (snorkel) grafts. This can also be used as a salvage maneuver in patients whereby proximal or distal branches are inadvertently covered.

- Chimney grafts are placed proximally in the innominate, left common carotid, and/or left subclavian arteries depending on the proximal extent of the graft (Fig. 10). These repairs have reintervention rates from 10% to 30%, depending on the number of chimneys performed, perioperative mortality of 5%, stroke rate of 4% [51,52].
- Periscope grafts can be placed distally into the celiac artery and superior mesenteric artery (SMA) to extend the distal seal for TEVARs (Fig. 11). Small case series have demonstrated technical success in the short term, although long-term data are lacking [53,54].

Physician-modified endografts (PMEGs) are another option for patients whereby branch coverage is necessary to obtain an adequate seal. In these repairs, fenestrations corresponding to the vessels needing coverage are created in the commercially available TEVAR endografts by the physician implanting the graft. The routine use of PMEGs requires FDA investigational device exemption (IDE) approval, but they can be performed outside of an IDE for compassionate use. In high volume centers, patients undergoing these repairs have excellent outcomes with similar freedom from reintervention, primary and secondary target vessel patency, and preservation of renal function compared with patients treated with commercially available devices, despite more complex aneurysm anatomy [55].

Spinal cord protection

One of the most important considerations for the repair of a DTAA is SCI. The incidence of paraplegia is lower with TEVAR compared with open repair, but

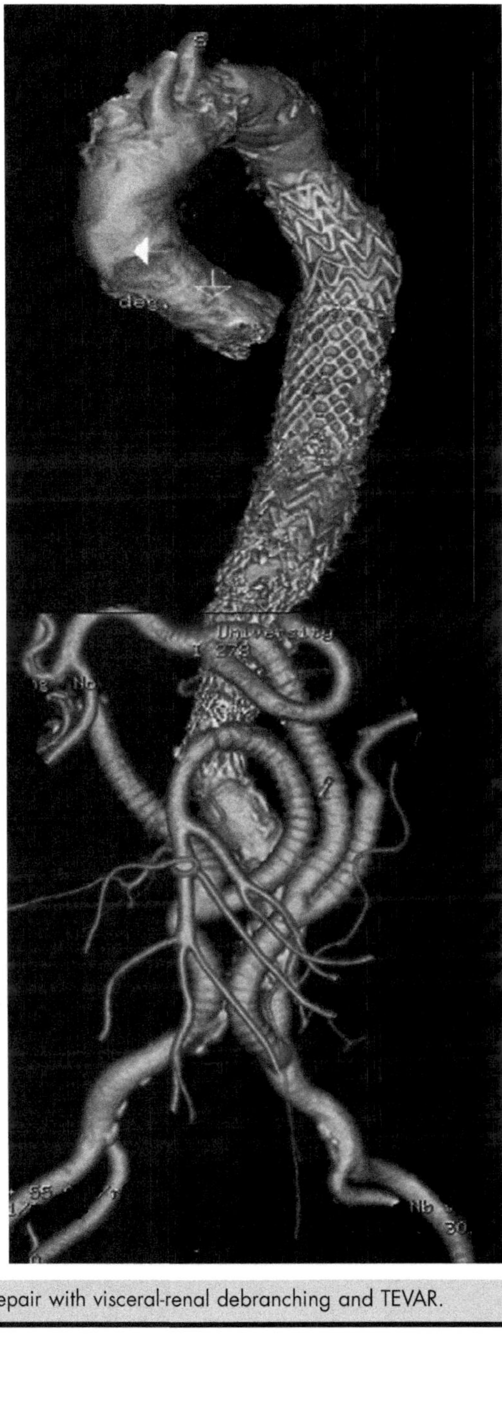

Fig. 9. Hybrid repair with visceral-renal debranching and TEVAR.

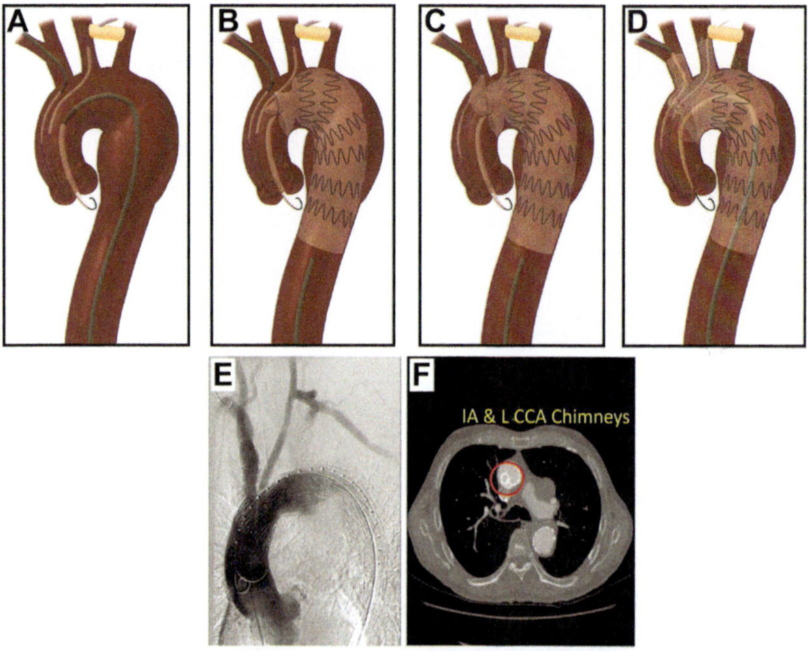

Fig. 10. Technical conduct of aortic arch chimney (AAC) stent graft placement during thoracic endovascular aortic repair (TEVAR) and post-TEVAR angiogram and CTA. (*A*) A patient with a proximal descending thoracic aneurysm requires a double chimney into the ascending aorta (zone 0). The carotid-subclavian bypass has been completed, and the left common carotid artery (LCCA) chimney, in this case, a Gore Viabahn is placed through the bypass graft. The innominate chimney stent, in this case an iliac limb device, has been delivered through the right axillary artery. The thoracic aortic endograft is also in place. Graft sizing is generally 30% greater than the outer-to-outer centerline aortic measurement at the anticipated landing zone (0%-10% in cases of dissection). Overlap between the chimney and thoracic stent grafts is generally 3 cm or greater (especially if there is significant arch curvature). (*B*) The device is partially deployed, with the proximal aspect still constrained while the chimney stents are deployed, which is demonstrated in (*C*). (*D*) Concomitant ballooning of all 3 stents, with a compliant balloon in both the innominate and aortic stent grafts and a noncompliant balloon in the LCCA stent graft. In this image, the left subclavian artery (LSA) has been embolized with a vascular plug. (*E*) Fluoroscopy image after the graft and chimney stents have been deployed with excellent flow through the stents as well as the TEVAR graft and no endoleak (*F*) Postoperative CTA demonstrating the stents alongside the TEVAR graft (red circle). (Adapted from [Voskresensky I, Scali ST, Feezor RJ, et al. Outcomes of thoracic endovascular aortic repair using aortic arch chimney stents in high-risk patients. J Vasc Surg. 2017;66(1):9–20.e3]; with permission [51]).

ranges from 1% to 4%, depending on the amount of aorta covered [11]. In patients who do have SCI, it is often a devastating complication with only 38% returning to normal function [56]. Additionally, in those with no functional improvement, 1-year mortality is up to 75% [57]. Given these poor outcomes

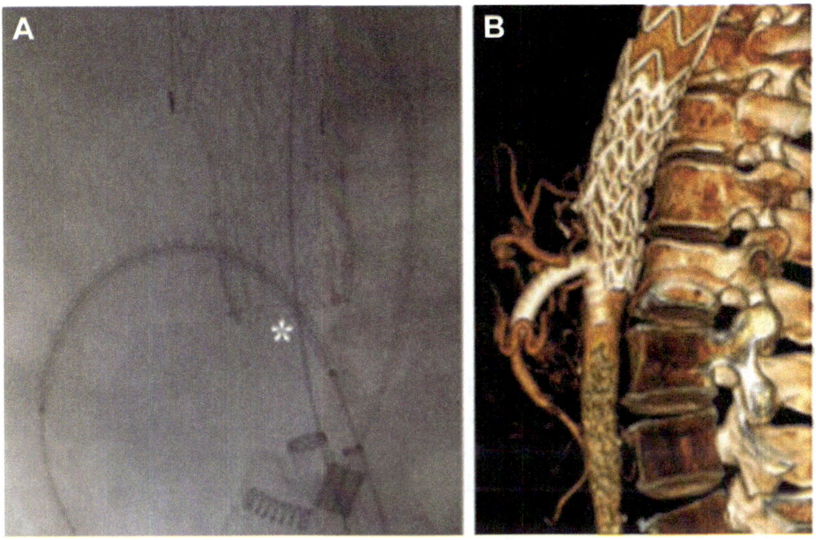

Fig. 11. Periscope into SMA to extend TEVAR distal seal. (*A*) Intra-operative fluoroscopy showing deployed GORE TAG endoprostheses and a preloaded VBX 8 × 79 mm with the distal part of the stent extending below the distal edge of the aortic endoprosthesis (*asterisk*). (*B*) Post-operative CTA reconstruction with the absence of endoleaks and patency of the superior mesenteric and renal arteries as well as good collateral flow to the celiac. (From [Manresa-Manresa F, Quintero-Pérez C, Mengíbar-Fuentes L. Periscope Technique for Superior Mesenteric Artery and Thoracic Stent Graft Extension for Type Ib Endoleak with Ruptured Thoracic Aortic Aneurysm. Eur J Vasc Endovasc Surg. 2021;61(3):519. doi:10.1016/j.ejvs.2020.11.002]; with permission).

with SCI, it is crucial that interventions to mitigate this risk be implemented including, when possible:

- Maintaining patency of the left subclavian and hypogastric arteries [58].
- Staging repairs for long-segment aortic coverage [59].
- Prophylactic CSF drainage [60].
- Permissive hypertension [60].
- Steroid therapy [60].
- Naloxone therapy [60].

In patients who develop SCI postoperatively, rescue protocols include increasing MAP to > 100 mm Hg, placement of CSF drain (if one is not in place), and dropping the CSF drain pressure, transfusion to Hgb greater than 10 mg/dL and steroids [11,61]. A multimodal approach with clear protocols for preoperative, intraoperative, and postoperative SCI prevention as well as rescue procedures for those who present with delayed SCI is imperative[11].

Indications for prophylactic CSF drainage catheter placement for TEVAR are evolving with some centers using them routinely and others placing them only in patients deemed high risk [11]. Risk factors for SCI after TEVAR include[11].

- Length of aortic coverage greater than 15 cm
- Previous TEVAR, EVAR, or open AAA repair
- Diseased or occluded internal iliac or vertebral arteries
- Planned LSA coverage

In these high-risk patients, the SVS recommends prophylactic CSF drainage [11].

Surveillance after thoracic endovascular aortic repair

Once a TEVAR graft has been implanted, it is imperative to follow patients with serial imaging. This surveillance is needed for the evaluation of complications requiring mitigation, including ongoing aneurysm expansion, stent migration, endoleak, device failure (fracture, migration or device component), stenosis, occlusion, and graft infection [11]. Long-term data for straightforward aneurysm repair whereby TEVARs are performed within the instructions for use of the TEVAR device suggest excellent outcomes with only 11% of patients requiring reintervention at 5 years [13]. Additionally, in patients treated for nonruptured aneurysms, the average time to any intervention was 28 months [64]. The SVS recommends CTA at 1 and 12 months after TEVAR and then yearly for life with more frequent imaging if any abnormalities are detected[11,62,63].

SUMMARY

DTAAs affect the elderly and have a significant morbidity and mortality if not treated. Repair should generally be performed when these aneurysms reach a diameter of 5.5 cm to mitigate the risk of rupture and other complications. Although there are no randomized control trials comparing open and endovascular repair with TEVAR, data from large administrative databases, as well as meta-analysis of smaller studies have demonstrated that TEVAR has lower morbidity and mortality and should be the primary method of repair for DTAAs. For these repairs, although the SCI rate is lower than with open repair, occurring in less than 4% of patients, it is a devastating complication and it is imperative to use a multimodal approach with defined protocols to mitigate this risk. TEVAR has changed the treatment paradigm for DTAAs and indications for endovascular repair of the thoracic aorta will undoubtedly continue to expand as technology evolves.

CLINICS CARE POINTS

- Although DTAAs are less common than AAAs, they are an important cause of morbidity and mortality in the elderly [1].
- Once detected, it is important to surveil DTAAs using either CTA or MRA with the following schedule (with the exception of patients with connective tissue disorder, who should be surveilled every 6 months regardless of aneurysm size):
  - 3 to 4 cm: every 2 years
  - 4 to 4.9 cm: yearly

- 5 to 6 cm: every 6 months

- Due to the rarer incidence of DTAAs compared with AAAs, data for treatment thresholds are not as clear. Based on the best available evidence, the SVS [11] recommends repair in:
  - Asymptomatic, low-risk patients at maximum aneurysm diameter ≥ 5.5 cm
  - Higher diameter for patients deemed high risk of death, renal failure, or paraplegia
- Although we still do not have long-term data comparing open and endovascular repair for DTAAs, thoracic endovascular aortic aneurysm repair (TEVAR) is associated with significantly lower morbidity, mortality and hospital stay [12]. Due to this, the SVS recommends TEVAR as the preferred approach for DTAAs with the exception of patients with connective tissue disorder and mycotic aortic aneurysms, whereby the data are much less clear[11].
- There are many endovascular and open adjuncts that can expand the use of TEVAR in patients who do not meet anatomic criteria for repair with TEVAR alone.
- There are multiple vessels that supply blood flow to the spinal cord that are at risk both during open and endovascular repair. The incidence of paraplegia is lower with TEVAR compared with open repair, but ranges from 1% to 4%, depending on the amount of aorta covered [11]. It is imperative to use a multimodal approach with defined protocols to mitigate this risk, including consideration for CSF drainage catheter placement. SVS recommends prophylactic CSF drainage in high-risk patients [11] including those with:
  - Length of aortic coverage greater than 15 cm
  - Previous TEVAR, EVAR, or open AAA repair
  - Diseased or occluded internal iliac or vertebral arteries
  - Planned left subclavian artery coverage

Once a TEVAR graft has been implanted, surveillance is needed for the evaluation of complications requiring mitigation, including ongoing aneurysm expansion, stent migration, endoleak, device failure (fracture, migration, or device component), stenosis, occlusion, and graft infection [11]. The SVS recommends CTA at 1 and 12 months after TEVAR and then yearly for life with more frequent imaging if any abnormalities are detected[11].

DISCLOSURE

The authors have nothing to disclose.

References

[1] Alsawas M, Zaiem F, Larrea-Mantilla L, et al. Effectiveness of surgical interventions for thoracic aortic aneurysms: a systematic review and meta-analysis. J Vasc Surg 2017;66(4):1258–68.

[2] Clouse WD, Hallett JW, Schaff HV, et al. Improved prognosis of thoracic aortic aneurysms: a population-based study. JAMA 1998;280(22):1926–9.

[3] Huang Y, Schaff HV, Dearani JA, et al. A population-based study of the incidence and natural history of degenerative thoracic aortic aneurysms. Mayo Clin Proc 2021;96(10):2628–38.

[4] Pleumeekers HJ, Hoes AW, van der Does E, et al. Aneurysms of the abdominal aorta in older adults. the rotterdam study. Am J Epidemiol 1995;142(12):1291–9.
[5] Cambria RA, Gloviczki P, Stanson AW, et al. Outcome and expansion rate of 57 thoracoabdominal aortic aneurysms managed nonoperatively. Am J Surg 1995;170(2):213–7.
[6] Crawford ES, DeNatale RW. Thoracoabdominal aortic aneurysm: observations regarding the natural course of the disease. J Vasc Surg 1986;3(4):578–82.
[7] Pressler V, McNamara JJ. Aneurysm of the thoracic aorta. J Thorac Cardiovasc Surg 1985;89(1):50–4.
[8] Juvonen T, Ergin MA, Galla JD, et al. Prospective study of the natural history of thoracic aortic aneurysms. Ann Thorac Surg 1997;63(6):1533–45.
[9] Griepp RB, Ergin MA, Galla JD, et al. Natural history of descending thoracic and thoracoabdominal aneurysms. Ann Thorac Surg 1999;67(6):1927–30, discussion 1953.
[10] Davies RR, Goldstein LJ, Coady MA, et al. Yearly rupture or dissection rates for thoracic aortic aneurysms: simple prediction based on size. Ann Thorac Surg 2002;73(1):17–27, discussion 27.
[11] Upchurch GR, Escobar GA, Azizzadeh A, et al. Society for vascular surgery clinical practice guidelines of thoracic endovascular aortic repair for descending thoracic aortic aneurysms. J Vasc Surg 2021;73(1S):55S–83S.
[12] Abraha I, Romagnoli C, Montedori A, et al. Thoracic stent graft versus surgery for thoracic aneurysm. Cochrane Database Syst Rev 2016;6:CD006796.
[13] Ziza V, Canaud L, Molinari N, et al. Thoracic endovascular aortic repair: a single center's 15-year experience. J Thorac Cardiovasc Surg 2016;151(6):1595–603.
[14] Chau KH, Elefteriades JA. Natural history of thoracic aortic aneurysms: size matters, plus moving beyond size. Prog Cardiovasc Dis 2013;56(1):74–80.
[15] Sidawy AN, Perler BA, editors. Rutherford's vascular Surgery and endovascular therapy editors. 9th edition. Elsevier; 2018.
[16] Dapunt OE, Galla JD, Sadeghi AM, et al. The natural history of thoracic aortic aneurysms. J Thorac Cardiovasc Surg 1994;107(5):1323–32, discussion 1332.
[17] Guo D-C, Papke CL, He R, et al. Pathogenesis of thoracic and abdominal aortic aneurysms. Ann N Y Acad Sci 2006;1085:339–52.
[18] Coady MA, Rizzo JA, Goldstein LJ, et al. Natural history, pathogenesis, and etiology of thoracic aortic aneurysms and dissections. Cardiol Clin 1999;17(4):615–35.
[19] Coady MA, Davies RR, Roberts M, et al. Familial patterns of thoracic aortic aneurysms. Arch Surg 1999;134(4):361–7.
[20] Elefteriades JA. Natural history of thoracic aortic aneurysms: indications for surgery, and surgical versus nonsurgical risks. Ann Thorac Surg 2002;74(5):S1877–80, discussion S1892.
[21] Fillinger MF, Greenberg RK, McKinsey JF, et al. Society for vascular surgery ad hoc committee on TEVAR reporting standards. reporting standards for thoracic endovascular aortic repair (TEVAR). J Vasc Surg 2010;52(4):1022–33, 1033.e15.
[22] Marrocco-Trischitta MM, Rylski B, Schofer F, et al. Prevalence of type III arch configuration in patients with type B aortic dissection. Eur J Cardiothorac Surg 2019;56(6):1075–80.
[23] Dumfarth J, Chou AS, Ziganshin BA, et al. Atypical aortic arch branching variants: a novel marker for thoracic aortic disease. J Thorac Cardiovasc Surg 2015;149(6):1586–92.
[24] Tanaka A, Milner R, Ota T. Kommerell's diverticulum in the current era: a comprehensive review. Gen Thorac Cardiovasc Surg 2015;63(5):245–59.
[25] Erben Y, Brownstein AJ, Velasquez CA, et al. Natural history and management of Kommerell's diverticulum in a single tertiary referral center. J Vasc Surg 2020;71(6):2004–11.
[26] Nijenhuis RJ, Leiner T, Cornips EMJ, et al. Spinal cord feeding arteries at MR angiography for thoracoscopic spinal surgery: feasibility study and implications for surgical approach. Radiology 2004;233(2):541–7.
[27] Colman MW, Hornicek FJ, Schwab JH. Spinal cord blood supply and its surgical implications. J Am Acad Orthop Surg 2015;23(10):581–91.

[28] Taterra D, Skinningsrud B, Pękala PA, et al. Artery of Adamkiewicz: a meta-analysis of anatomical characteristics. Neuroradiology 2019;61(8):869–80.
[29] Olsson C, Thelin S, Stahle E. Thoracic aortic aneurysm and dissection: Increasing prevalence and improved outcomes reported in a nationwide population-based study of more than 14,000 cases from 1987 to 2002. J Vasc Surg 2007;46(3):609.
[30] Cooper MA, Upchurch GR. Duplex ultrasound screening for abdominal aortic aneurysm. In: AbuRahma AF, Perler BA, editors. Noninvasive vascular diagnosis: a practical textbook for clinicians. Springer International Publishing; 2020. p. 1–16.
[31] Writing Committee Members, Hiratzka LF, Bakris GL, et al. ACCF/AHA/AATS/ACR/ASA/SCA/SCAI/SIR/STS/SVM guidelines for the diagnosis and management of patients with thoracic aortic disease: executive summary. Circulation 2010;121(13):1544–79.
[32] Patel HJ, Sood V, Williams DM, et al. Late outcomes with repair of penetrating thoracic aortic ulcers: the merits of an endovascular approach. Ann Thorac Surg 2012;94(2): 516–22, discussion 522.
[33] Ganaha F, Miller DC, Sugimoto K, et al. Prognosis of aortic intramural hematoma with and without penetrating atherosclerotic ulcer: a clinical and radiological analysis. Circulation 2002;106(3):342–8.
[34] Chou AS, Ziganshin BA, Charilaou P, et al. Long-term behavior of aortic intramural hematomas and penetrating ulcers. J Thorac Cardiovasc Surg 2016;151(2):361–72, 373.e1.
[35] Evangelista A, Czerny M, Nienaber C, et al. Interdisciplinary expert consensus on management of type B intramural haematoma and penetrating aortic ulcer. Eur J Cardiothorac Surg 2015;47(2):209–17.
[36] Ota T, Okada K, Takanashi S, et al. Surgical treatment for Kommerell's diverticulum. J Thorac Cardiovasc Surg 2006;131(3):574–8.
[37] Macedo TA, Stanson AW, Oderich GS, et al. Infected aortic aneurysms: imaging findings. Radiology 2004;231(1):250–7.
[38] Cowan JA, Dimick JB, Henke PK, et al. Surgical treatment of intact thoracoabdominal aortic aneurysms in the United States: hospital and surgeon volume-related outcomes. J Vasc Surg 2003;37(6):1169–74.
[39] Barbato JE, Kim JY, Zenati M, et al. Contemporary results of open repair of ruptured descending thoracic and thoracoabdominal aortic aneurysms. J Vasc Surg 2007;45(4): 667–76.
[40] Coselli JS, LeMaire SA, Miller CC, et al. Mortality and paraplegia after thoracoabdominal aortic aneurysm repair: a risk factor analysis. Ann Thorac Surg 2000;69(2):409–14.
[41] Qato K, Conway A, Lu E, et al. Outcomes of thoracic endovascular aneurysm repair (TEVAR) in patients with connective tissue disorders. Vasc Endovascular Surg 2020;54(8):676–80.
[42] Dake MD, Miller DC, Semba CP, et al. Transluminal placement of endovascular stent-grafts for the treatment of descending thoracic aortic aneurysms. N Engl J Med 1994;331(26): 1729–34.
[43] Jaffan AAA, Prince EA, Hampson CO, et al. The preclose technique in percutaneous endovascular aortic repair: a systematic literature review and meta-analysis. Cardiovasc Intervent Radiol 2013;36(3):567–77.
[44] Bensley RP, Hurks R, Huang Z, et al. Ultrasound-guided percutaneous endovascular aneurysm repair success is predicted by access vessel diameter. J Vasc Surg 2012;55(6): 1554–61.
[45] de Souza LR, Oderich GS, Banga PV, et al. Outcomes of total percutaneous endovascular aortic repair for thoracic, fenestrated, and branched endografts. J Vasc Surg 2015;62(6): 1442–9.e3.
[46] Matsumura JS, Rizvi AZ. Society for vascular surgery. left subclavian artery revascularization: society for vascular surgery Practice Guidelines. J Vasc Surg 2010;52(4):65S–70S.
[47] Holt PJ, Johnson C, Hinchliffe RJ, et al. Outcomes of the endovascular management of aortic arch aneurysm: implications for management of the left subclavian artery. J Vasc Surg 2010;51(6):1329–38.

[48] Leon LR, Mills JL, Jordan W, et al. The risks of celiac artery coverage during endoluminal repair of thoracic and thoracoabdominal aortic aneurysms. Vasc Endovascular Surg 2009;43(1):51–60.

[49] Arnaoutakis DJ, Scali ST, Beck AW, et al. Comparative outcomes of open, hybrid, and fenestrated branched endovascular repair of extent II and III thoracoabdominal aortic aneurysms. J Vasc Surg 2020;71(5):1503–14.

[50] Patel HJ, Upchurch GR, Eliason JL, et al. Hybrid debranching with endovascular repair for thoracoabdominal aneurysms: a comparison with open repair. Ann Thorac Surg 2010;89(5):1475–81.

[51] Voskresensky I, Scali ST, Feezor RJ, et al. Outcomes of thoracic endovascular aortic repair using aortic arch chimney stents in high-risk patients. J Vasc Surg 2017;66(1):9–20.

[52] Moulakakis KG, Mylonas SN, Dalainas I, et al. The chimney-graft technique for preserving supra-aortic branches: a review. Ann Cardiothorac Surg 2013;2(3):339–46.

[53] Varu V, Chandra V, Dake MD, et al. The "periscope" technique successfully lengthens the distal landing zone during TEVAR. J Vasc Surg 2013;58(2):556.

[54] Manresa-Manresa F, Quintero-Pérez C, Mengíbar-Fuentes L. Periscope technique for superior mesenteric artery and thoracic stent graft extension for type ib endoleak with ruptured thoracic aortic aneurysm. Eur J Vasc Endovasc Surg 2021;61(3):519.

[55] Oderich GS, Ribeiro MS, Sandri GA, et al. Evolution from physician-modified to company-manufactured fenestrated-branched endografts to treat pararenal and thoracoabdominal aortic aneurysms. J Vasc Surg 2019;70(1):31–42.

[56] DeSart K, Scali ST, Feezor RJ, et al. Fate of patients with spinal cord ischemia complicating thoracic endovascular aortic repair. J Vasc Surg 2013;58(3):635–42.

[57] Buth J, Harris PL, Hobo R, et al. Neurologic complications associated with endovascular repair of thoracic aortic pathology: Incidence and risk factors. a study from the European Collaborators on Stent/Graft Techniques for Aortic Aneurysm Repair (EUROSTAR) registry. J Vasc Surg 2007;46(6):1103–10, discussion 1110.

[58] Eagleton MJ, Shah S, Petkosevek D, et al. Hypogastric and subclavian artery patency affects onset and recovery of spinal cord ischemia associated with aortic endografting. J Vasc Surg 2014;59(1):89–94.

[59] O'Callaghan A, Mastracci TM, Eagleton MJ. Staged endovascular repair of thoracoabdominal aortic aneurysms limits incidence and severity of spinal cord ischemia. J Vasc Surg 2015;61(2):347–54.

[60] Acher CW, Wynn MM, Hoch JR, et al. Combined use of cerebral spinal fluid drainage and naloxone reduces the risk of paraplegia in thoracoabdominal aneurysm repair. J Vasc Surg 1994;19(2):236–46, discussion 247.

[61] Estrera AL, Sheinbaum R, Miller CC, et al. Cerebrospinal fluid drainage during thoracic aortic repair: safety and current management. Ann Thorac Surg 2009;88(1):9–15, discussion 15.

[62] von Allmen RS, Anjum A, Powell JT. Outcomes after endovascular or open repair for degenerative descending thoracic aortic aneurysm using linked hospital data. Br J Surg 2014;101(10):1244–51.

[63] Riesenman PJ, Farber MA, Mendes RR, et al. Coverage of the left subclavian artery during thoracic endovascular aortic repair. J Vasc Surg 2007;45(1):90–4, discussion 94.

[64] Kuratani T. Best surgical option for arch extension of type B dissection: the endovascular approach. Ann Cardiothorac Surg 2014;3(3):292–9.

Advances in Surgery 56 (2022) 151–168

ADVANCES IN SURGERY

What Surgeons Need to Know About Gene Therapy for Cancer

Shanmugappiriya Sivarajah, MD MPH[a], Kevin Emerick, MD[a], Howard L. Kaufman, MD[b,*]

[a]Department of Otolaryngology, Massachusetts Eye and Ear Infirmary, 243 Charles Street Boston, MA 02114 USA; [b]Division of Gastrointestinal and Oncologic Surgery, Massachusetts General Hospital, 55 Fruit Street, Yawkey 7E, Boston, MA 02114, USA

Keywords

• Cancer • Cell therapy • Gene editing • Gene therapy • Immunotherapy • Oncolytic viruses

Key points

- Advances in gene therapy have led to numerous emerging therapeutic approaches for patients with cancer.
- Understanding the basic rationale for these approaches is important for managing patients and their tissues to optimize therapeutic benefit.
- The clinical surgeon plays a pivotal role in managing patients with cancer and should be aware of these new therapeutic approaches.
- Surgeons can help optimize gene therapy and improve clinical outcomes for gene therapy in the treatment of human cancer.

INTRODUCTION

On June 26, 2000, then US President Bill Clinton and Dr Craig Ventner, CEO of Celera Genomic Corporation released a statement from the White House reporting the completion of the first survey of the entire human genome. This major milestone in biomedical research opened a new era for both understanding complex disease, such as cancer, as well as providing a basis for new therapeutic strategies. Yet, the impact on patients with cancer would await nearly another 15 years, as academic and pharmaceutical investigators learned

*Corresponding author: Division of Gastrointestinal and Oncologic Surgery, Massachusetts General Hospital, 55 Fruit Street, Yawkey 7E, Boston, MA 02114 USA, *E-mail address:* HLKaufman@mgh.harvard.edu

https://doi.org/10.1016/j.yasu.2022.02.006

how to interpret and apply genomic data to individual patients suffering from cancer. A major advance was the evolution of big data management, now being replaced by artificial intelligence programs, that can deal with large data sets and more rapidly identify clinically meaningful associations. For example, although mutations in the gene encoding BRAF was recognized in nearly 50% of all patients with cutaneous melanoma, and drug developers identified effective BRAF inhibitors, early clinical studies did not test for BRAF mutation status in patients before study enrollment. Today, it is clear that only very specific mutations, namely mutations replacing the amino acid valine at position 600 within the BRAF protein with a glutamic acid (V600E) or lysine (V600K) respond to BRAF inhibition. Today, it has become standard to test for BRAF mutations in patients with melanoma before treatment planning, and there is an emerging area of drug development focusing on non-V600E/K mutations to extend the benefit of targeted therapy to a large number of patients with BRAF-mutated melanoma.

Another area that has benefitted greatly from advances in genomic analysis is cancer immunotherapy. In fact, the evolution of RNA sequencing to include single-cell evaluation is revolutionizing our understanding of how cancer cells interact with immune system. Despite having the human genome sequences in 2000, understanding of the cancer immunity cycle was incomplete. New data suggest that molecular factors comprising the intracellular interferon pathway in cancer cells may be defective, and this short circuits cancer immunosurveillance. These findings have also provided new strategies for immunotherapy of cancer. Immunotherapy has achieved considerable success largely with the success of immune checkpoint blockade that blocks negative regulators of T-cell responses, such as cytotoxic T-lymphocyte antigen 4 and programmed cell death 1 (PD-1) pathways. In addition, chimeric antigen receptor (CAR) T cells have shown significant promise in a range of hematologic malignancies. Perhaps one of the most important advances has been the elucidation of biomarkers associated with therapeutic response to immunotherapy; this includes the presence of tumor-infiltrating lymphocytes, expression of the PD-1 ligand, PD-L1 by tumor cells, and a high tumor mutation burden (TMB). Overall, tumors with high TMB have been more responsive to immunotherapy, and thus knowledge of the genomic status of individual cancers is mandatory for appropriate treatment planning. Further enthusiasm is high for the potential use of adoptive T-cell transfer using lymphocytes derived from metastatic tumors, and the development of personalized cancer vaccines may be feasible from rapid assessment of genomic mutations within an individual tumor.

Another major barrier to effective gene therapy was the potential for insertional mutagenesis. When DNA is inserted into a cell it enters the nucleus and becomes incorporated in the cellular genome for transcription. Until recently, the site for genetic insertions was random and sometimes this could result in altering normal genome transcription, resulting in truncated proteins or, in rare cases, neoplastic transformation. The advent of gene editing technologies has now provided a pathway for more targeted gene delivery to host cells and is expanding the potential strategies for gene therapy while also adding an important safety component to such approaches.

Surgeons need to be familiar with the advances in molecular genomics and immunotherapy for several reasons. First, for most patients with cancer they will enter the health care system through surgical management. Because surgeons may be the first health care providers to see patients, it is important to ensure that initial biopsy is done appropriately to optimize both histologic and molecular data that are needed for tumor staging, diagnostic and prognostic information, and treatment planning. Further, surgeons are increasingly being called on to assist in therapeutic management for patients with cancer. Injections of oncolytic viruses and other intratumoral agents often requires access to tissue not easily accessible by clinical palpation or endoscopic visualization. Harvesting of lymphocytes from tumors for adoptive cell therapy also requires surgeons understand how to select metastatic lesions for optimal cell recovery and how to preserve biospecimens for diagnostic and therapeutic assays. In this review, the authors describe the modern definition of cancer gene therapy, discuss some of the promising approaches in clinical use and development, and finally highlight what the surgeon needs to know to ensure optimal management for the patient with cancer.

What is gene therapy of cancer?

Gene therapy is broadly defined as the "treatment of disease by introducing a gene with therapeutic effect or by manipulating the disease-related gene" [1]. As such, gene therapy can refer to a wide range of treatments that use genetic material (DNA or RNA) to modify cells [2]. The potential to treat disease at its genetic roots is an alluring concept; however, there are several hurdles to the application of gene therapy. Gene transfer must overcome complex cellular and tissue barriers to deliver genetic information without disrupting cellular regulatory mechanisms [3]. In addition, the gene-corrected cells must be present in large enough quantities to reverse the condition while going undetected by the host immune system and to transfer the altered genes onto progeny to prevent further hereditary transmission [3].

Cancer is a major cause of mortality worldwide. There are numerous available treatment modalities, including surgery, radiation, and systemic therapies such as hormonal therapy, targeted therapy, chemotherapy, and immunotherapy [4]. Promising treatments using gene therapy can target cancers that have poor treatment responses to existing treatments and survival outcomes. In addition, gene therapy offers the potential to reduce debilitating side effects associated with conventional treatments. Because cancer is a disease caused by genetic mutations that lead to aberrations in cellular growth and apoptosis, it seems logical that gene therapies may have a role in treatment [4]. The interaction of cancer cells with their microenvironment (ie, the extracellular matrix, host immune cells, and angiogenetic growth factors) is apotential target for cancer gene therapy [4].

Gene replacement therapy

There are 2 broad categorizations for cancer gene therapy (Table 1) [5]. The first encompass strategies to kill or slow the growth of the tumor, and this can be accomplished by directly targeting either tumor cells or the host. The second is the development of vectors and delivery systems for efficient gene transfer. The greatest challenge of this strategy involves safely transferring the desired gene into the target tissue, without encountering the host immune system (ie, phagocytes or nucleases) [4]. In addition, gene transfer must be directed to specific cells, such as cancer and not normal cells or tumor-specific effector immune cells but not normal tissues. The term vector refers to the gene delivery vehicle or molecular carrier, which facilitates the release of the gene into the cell and its successful expression [4]. Vectors may be viral or nonviral. Viral vectors are favorable, as they target both dividing and nondividing cells; however, viral vectors must also overcome issues related to host immunogenicity [4]. Nonviral vectors such as physical methods of gene delivery, and chemical-based nanoparticles, illicit little to no host immune response but are less efficient in gene transfer compared with viral vectors [4]. Vectors are being developed for a variety of applications for cancer gene therapy, including immunotherapy, suicide gene therapy, microRNA (miRNA)-targeted therapy, CAR T-cell therapy and engineered adoptive T-cell therapy, oncogene

Table 1
Types of cancer gene therapy

Strategy	Approaches
Directed to tumor	• Tumor suppressors • Dominant-negative genes • Apoptosis induction • Tumor-specific viruses • Tumor-specific gene expression • Sensitization to radiation and chemotherapy
Directed to host	• Angiogenesis inhibition • Confer drug resistance on sensitive tissues, especially bone marrow • Immunotherapy
Viral vectors	• Adenoviruses • HSV-1 • SV40 • Newcastle disease virus • Retroviruses (eg, lentivirus, reovirus) • Vaccinia virus
Nonviral vectors	• Lipofection • Bacteria • Nucleotides (antisense, ribozymes, siRNA) • Monoclonal antibodies • Proteins/peptides

Adapted from Gottesman M. Cancer gene therapy: an awkward adolescence. Cancer Gene Ther. 2003; 10(7): 501-508; with permission..

silencing, and CRISPR/Cas9 gene editing. In addition, monoclonal antibodies and other proteins have been successfully delivered to tumors where they may exert functional antitumor activity while avoiding systemic toxicity. The general strategy for direct tumor cell gene therapy is shown in Fig. 1.

Tumor suppressor gene products that are inactivated in certain tumors are often associated with tumorigenesis, and replacing tumor suppressor genes is one way of targeting growth regulation in cancer cells. The p53 gene regulates diverse cellular processes, including cell-cycle arrest, senescence, apoptosis, and autophagy [6]. It is frequently inactivated by somatic mutations, present in approximately 50% of all types of human cancers. Li Fraumeni syndrome is a complex hereditary cancer predisposition disorder, associated with germline mutations of p53. Tumor cells with impaired p53 function often demonstrate refractory responses to conventional chemoradiotherapy. Therefore, several different viral vectors have been constructed to restore wild-type p53 function in tumors (specifically adenoviral vectors or Adp53). These vectors aim to increase p53 levels, resulting in cessation of cell growth or induction of apoptosis in synergy with chemotherapy agents. Several preclinical in vitro and in vivo experiments have investigated the role of a p53-expressing replication-deficient adenovirus vector (Ad-p53) in non–small-cell lung cancer, head and neck cancer, malignant brain tumors, ovarian cancer, bladder cancer, cervical cancer, colorectal cancer, and esophageal cancer [7–10]. Gendicine (recombinant human p53 adenovirus), developed by Shenzhen SiBiono GeneTech Co. Ltd., was approved in 2003 by the China Food and Drug Administration (FDA) as the first gene therapy product in China to treat head and neck cancer. It entered the commercial market in 2004 but has not been approved for use outside of China. Gene therapy targeting p53 can also be offered in combination with chemotherapeutic agents. Tamura and colleagues combined p53 gene therapy (with the AdRGD-Pgp53 vector that offers autoregulated expression of p53) with cabazitaxel (a chemotherapeutic agent) in a xenograft mouse model and showed a statistically significant reduction in prostate tumor volume [11]. Table 2 summarized currently approved gene therapy agents.

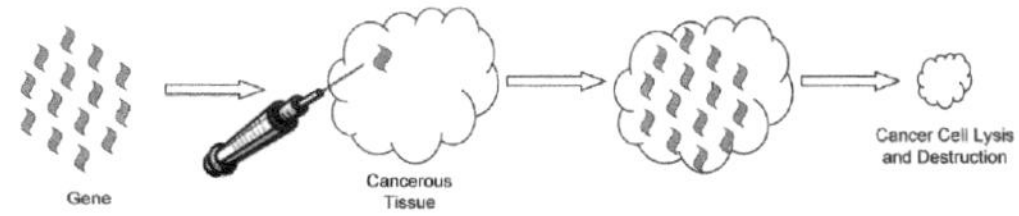

Fig. 1. Gene transfer therapy. In its simplest form, gene therapy involves introduction of a gene encoding protein with anticancer functions by directly injecting the gene into an established tumor cell. A variety of vectors, such as viruses, bacteria, plasmids, and RNA preparations, have been used for gene delivery. In addition, monoclonal antibodies, whole proteins, and functional peptides have also been evaluated for direct tumor cell injection. These approaches can deliver high doses of anticancer agents while avoiding systemic toxicity from on-target, off-tumor effects. Reproduced [or adapted] with permission. Cross D, Burmester K. Gene therapy for cancer treatment: past, present and future. Clin Med Res. 2006 Sept; 4(3): 218-27. Copyright 2006 Marshfield Clinic. All rights reserved.

Table 2
Gene therapies approved in the western world

Drug name		Indication	Comments
Alipogene tiparvovec	Glybera	Lipoprotein lipase deficiency	• AAV-based therapy • For treatment of familial lipoprotein lipase deficiency • Conditional marketing approval by EMA in 2012 • Withdrawn in 2017
Sipuleucel-T	Provenge	Prostate cancer	• Autologous dendritic cell encoding human GM-CSF and PAP • Indicated for asymptomatic or minimally symptomatic metastatic prostate cancer resistant to hormone therapy • FDA approved in 2008
Talimogene laherparepvec (T-VEC)	Imlygic	Melanoma	• Genetically modified HSV-1 encoding GM-CSF • Local treatment of tumors that recur after surgery • Approved by the FDA in 2015
Strimvelis	Strimvelis	Adenosine deaminase deficiency	• γ-retrovirus–based therapy • Treatment of severe combined immunodeficiency due to adenosine deaminase deficiency (ADA-SCID) • EMA approval in 2016 • Not approved by FDA
Tisagenlecleucel	Kymriah	DLBCL ALL	• CD19-directed genetically modified autologous CAR T cell • For treatment of DLBCL lymphoma and ALL patients $\leq$ 25 years • FDA approval in 2017
Axicabtagene ciloleucel	Yescarta	DLBCL Follicular lymphoma	• CD19-directed genetically modified autologous CAR T-cell immunotherapy • For treatment of non-Hodgkin lymphoma FDA approval in 2017
Voretigene neparvovec	Luxterna	Inherited retinal disease	• AAV-based gene therapy • For treatment of bi-allelic RPE65 mutation-associated retinal dystrophy • Requires sufficient residual retinal cells

Abbreviations: AAV, adeno-associated virus; ALL, acute lymphoblastic leukemia; DLBCL, diffuse large B-cell lymphoma; EMA, european medicines agency; FDA, US Food and Drug Administration; GM-CSF, granulocyte-macrophage colony-stimulating factor; PAP, prostate acid phosphatase; RPE65, gene encoding retinoid isomerohydrolase.

Cancer vaccines

Unlike its impact against infectious diseases, vaccines have not had the desired effect against cancers. Vaccines attempt to induce an in vivo adaptive immune response against defined antigenic markers and to target such cells for lysis [12]. Adaptive immunity is antigen dependent and antigen specific, generating memory T and B cells to mount a more rapid and efficient immune response [13]. Antigen needs to be proceeded by professional antigen-presenting cells, such as dendritic cells (DCs), which can present processed peptides on major histocompatibility complex (MHC) class II molecules to trigger CD4+ helper T-cell responses and via MHC class I molecules to generate cytotoxic CD8+ effector T cells. Before 2000 most cancer vaccines used defined tumor-associated antigens that were shared across patients with similar tumors, such as prostate specific antigen or carcinoembryonic antigen [14]. Although such vaccines were not effective in clinical trials, vaccination against cancer-associated viral antigens, such as human papillomavirus (HPV) has been effective when used as preventative vaccines. The ability to rapidly identify mutations within a tumor has resulted in new interest for using mutated antigens as potential targets for vaccine development [15]. These so-called personalized vaccines require tumor tissue for mutation analysis, ex vivo assessment of MHC binding affinity and avidity by putative peptides and construction of a vaccine formulation for delivery back to patients. Although this has been tested in early phase clinical studies with evidence of immune responses, the time required from biopsy to vaccine preparation is still unacceptably long. Surgeons should be aware of this trend, as artificial intelligence and other bioinformatic advances may improve the clinical feasibility of this approach, which will likely require careful biopsy and rebiopsy of tumors to optimize antigen selection for individual patients. Another approach that has been tested in patients has been the use of irradiated whole tumor cell vaccines that precludes the need to a priori identify the antigenic repertoire, but these have thus far not demonstrated therapeutic benefit.

To date, only 2 cancer vaccines have been approved worldwide. In April 2010, the US FDA approved the first and only cancer treatment vaccine in the United States, sipuleucel-T (Provenge), for treating men with metastatic hormone-refractory prostate cancer with minimal or no clinical symptoms. Sipuleucel-T is an autologous DC vaccine modified ex vivo to express a fusion protein composed of prostatic acid phosphatase (PAP) and granulocyte-macrophage colony-stimulating factor (GM-CSF) [15]. PAP antigens are nearly universally expressed in prostate cancer cells, serving as a robust target marker for tumor cells. Antigen-presenting DC are procured from the patient and sent to a production facility where they are coincubated with the fusion protein, which is taken up and presented on the cell surface. The activated antigen-presenting DCs are readministered to the patient via 3 treatments over a period of 6 weeks, to trigger an immune response against PAP-positive prostate cancers. Clinical trials in patients with advanced prostate cancer showed that sipuleucel-T safely improved overall survival of patients for an average of 4 months [16].

Oncophage is a vaccine that is made by eluting the gp96-heat shock protein-peptide complex from autologous tumor cells and is used for vaccination. Although not approved in the United States, Oncophage has been approved in Russia since 2008 for the treatment of early stage renal cell carcinoma.

Randomized studies of Oncophage have failed to demonstrate a therapeutic benefit in Western countries.

Oncolytic virus therapy for cancer

An oncolytic virus is defined as a genetically engineered or naturally occurring virus that can selectively replicate in and kill cancer cells without harming normal tissues [16]. In gene therapy, the virus is used as a carrier for gene transfer; however, in oncolytic virus therapy, the virus itself is used as an active drug reagent [17]. It was first observed more than a century ago that tumor regression was observed in patients with cancer who were infected with certain viruses [17,18]. Early clinical trials were performed in an attempt to treat pateints with cancer with wild-type or naturally attenuated viruses, harnessing infections with hepatitis, West Nile virus, yellow fever, dengue fever, and adenoviruses. However, these viruses were not deemed appropriate candidates for virotherapy, due to insufficient control of selective virulence in infected patients [17].

Protective mechanisms against viral infection (eg, interferon [IFN] signaling pathway) are impaired in cancer cells. Type I IFNs (IFN α/β) are antiviral cytokines that are produced when viral components are detected by host pattern recognition receptors [19]. The defects in interferon signaling in cancer cells likely explains why oncolytic viruses preferentially replicate in cancer cells (Fig. 2). Several strategies have been used to identify clinically appropriate oncolytic viruses, including selection of minimally pathogenic native viruses shown to replicate in tumor cells in vitro but not in normal cells. Alternatively, viruses may be attenuated to reduce pathogenicity and improve selective tumor cell replication. The latter strategy allows for stricter control of viral replication. In 1991, Martuza and colleagues demonstrated that a genetically engineered herpes simplex virus type I (HSV-1) with a mutation in the thymidine kinase gene replicated selectively in cancer cells in glioma cell lines [18]. Oncolytic viruses cause lysis in tumor cells, and this results in an immunogenic cell death with release of tumor-associated antigens as well as viral-induced danger signals that cooperate to prime host immune responses against the cancer cells. Although oncolytic viruses may enter normal cells, they usually cannot replicate efficiently and so immunogenic cell death does not occur. Importantly,

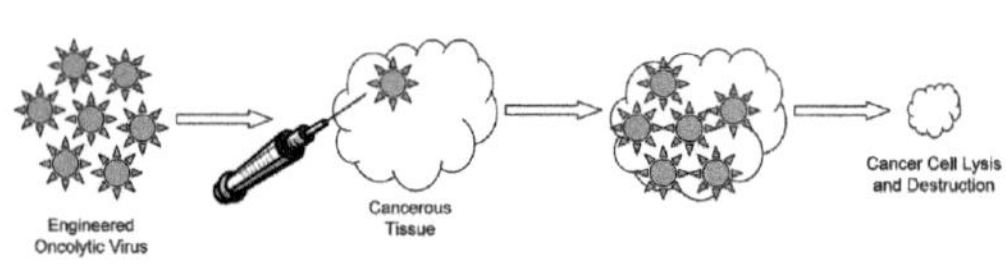

Fig. 2. Oncolytic virus therapy for cancer. Oncolytic viruses enter cancer cells and replicate, resulting in lysis and immunogenic cell death. The release of tumor-associated antigens and viral-induced danger signals promotes host immunity against both the virus and tumor cells. Although oncolytic viruses may enter normal cells, they undergo abortive replication and do not kill the cells, providing a highly tumor-specific treatment approach.

clinical trials for oncolytic virus therapies have been numerous, and overall, these agents have exhibited a very tolerable and similar safety profile [20]. Mild constitutional symptoms such as fatigue, fever, chills, nausea, and local injection site reactions are the most common adverse events reported with oncolytic virus treatment [20].

The most common viruses to be used in oncolytic viral therapy are adenoviruses, HSV-1 and poxviruses [20]. Ongoing research suggests that other viruses, including coxsackievirus, reovirus, Newcastle disease virus, measles virus, and others, may also play a role in oncolytic virus therapy. To date, one native virus and 2 genetically engineered oncolytic viruses have been approved for cancer treatment globally. Rigvir is a live, nonpathogenic enterovirus (ECHO group, type 7) that has been approved for the treatment of melanoma in several Eastern European countries [20]. Oncorine (H101, the same construct as ONYX-015) is an E1B-deleted oncolytic adenovirus, which was approved in China for head and neck cancer and esophageal cancer in 2005. The other genetically modified oncolytic virus is talimogene laherparepvec (T-VEC; Imlygic; formerly OncoVex^{GM-CSF}), which was approved by the US FDAFDA for melanoma treatment in October 2015. The virus was subsequently approved in Europe, Australia, and Israel. T-VEC is discussed in more detail, as this agent was largely developed in collaboration with surgical investigators and is being used in surgical practice.

Talimogene laherparepvec

T-VEC was derived from an attenuated and tumor cell replication selective HSV-1 virus initially derived from an oral fever blister. T-VEC contains deletions in the γ34.5 and α47 viral genes. In normal cells, viral replication is blocked by activation of protein kinase R (PKR) and subsequent phosphorylation of eukaryotic initiation factor 2 (eIF2) [17]. In cancer cells, this PKR-eIF2 pathway is disrupted, leading to uncontrolled cellular proliferation. The γ34.5 gene causes dephosphorylation of eIF2 and blocks PKR-induced disruption of protein synthesis. Inactivation of the γ34.5 gene renders the virus incapable of replicating in normal cells and also reduces the neuropathogenicity associated with native HSV-1. The viral α47 gene normally functions to block host immune responses by interfering with viral peptide loading onto infected cell MHC class I molecules. Deletion of the α47 gene increases tumor antigen presentation by infected cancer cells and hence acts to enhance host antitumor immunity. In addition, T-VEC that encodes 2 copies of the human GM-CSF gene is inserted into the deleted γ34.5 loci. GM-CSF is thought to promote host immune responses by recruiting and activating DCs that can then prime T cells against viral and tumor-associated antigens.

A phase I clinical trial of T-VEC was conducted in 2006 [21]. The virus was administered in 13 patients with breast, head and neck, and gastrointestinal cancers and malignant melanoma. The virotherapy was generally well tolerated, the most common side effects of which were local inflammation, erythema, and febrile responses; this was followed by a multiinstitutional phase

II study that enrolled 50 patients with unresectable melanoma treated with intratumoral T-VEC every 3 weeks (regional disease stage IIIc, n = 10; skin or lymph node metastases, stage IV M1a, n = 16; lung-only metastases, stage IV M1b, n = 4; and visceral involvement, stage IV M1c, n = 20) [22]. Most patients (74%) had received prior systemic therapies. Among the 50 patients treated, an objective response rate of 26% was seen with 8 patients achieving a complete response, whereas 5 patients achieved a partial response, including regression of distant, noninjected lesions.

A randomized phase III trial was performed in patients with unresectable stage IIIB-IV melanoma (OPTiM; NCT00769704) [23]. Four hundred thirty-six patients were randomly assigned in a 2:1 ratio to intratumoral T-VEC or subcutaneous GM-CSF treatment arms. At the primary analysis, 290 deaths had occurred (T-VEC, n = 189; GM-CSF, n = 101). The durable response rate (defined as an objective response lasting continuously for 6 months or longer) was significantly higher in the T-VEC arm (16.3%) compared with the GM-CSF arm (2.1%). The overall response rate (ORR) was also higher in the T-VEC arm (26.4 vs 5.7%). The treatment showed profound efficacy in patients with stage IIIB, IIIC, or IV M1a. The most common adverse effects of T-VEC were fevers, chills, and fatigue, with greater than 2% of patients experiencing cellulitis (the only grade 3 or 4 treatment-related adverse event). There were no fatalities related to treatment administration. In a final analysis after median follow-up of 49 months, the objective response rate was 31.5% for patients treated with T-VEC compared with 6.4% for GM-CSF treatment. In addition, the median overall survival was 23.3 months for T-VEC-treated patients compared with 18.9 months for GM-CSF treatment (unstratified hazard ratio 0.79; 95% confidence interval, 0.62–1.00; $P = 0.049$). The successes of this clinical trial resulted in T-VEC approval for local treatment of unresectable cutaneous, subcutaneous, and nodal lesions in patients with melanoma that recurs after initial surgery. Several real-world reports have suggested higher response rates when T-VEC is used for more limited disease, such as recurrent in-transit metastases, which supports treatment at earlier stages of disease.

Cellular therapy of cancer

Genetically modified immune cells expressing either CARs or T-cell receptors (TCRs) isolated from tumor-reactive T cells has shown potential for treatment of certain types of cancer. Both therapies require isolation of T cells from the patient through apheresis, gene transfer (usually via retro- or lentiviral vectors), ex vivo T-cell expansion, and host conditioning before the cells are reintroduced back into the host [24]. CAR T-cell therapy has significantly changed the landscape for treatment of lymphoid malignancies. Although studies of CAR T cells are being pursued in solid tumors, the use of tumor-infiltrating T lymphocytes (TILs) has shown more promise in solid tumors, and regulatory approval of TILs in melanoma is anticipated in 2022.

CAR T cells are created by transducing a genetically engineered CAR fusion protein by means of a retrovirus or lentivirus into autologous T cells (Fig. 3). A

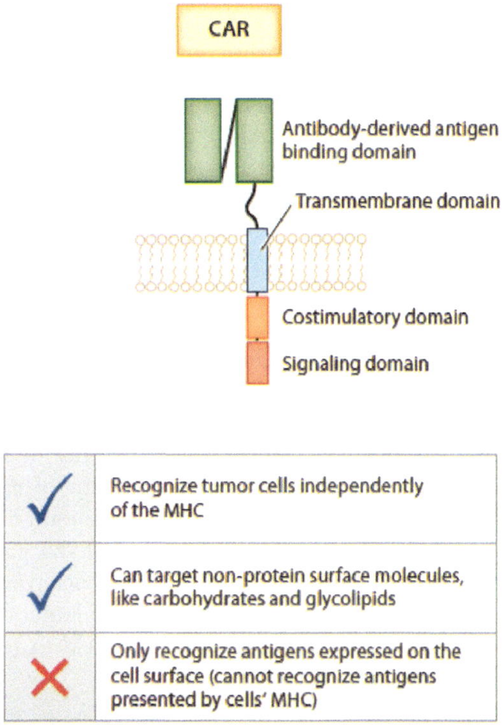

Fig. 3. Chimeric antigen receptors (CARs). T cells collected from peripheral blood are transduced with the CAR, which provides MHC-independent recognition of tumor cell surface targets, such as CD19 in B-cell malignancies. Many CAR products also contain accessory T-cell signaling apparatus, such as 4-1BB, to provide additional T-cell co-stimulation. CARs can be expressed in other cells, and CAR-NK and CAR-macrophages are in clinical development. *Adapted from* Anguela XM, High KA. Entering the modern era of gene therapy. Annu Rev Med. 2019; 70:273-288; with permission.

CAR construct is usually formed by linking a single-chain variable fragment derived from an antibody to intracellular signaling chains (ie, TCR-derived CD3ζ domain and one or more intracellular costimulatory domains) [24]. The CAR T cells are infused into patients following a lymphodepleting protocol, such as fludarabine and cyclophosphamide [25].

CAR-based technology has centered around CD19, an antigen highly expressed on the cell surface by most B-cell malignancies but absent in normal tissues, except normal B cells. Early studies in 2010 and 2011 on CAR T-cell therapies showed unprecedented antitumor activity in patients with diffuse large B-cell lymphoma, chronic lymphocytic leukemia, and B-cell acute lymphoblastic leukemia occurring in children and young adults [24]. The phase II multicenter ELIANA trial evaluated tisagenlecleucel-T (or Kymriah) for B-cell lymphoblastic leukemia and demonstrated 60% complete remission (CR) rate and 81% ORR in 75 children and young adults [26]. Treatment-related toxicities were frequent, with 73% of patients experiencing severe (grade 3 or higher) adverse events. Similarly, the phase II multicenter ZUMA-1 trial on axicabtagene ciloleucel (YESCARTA) studied 101 patients with refractory aggressive lymphomas and demonstrated an 83% ORR and a 58% CR rate [27]; this led to the FDA approval of these 2 CAR T-cell therapies in 2017, for the treatment of relapsed and refractory large B-cell lymphoma. KYMRIAH was also approved for the treatment of relapsed and refractory B-cell acute lymphoblastic leukemia in pediatric and young adult patients aged 25 years or younger.

CAR T-cell infusions are associated with several potentially severe toxicities, including cytokine release syndrome (CRS), neurotoxicity or CAR T-cell–related encephalopathy syndrome, macrophage activation syndrome, and tumor lysis syndrome [27,28]. Severe CRS and neurotoxicity typically occurs with a frequency of 10% to 50%. CRS presents with fever, hemodynamic instability, hypoxia, and end-organ dysfunction. The severity of CRS presentation may correlate with CAR T-cell infusion dose, extent of expansion of cells in vivo, and amount of tumor burden. CRS may respond to tocilizumab, an anti-interleukin-6 receptor antagonist but requires intensive patient monitoring. The costs of CAR T-cell therapy have also been a deterrent to more widespread availability with treatment usually restricted to larger academic medical centers. There is currently several research in this field to refine the CAR T cells to reduce both cost and toxicity.

Gene editing

The development of Clustered Regularly Interspaced Short Palindromic Repeats (CRISPR)-Cas9-mediated genome editing technology has completely revolutionized the landscape of gene therapy. These technologies allow genetic material to be added, removed, or altered at specific locations in the genome. Based on an ancient bacterial immune defense system, CRISPR/Cas9 consists of the Cas9 endonuclease and a short noncoding guide RNA (gRNA) that has 2 components: a target-specific CRISPR RNA (cRNA) and a helper trans-activating RNA. The gRNA unit guides Cas9 to a specific genome locus with base pairing between the cRNA sequence and the target sequence [29,30]. The target DNA sequence, known as the "protospacer," must be complementary to the gRNA and contain a 3-nucleotide protospacer adjacent motif (PAM) on the 5′ end of the target strand. On binding to the target sequence, the Cas9 endonuclease induces specific double-stranded breaks (DSBs) at approximately −3 nucleotides before the PAM sequence that are repaired by cellular DNA repair machinery via the less frequent and less efficient homology-directed repair or the predominantly used, highly efficient nonhomologous end joining mechanism. Simple alterations of the gRNA sequence and the simultaneous expression of different gRNAs allows researchers to re-target new DNA sequences and introduce multiple DSBs.

The implications of this are far-reaching. For instance, the CRISPR-Cas9 system has potential for combatting carcinogenic viral infections, such as

HPV in cervical and head and neck cancers, hepatitis B virus and hepatitis C virus in liver cancer, and Epstein-Barr virus in nasopharyngeal carcinoma, Hodgkin lymphoma, and Burkitt lymphoma. It is possible to use CRISPR-Cas9 technology to target viral oncogenes using viral genome-specific Cas9-gRNA, suppress viral oncogene expression, and induce cancer cell death [30]. For instance, HPV infection is mediated by oncoproteins E6 and E7, which induce malignant transformation. E6 targets the cellular tumor suppressor p53, whereas E7 destabilizes the retinoblastoma (Rb) protein, which typically induces cell-cycle arrest and senescence. Kennedy and colleagues demonstrated that introduction of a bacterial Cas9 RNA-guided endonuclease, together with single-guide RNAs specific for E6 or E7, induced cleavage of the HPV genome, leading to induction of p53 or Rb and subsequent cell-cycle arrest and eventual cell death [31]. HPV16 E6+ E7- CRISPR/Cas9 has also been shown to be a chemosensitizer of cisplatin in the treatment of cervical cancer [32]. Other applications of CRISPR-Cas9 technology are illustrated in Fig. 4. Although promising, the clinical implication of gene editing awaits future clinical trials.

The surgeon's role in gene therapy of cancer

The advances in identifying abnormal genes and gene mutations in cancer have resulted in new insights into the disease as well as new therapeutic approaches. Surgeons need to be aware of these advances, as they have been pivotal in the early studies of gene therapy in oncology as well as being often the first and often only health care provider engaged in the management of the patient with cancer. The authors review the role for surgeons as basic scientists, clinical investigators, technical experts, and academic authorities for gene therapy in patients with cancer.

Surgeons have played a critical role in many human disease processes and in developing innovative treatment options. Indeed, surgeons were at the forefront of developing adoptive cell therapy for patients with cancer as driven by the outstanding work in the Surgery Branch at the National Cancer Institute. In addition, surgeons have been the primary drivers of research in cancer vaccines, oncolytic viruses, antiangiogenesis therapy, and biomarker analyses. The arena of gene therapy is ripe for new ideas and insights into how to use the emerging technologies around oncolytic viral immunogenicity, optimizing T cells and other immune cells for therapeutic purposes, and bringing gene editing to surgical and oncologic problems. Indeed, residents in surgical training should be encouraged to spend time in basic research laboratories in these areas. Although some may pursue academic surgery and be interested in maintaining a basic science laboratory as part of their professional development, others may gain insights into new approaches and will be better positioned to participate in novel clinical trials and integrate new strategies into the treatment plans for their patients.

Large clinical trials are the stepping stone for establishing treatment outcomes, formulating guidelines and directing further research. Challenges in

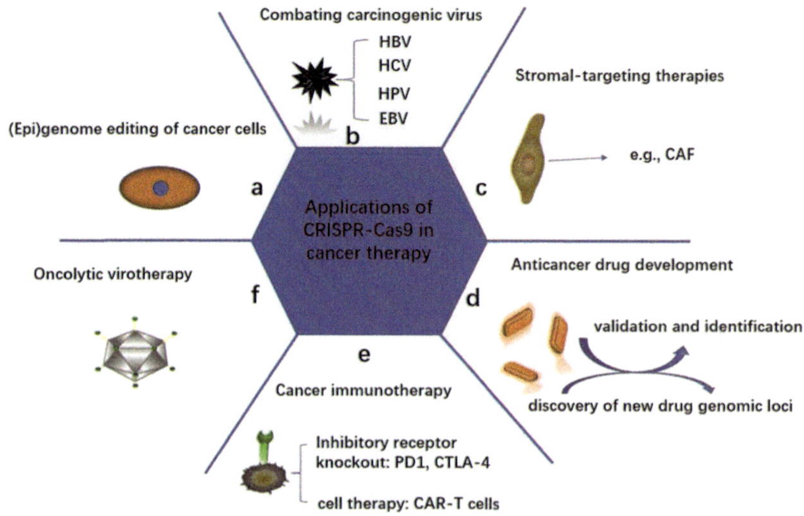

Fig. 4. Applications of CRISPR-Cas9 technology for therapeutic gene editing. (*A*) Genes may be added or deleted from cancer cells in a sequence-specific manner to replace tumor suppressor or silence oncogenes. (*B*) Integrated carcinogenic viral genes may be deleted. (*C*) In addition to cancer cell, stromal cells such as cancer-associated fibroblasts (CAF) may be targeted. (*D*) Genome changes may be used to alter drug kinetics and potency within cancer cells. (*E*) Immune suppressive gene expression can be inhibited, and immune cells can be manipulated to increase their anticancer activity. (*F*) Viruses can be targeted for improved oncolytic and antitumor immune activity. *From* Minjiang Chen, Aiwu Mao, Min Xu, Qiaoyou Weng, Jianting Mao, Jiansong Ji, CRISPR-Cas9 for cancer therapy: Opportunities and challenges, Cancer Letters, 447, 2019, 48-55 (HYPERLINK "https://nam11.safelinks.protection.outlook.-com/?url=https%3A%2F%2Fdoi.org%2F10.1016%2Fj.canlet.2019.01.017&data=05%7C01%7CJ.Surendrakumar%40elsevier.com%7Ce923f2aa00cb47ec946108da553c392d%7C9274ee3f94254109a27f9fb15c10675d%7C0%7C0%7C637916014392703281%7CUnknown%7CTWFpbGZsb3d8eyJWIjoiMC4wLjAwMDAiLCJQIjoiV2luMzIiLCJBTiI6Ik1haWwiLCJXVCI6Mn0%3D%7C3000%7C%7C%7C&sdata=CZCi17vNq5%2BD517mYZZ-Ko5WkTqoxMl%2FectMytdNJ77g%3D&reserved=0" https://doi.org/10.1016/j.canlet.2019.01.017).

organizing clinical trials lie within their decentralized nature, the involvement of multiple clinical sites with different degrees of specialization, the standardization of tissue procurement, and funding opportunities. Surgeons are well trained to assume a principal investigator role in cancer clinical trials where tissue collection and processing are essential components of the treatment approach or correlative monitoring. In addition, the recent approval of multiple new targeted therapy and immunotherapy agents for patients with metastatic disease has led to interest in moving such agents into earlier stages of disease. Indeed, adjuvant targeted therapy and immunotherapy are now approved in the adjuvant setting for patients with stage IIIB and IIIC melanoma, and pembrolizumab was just approved for the adjuvant treatment of renal cell carcinoma. [33,34]. There is considerable enthusiasm for pursuing intratumoral therapy in the neoadjuvant setting. For most intratumoral agents the presence of an established tumor is needed and this may help immunize patients with in situ tumor antigens when immune responses are desired or may be needed to alter known tumorigenic profiles. Neoadjuvant therapy is also helpful in promoting understanding of drug mechanisms by providing tissue for more complete biomarker analyses. Surgeons are critical to conducting such studies as surgery, and the timing of surgery in experimental and control arms remains controversial.

The study of cancer pharmacology must take into consideration the considerable intrapatient and interpatient tumor heterogeneity. Studies investigating antitumor immunity depend on the efficient collection of tumor tissue. The quality of tissue collection can be affected by various factors, including the anatomic location of tissue, time from tissue isolation to processing, processing sterility, tumor processing methods, storage conditions, and temperatures. Surgeons are increasingly being asked to serve as technical experts in the collection and processing of tissue. In the case of adoptive TIL therapy, surgical resection of metastatic tumors for cell generation is required. Surgeons need to consult with medical oncologists and immunologists on how to identify the best tumor for harvesting; this may include considerations such as the size of the tumor to ensure sufficient cell yield, the anatomic location to limit postoperative morbidity, and the kinetics of tumor growth to select the tumors most likely to contain immune relevant cells. In addition, depending on the cell product being developed, specific storage in proprietary fluids and collection containers to ensure cell viability and sterility are mandatory. A similar strategy may be needed for collection of tumors to identify neoantigens for personalized vaccine development.

In addition to cell harvesting, surgeons may be called on to inject oncolytic viruses, nonviral agents, and gene editing compounds into tumor cells. Although this may be done via direct palpation for superficial tumors, or via endoscopic or interventional radiology imaging techniques, some tumors may require surgical intervention. For example, many brain tumors are not easily accessible except through craniotomy. In-dwelling catheters may be inserted to provide for repeat injections over time. Similar strategies have been used for isolated liver perfusion or intraperitoneal delivery of various agents. Surgeons are often skilled at performing bedside ultrasound, and this has been a useful technique for many oncolytic virus studies where tumors are not palpable or become smaller during treatment but may still be present and require size assessment before treatment to determine and/or visualization for intralesional drug administration. Further, the collection of tumor tissue for biomarker analysis is very important, and surgeon should be included early in studies that require tissue collection and processing to ensure optimal condition of the specimen for laboratory analyses. For example, when viable cells are needed it is critical to collect the specimen in a sterile manner, and the specimen may need to be placed in storage medium that promotes cell viability, depending on the assays being conducted. Thus, communication between pathologist or immunologist and surgeon is essential before tissue collection. In general, surgeons should be included in early consultation for products that may require surgical input or patient management.

Progress in cancer drug development has accelerated and resulted in major advances over the last decade. As the pace of drug discovery and evaluation increases, surgeons should also be expected to play an increasing role in updating tumor staging, redirecting diagnostic and therapeutic procedures and included as expert authorities in the evaluation and implementation of new strategies for patients with cancer.

SUMMARY AND FUTURE DIRECTIONS

Since the cloning of the human genome in 2000, the application of gene therapy to cancer has only recently been realized; this has evolved from advances in understanding the genetic mutations in patient's cancer cells as well as more rapid diagnostic testing capabilities allowing detection of the genetic landscape of individual tumors. In addition, advances in cancer immunology have resulted in several new drugs, including checkpoint inhibitors, vaccines, oncolytic viruses, and CAR T-cell therapies that have had a significant impact on patient outcomes across almost all types of cancer. Additional advances in gene editing, neoantigen-based cancer vaccines, and adoptive T-cell therapy are anticipated to bring further progress to the field over the next few years. Rapid access to genomic data, as through artificial intelligence and deep learning pathways, will also help bring gene therapy to the clinic in a more feasible manner. Further basic research to better understand the complex interplay between cancer genome alterations and the host immune response are likely to give rise to new therapeutic paradigms and combination regimens that will require clinical trials to validate. The advances in laboratory genomics, including single-cell RNA sequencing capabilities, demands that tissue be collected carefully in a standardized manner and be safeguarded to maximize the information gained for individual patients as well as society. For this reason, surgeons need to know about advances in gene therapy for cancer.

CLINICS CARE POINTS

- Surgeons are increasingly being asked to obtain tissue for diagnostic, therapeutic, and biomarker purposes for patients treated with gene therapy.
- Early consultation with pathologists and medical oncologist to ensure proper selection of tumor samples, surgical procedure, tissue handling, and specimen processing is important before operation.
- Surgeons may also be asked to provide access to tissue for gene therapy delivery using open, laparoscopic, and endoscopic approaches.

DISCLOSURE

H.L. Kaufman is an employee of Ankyra Therapeutics and served on clinical advisory board for Castle Biosciences and Marengo Therapeutics. The other authors have no financial disclosures.

References

[1] Yamamoto M, Curiel DT. Cancer gene therapy. Technol Cancer Res Treat 2005;4(4): 315–30.
[2] Cross D, Burmester K. Gene therapy for cancer treatment: past, present and future. Clin Med Res 2006;4(3):218–27.
[3] Naldini L. Gene therapy returns to centre stage. Nature 2015;526(7573):351–60.
[4] Singh V, Khan N, Jayandharan G. Vector engineering, strategies and targets in cancer gene therapy. Cancer Gene Ther 2021; https://doi.org/10.1038/s41417-021-00331-7.
[5] Gottesman M. Cancer gene therapy: an awkward adolescence. Cancer Gene Ther 2003;10(7):501–8.
[6] Tazawa H, Kagawa S, Fujiwara T. Advances in adenovirus-mediated p53 cancer gene therapy. Expert Opin Biol Ther 2013;13(11):1569–83.
[7] Lara-Guerra H, Roth J. Gene therapy for lung cancer. Crit Rev Oncog 2016;21(1–2): 115–24.
[8] Saleh A, Perets R. Mutated p53 in HGSC- from a common mutation to a target for therapy. Cancers (Basel) 2021;13(14):3465.
[9] Hayashi T, Fujita K, Hayashi Y, et al. Mutational landscape and environmental effects in bladder cancer. Int J Mol Sci 2020;21(17):6072.
[10] Michel M, Kaps L, Maderer A, et al. The role of p53 dysfunction in colorectal cancer and its implication for therapy. Cancers (Basel) 2021;13(10):2296.
[11] Tamura RE, Lana MG, Costanzi-Strauss E, et al. Combination of cabazitaxel and p53 gene therapy abolishes prostate carcinoma tumor growth. Gene Ther 2020;27(1–2):15–26.
[12] Vermaelen K. Vaccine strategies to improve anti-cancer cellular immune responses. Front Immunol 2019;10:8.
[13] Marshall JS, Warrington R, Watson W, et al. An introduction to immunology and immunopathology. Allergy Asthma Clin Immunol 2018;14(2):49.
[14] Neek M, Kim T Il, Wang S. Protein-based nanoparticles in cancer vaccine development. Nanomedicine 2019;15(1):164–74.
[15] Thomas S, Prendergast GC. Cancer vaccines: a brief overview. Methods Mol Biol 2016;1403:755–61.
[16] Kantoff PW, Higano CS, Shore ND, et al. Sipuleucel-T immunotherapy for castration-resistant prostate cancer. N Engl J Med 2010;363(5):411–22.
[17] Fukuhara H, Ino Y, Todo T. Oncolytic virus therapy: a new era of cancer treatment at dawn. Cancer Sci 2016;107(10):1373–9.
[18] Martuza RL, Malick A, Markert JM, et al. Experimental therapy of human glioma by means of a genetically engineered virus mutant. Science 1991;252:854–6.
[19] Richards K, Macdonald A. Putting the brakes on the anti-viral response: negative regulators of type I interferon (IFN) production. Microbes Infect 2011;13(4):291–302.
[20] Mondal M, Guo J, He P, et al. Recent advances of oncolytic virus in cancer therapy. Hum Vaccin Immunother 2020;16(10):2389–402.
[21] Hu JC, Coffin RS, Davis CJ, et al. A phase I study of OncoVEXGM-CSF, a second-generation oncolytic herpes simplex virus expressing granulocyte macrophage colony-stimulating factor. Clin Cancer Res 2006;12(22):6737–47.
[22] Senzer NN, Kaufman HL, Amatruda T, et al. Phase II clinical trial of a granulocyte-macrophage colony-stimulating factor-encoding, second-generation oncolytic herpes virus in patients with unresectable metastatic melanoma. J Clin Oncol 2009;27(34):5763–71.
[23] Andtbacka RH, Kaufman HL, Collichio F, et al. Talimogene Laherparepvec improves durable response rate in patients with advanced melanoma. J Clin Oncol 2015;33(25):2780–8.

[24] Anguela XM, High KA. Entering the modern era of gene therapy. Annu Rev Med 2019;70: 273–88.
[25] Hay KA, Turtle CJ. Chimeric antigen receptor (CAR) T cells: lessons learned from targeting of CD19 in B cell malignancies. Drugs 2017;77(3):237–45.
[26] Maude SL, Laetsch TW, Buechner J, et al. Tisagenlecleucel in children and young adults with B-cell lymphoblastic leukemia. N Engl J Med 2018;378:439–48.
[27] Neelapu SS, Locke FL, Bartlett NL, et al. Axicabtagene ciloleucel CAR T-cell therapy in refractory large B-cell lymphoma. N Engl J Med 2017;377:2531–44.
[28] Yanez L, Sanchez-Escamilla M, Perales M, et al. Cell toxicity: current management and future directions. Hemasphere 2019;3(2):e186.
[29] Memi F, Ntokou A, Papangeli I. CRISPR/Cas9 gene-editing: research technologies, clinical applications and ethical considerations. Semin Perinatol 2018;42(8):487–500.
[30] Chen M, Mao A, Xu M, et al. CRISPR-Cas9 for cancer therapy: opportunities and challenges. Cancer Lett 2019;447:48–55.
[31] Kennedy EM, Kornepati AVR, Goldstein M, et al. Inactivation of the human papillomavirus E6 or E7 gene in cervical carcinoma cells by using a bacterial CRISPR/Cas RNA-guided endonuclease. J Virol 2014;88(20):11965–72.
[32] Zhen S, Lu J, Wang L, et al. In Vitro and In vivo synergistic therapeutic effect of cisplatin with human papillomavirus16 E6/E7 CRISPR/Cas9 on cervical cancer cell line. Transl Oncol 2016;9(6):498–504.
[33] Eggermont AMM, Blank CU, Mandala M, et al. Adjuvant pembrolizumab versus placebo in resected stage III melanoma. N Engl J Med 2018;378(19):1789–801.
[34] Choueiri TK, Tomczak P, Park SH, et al. Adjuvant pembrolizumab after nephrectomy in renal-cell carcinoma. N Engl J Med 2021;385(8):683–94.

Advances in Surgery 56 (2022) 169–204

ADVANCES IN SURGERY

Is There a Place for Hyperbaric Oxygen Therapy?

Kinjal N. Sethuraman, MD, MPH[a], Ryan Smolin, BS, MS[b], Sharon Henry, MD[c,*]

[a]University of Maryland Medical Center, Hyperbaric and Dive Medicine, 22 South Greene Street, Baltimore, MD 2120, USA; [b]University of Maryland School of Medicine, 685 West Baltimore Street, Suite 150, Baltimore, MD 21201, USA; [c]University of Maryland Medical Center, R A Cowley Shock Trauma Center, Room T1R59, 22 South Greene Street, Baltimore, MD 21201, USA

Keywords

• Hyperbaric oxygen therapy • Inhalation • Hyperbaric chamber • Hypoxia

Key points

- Hyperbaric oxygen therapy (HBOT) is an approved treatment of a host of clinical diagnoses and conditions. The physiologic changes attributed to this treatment are the rationale supporting its use.
- HBOT results in increased tissue oxygenation, vasoconstriction, activation of fibroblast, downregulation of inflammatory cytokines, upregulation of growth factors, potentiation of antibiotic efficacy, and reduction of leukocyte chemotaxis. These effects make it an attractive adjunct to improve healing of problem wounds, control severe soft tissue infections, and to decrease edema and improve tissue oxygenation in crush and compartment syndromes.
- Many of the data supporting the use of HBOT derive from animal studies because there have been few randomized controlled trials. Case series and some randomized controlled trials provide an additional level of support for some acute indications.

INTRODUCTION

Hyperbaric oxygen therapy (HBOT) involves treating patients by providing 100% oxygen through inhalation while they are inside a treatment chamber pressurized to more than 1.4 absolute atmospheres (ATA) [1]. Oxygen can be thought of as a drug and the hyperbaric chamber as the dosing device.

*Corresponding author. 22 South Greene Street, Room T1R59, Baltimore, MD 21201. *E-mail address:* sharon.henry@som.umaryland.edu

https://doi.org/10.1016/j.yasu.2022.02.011

The effect of hyperbaric hyperoxia is dose dependent and, therefore, treatment depth and duration are important when considering its use.

HBOT can either be the primary method of treatment or used adjunctively to medications or surgical techniques. The indications for HBOT according to the latest publication by the Undersea and Hyperbaric Medical Society include a variety of diagnoses, as listed in Box 1 [1]. Many indications are approved by private and federal insurance programs [2]. Despite the diverse conditions for which HBOT has been used, the underpinning physiology is to bring oxygen-rich plasma to hypoxic tissue, preventing reperfusion injury, strengthening immune responsiveness, and encouraging new collagen deposition as well as endothelial cell formation. More than half of the approved diagnoses for which HBOT is used are relevant to surgeons. Familiarity with the potential indications and utility is therefore valuable.

OVERVIEW

HBOT provides increased oxygen delivery to tissues and decreases the gas bubbles present in tissues. Principles founded in physics explain the theoretic framework and the clinical experience, both positive and negative. Boyle's

Box 1: Fourteen approved diagnoses for hyperbaric oxygen therapy according to the Undersea and Hyperbaric Medical Society

Air or gas embolism
Arterial insufficiencies[a]
Central retinal artery occlusion
Selected problem wounds[a]
Carbon monoxide poisoning
Clostridial myonecrosis (gas gangrene)[a]
Compromised grafts and flaps[a]
Acute traumatic ischemias (crush and compartment syndromes)[a]
Decompression sickness
Delayed radiation injuries (soft tissue and bony necrosis)
Sudden sensorineural hearing loss
Intracranial abscess
Necrotizing soft tissue infections[a]
Refractory osteomyelitis[a]
Severe anemia
Thermal burns[a]

[a]Indications of interest to surgeons.
Based on Moon, R.E. *UHMS hyperbaric oxygen therapy indication*, 14th ed. Best Publishing Company, North Palm Beach, Florida, USA, 2019.

law tells us that, at a given temperature, a volume of gas is inversely proportional to its pressure. Trapped gas expands during decompression. Charles' law states that, with a constant volume, pressure and temperature vary. Thus, temperatures increase during compression and decrease with decompression. One absolute atmosphere (ATA) or 760 mm Hg represents the pressure the air above the ground exerts on the surface of the Earth. Dalton's law tells us the total pressure of a mixture of gases is equal to the sum of the partial pressures of each component gas. The pressure a gas exerts changes if the pressure changes or the concentration of gas in the mixture changes [3]. Henry's law refers to gases dissolved in solution. The concentration of a gas in solution depends on its solubility and its partial pressure [3]. Under normal circumstances, hemoglobin is about 97% saturated with oxygen and a small fraction of oxygen is dissolved in plasma, 3 mL of oxygen per liter of blood. Breathing 100% oxygen increases this to 15 mL per liter of blood and, during HBOT at 2.5 ATA, 60 mL of oxygen is dissolved in each liter. This oxygen level is sufficient to support resting tissue metabolism without any contribution from the oxygen saturated on hemoglobin [4]. At the capillary level, oxygen reaches cells by diffusion. Oxygen delivery is inversely proportional to the distance squared and proportional to the oxygen level at the capillary. Tissues with high metabolic rates have denser distribution of capillaries, whereas tissues such as subcutaneous fat, tendon, and fascia with lower metabolic rates have a scanter distribution [5].Under hyperbaric conditions, the diffusion distance is augmented 3-fold by the higher Po_2 at the capillary [6]. Exposure to hyperbaric oxygen produces several reliable physiologic responses in the body. They are listed in Box 2 [6].

There are broadly 2 types of hyperbaric chamber, monoplace and multiplace. Monoplace chambers are the most prevalent. They are mobile and constructed with acrylics to allow visualization of the patient. They can be equipped to accommodate ventilated patients and with intravenous pass-through ports to allow continuous infusions. They can be pressurized with oxygen, so patients are able to breathe freely or air with the patients breathing oxygen through a mask. Multiplace chambers permit multiple patients to be treated simultaneously. These chambers are pressurized with air and individual patients receive 100% oxygen through a hood or a ventilator (Figs. 1 and 2). Staff can be present within the chamber to troubleshoot problems that may arise during the treatment, which is essential for critically ill patients. . Critically ill patients can be managed in these larger chambers because there is sufficient space for a stretcher and chamber-approved equipment, including ventilators and intravenous pumps.

The precise dose/treatment varies depending on the indication but broadly ranges from 2.0 to 3.0 ATA for 90 to 120 minutes up to 3 times daily. Air breaks are given to decrease the risk of oxygen toxicity. Compression and decompression occur over a defined time and are prescribed as treatment tables.

Box 2: Physiologic effects of hyperbaric oxygen therapy

Cardiovascular

- Bradycardia
- Decreased cardiac output
- Decreased cerebral blood flow
- Increased risk of arrhythmias
- Increased systolic blood pressure
- Decreased diastolic blood pressure

Respiratory

- Depressed ventilation caused by stimulation of aortic and carotid baroreceptors
- Washout of nitrogen with potential atelectasis

Peripheral vessels

- Increased peripheral resistance
- Vasoconstriction

Blood/coagulation

- Stimulation of fibrinolysis hours after exposure
- Decreased platelet aggregation
- Increase red blood cell elasticity

Metabolism

- Altered cerebral glucose metabolism

Oxygen metabolism

- Decreased reliance on oxygen bound to hemoglobin

Modified from HBOT Londahl M. Hyperbaric oxygen therapy as Adjunctive treatment of Diabetic foot ulcers. Medical clinics of North America, 2013; 97(5): 957-980.

CONTRAINDICATIONS AND COMPLICATIONS

HBOT infrequently results in severe complications. There are only a few absolute contraindications to HBOT. The presence of an untreated pneumothorax is an absolute contraindication to HBOT because additional oxygen transfer or diffusion outside the lung during decompression has the potential to produce tension physiology. The other absolute contraindication is related to the use of certain medications. Cisplatin use with HBOT can result in delayed wound healing. Historical or concurrent use of bleomycin in combination with HBOT can result in interstitial pneumonitis. HBOT enhances the cardiotoxicity of doxorubicin [7]. Several relative contraindications exist and are listed in Box 3. The potential benefit of HBOT must be weighed against the problems associated with the relative contraindications. Table 1 [8–12] lists the common complications associated with HBOT and their relative frequencies [8]. The most worrisome risk of HBOT is fire. High concentrations

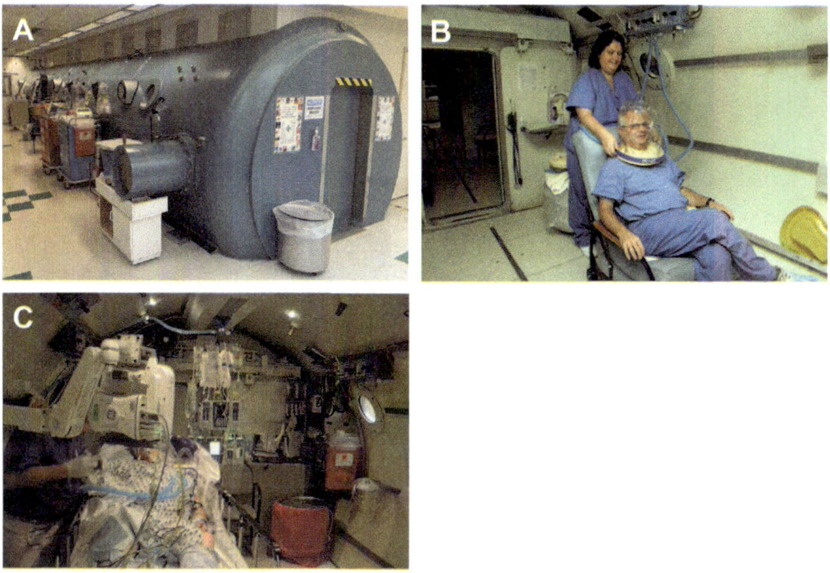

Fig. 1. (*A*) External view of multiplace hyperbaric chamber. (*B*) Interior view of multiplace chamber. Patients can be placed in chairs or on stretchers. Patients wear hoods to inhale 100% oxygen while the chamber is pressurized with air. (*C*) Multiplace hyperbaric chamber with critically ill patient. Equipment must be compatible with pressurization.

of oxygen under pressure make this environment highly flammable. Rigorous attention to what is brought into the chamber is important. Electrical equipment, makeup, lotions, grease, newspapers, and certain clothing are prohibited [10].

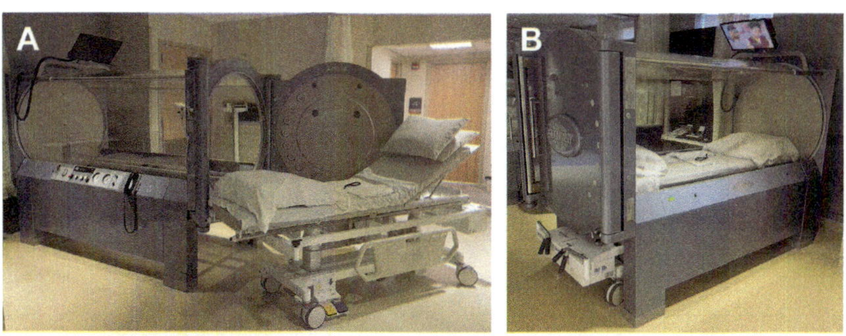

Fig. 2. (*A*) Monoplace chamber with stretcher outside. Acrylic walls enable visualization of patient for monitoring. (*B*) Monoplace chamber with stretcher inside. Television can be visualized through clear walls.

Box 3: Relative contraindications to hyperbaric oxygen therapy

Upper respiratory infection
Allergic rhinitis
Chronic sinusitis and otitis
Chronic obstructive pulmonary disease with emphysema or CO_2 retention
History of pneumothorax or thoracic surgery
History of ear, nose, or throat surgery
Epilepsy
Optic neuritis
Uncontrolled hypertension
Uncontrolled heart failure
Claustrophobia
Dangerous behavior

Potential adverse reactions to treatment with HBOT should be considered when initiating therapy. The most common adverse events associated with HBOT are benign and can be managed with accommodations. The incidence of adverse events is reported as 2%, with 0.44% reported as the per-treatment

Table 1
The most common adverse effects of hyperbaric oxygen therapy

Event	Frequency
Otic/sinus barotrauma	0.37%
Confinement anxiety	0.16%
Hypoglycemia	0.08%
Seizure	0.02%
Shortness of breath	0.05%
Oxygen toxicity	0.3% - 0.17%
Pneumothorax	1 in 1.5 million treatments
CHF exacerbation	1 in 300 [12]
Progressive myopia	—
Pulmonary edema	—
Accelerated maturation of cataracts	—
Ear pain	17% [11]
Myopia	1 in 50,000–60,000 treatments [11]
Fires	Rare but frequently fatal [10]

Table revised from Jokinen-Gordon H, Barry RC, Watson B and Covington DS. A retrospective Analysis of Adverse Events in Hyperbaric Oxygen Therapy (2012-2015): Lessons learned from 1.5 million treatments. Advances in Skin and Wound Care, 2017; 20(3):125-129 and Lam G, Fontaine R, Ross FL and Chiu ES. Hyperbaric Oxygen therapy: Exploring the Clinical Evidence. Advances in Skin and Wound Care, 2017; 30(4):181-190; and *Data from* Refs. [10–12].

rate [8]. A recent retrospective review of multiple advanced wound care and hyperbaric medicine centers across the United States found 99.3% of hyperbaric oxygen treatments occurred without an adverse event recorded [8]. The most common events were otic/sinus barotrauma and confinement anxiety [10]. Confinement anxiety is intolerable to some but can be managed with small doses of anxiolytics in others. Most patients can equalize the pressure within the middle ear and paranasal sinuses. Sedated patients, those with altered mental status, or awake patients unable to equalize pressures may need myringotomy or myringotomy tubes. Decreased vital capacity and myopia are reversible side effects that can occur with prolonged treatment. Neurotoxicity resulting in seizures can occur. Seizures usually occur in patients with poorly controlled underlying seizure disorders. Severe events such as seizures or pulmonary barotrauma occurred in fewer than 2 episodes in 10,000 treatments [8]. Adverse reactions occurred more commonly at higher pressures.

CLINICAL INDICATIONS

Problem wounds

Problem wounds fail to heal with standard medical and surgical treatment in a reasonable time frame. They have been described as a silent epidemic affecting large segments of the world's population. Given the ambiguous definition, determining prevalence and incidence is challenging. It is estimated that 1% to 2% of the population have a chronic wound in their lifetimes [13,14]. In normal acute wound healing, an organized process leads to predictable repair of the tissues with platelets, keratinocytes, immune cells, microvascular cells, and fibroblast all playing key roles in the restoration of tissue integrity and function. Chronic wounds have a substantial impact on quality of life and health care costs. It is estimated that 6.5 million patients in the United States are affected, and more than $25 billion are expended annually in treating wounds and wound-related complications [15].

PATHOPHYSIOLOGY

Patients affected by chronic wounds are rarely healthy. They nearly uniformly are affected by conditions that substantially hinder the ordered process of wound healing. Most chronic wounds begin as trivial traumatic injuries. Simple scratches in dry skin, insect bites, or minor penetrating injuries can lead to a problem wound in patients with underlying pathologic conditions. Chronic wounds are broadly classified by cause as venous, arterial, diabetic, or pressure related. These wounds are usually mired in an extended inflammatory phase that may result from persistent infection or biofilm formation and/or the inability of dermal or epidermal cells to respond to reparative stimuli. Inflammatory cells are excessively recruited to the wound bed often because of infection. Expression of adhesion molecules allows these cells to become resident in the wound bed [16]. Inflammatory cells produce reactive oxygen species (ROS) that can damage the extracellular matrix (ECM) and produce premature senescence of the wound. Proinflammatory cytokines lead to the production of serine proteinases and matrix metalloproteases (MMPs) that degrade the ECM and inactivate growth factors. Inhibitors to the proteinases are also inactivated, amplifying the negative impact on healing [17] (Fig. 3).

Oxygen plays a vital role as a nutrient required for successful wound healing. Oxygen regulates migration and proliferation of fibroblasts. Bacteria are controlled through the oxidative processes of leukocytes. Leukocytes are ineffective in hypoxic conditions [13]. Angiogenesis requires oxygen, and collagen production depends on oxygen.

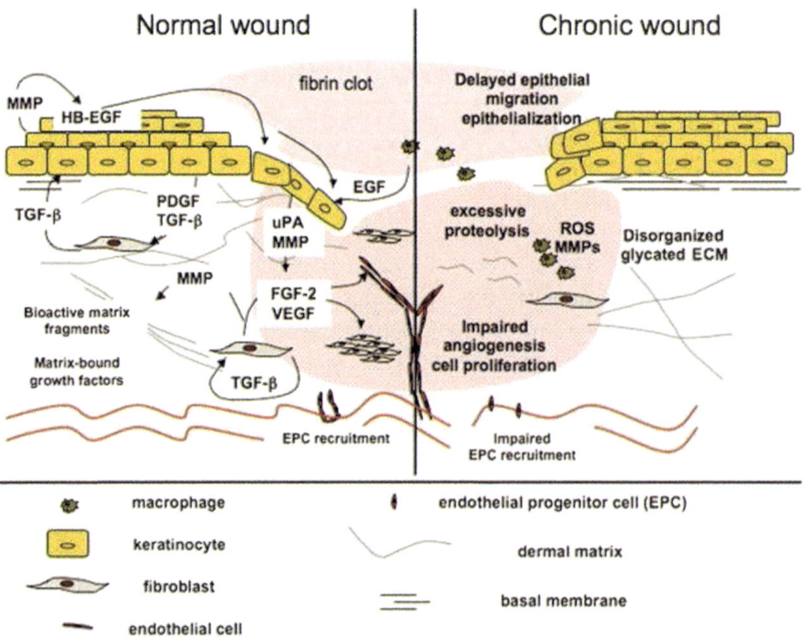

Fig. 3. Normal and disordered wound healing. (*Left*) Normal wound healing. There are multiple growth factors. The extracellular matrix is well organized, and the cells present in the wound respond appropriately to stimuli. Synthesis of the wound's ECM is occurring at a higher rate than its degradation. This activity is regulated by tissue inhibitors of matrix metalloproteinases. Angiogenesis is occurring through development of new blood vessels from existing vessels and bringing in endothelial progenitor cells (EPC). (*Right*) The disordered process occurring in the chronic wound. There may be high levels of bacteria in biofilms fueling persistent inflammation and the breakdown of critical growth factors, receptors, and the ECM. Cells cannot proliferate or migrate effectually. New blood vessels do not develop sufficiently, leading to insufficient oxygen and nutrient availability to cells in the wound bed and stalling wound healing. EGF, epidermal growth factor; FGF, fibroblast growth factor; TGF, transforming growth factor; uPA, urokinase-type plasminogen activator. (Demidova-Rice TN, Hamblin MR, Herman IM. Acute and impaired wound healing: pathophysiology and current methods for drug delivery, part 1: normal and chronic wounds: biology, causes, and approaches to care. Advances in Skin & Wound Care. 2012 Jul;25(7):304-314. https://doi.org/10.1097/01.asw.0000416006.55218.d0. PMID: 22713781; PMCID: PMC3428147.)

WHY IT WORKS

HBOT has been used to treat chronic wounds since 1968 [18]. The primary objective of treating a chronic wound with HBOT is to correct wound hypoxia. Intermittently providing hypoxic tissue with supranormal oxygen levels may permit normal wound healing to resume. HBOT results in increased tissue oxygenation, vasoconstriction, activation of fibroblast, downregulation of inflammatory cytokines, upregulation of growth factors, potentiation of antibiotic efficacy, and reduction of leukocyte chemotaxis. The upregulation of vascular endothelial growth factor (VEGF) and release of platelet-derived growth factor (PDGF) may produce a persistent improvement in wound healing [17]. Intracellular adenosine triphosphate (ATP) is preserved, supporting the increased metabolism of the wound [17]. In addition, nitric oxide synthase 3 (NOS-3), required for mobilization of circulating stem progenitor cells, is stimulated in the bone marrow by HBOT [19]. These physiologic changes theoretically support the use of hyperbaric oxygen in problem wounds (Fig. 4).

EVIDENCE FOR PROBLEM WOUNDS

The scientific support for improvement in wound outcomes is less straightforward. Early studies were mostly case series and retrospective analyses that showed promising associations with improved healing, decreased amputation, and decreased mortality with the use of hyperbaric oxygen. Small uncontrolled studies often with heterogeneous populations and poorly defined outcome measures have formed the basis of the literature both supporting and denouncing the use of HBOT in treating chronic wounds. Most of the data in problem wounds are from the treatment of diabetic foot ulcers (DFUs). The first prospective controlled study evaluating the effect of HBOT on patients with DFUs was published in 1987 by Baroni and colleagues [20]. Eighteen patients with Wagner grade 3 and 4 ulcers were treated with HBOT. They were matched with patients with similar wounds and severity of diabetes. Attending surgeons blinded to the treatment group made decisions regarding the need for amputation. Sixteen patients in the HBOT group healed and 2 underwent amputation, whereas 1 healed and 4 required amputations in the control group [20]. Several other randomized trials have since followed with varied outcomes (Table 2). A 2010 study included 49 patients in the treatment group and 45 in the control group. One-year follow-up of the per-protocol analysis found ulcer healing in 61% in the treatment group and 27% in the control group, with 3% in both groups requiring amputation [21]. A large, longitudinal database study using propensity matching failed to show any benefit from the use of HBOT in either preventing amputation or augmenting wound healing; however, this study included all wound classes and severity and all patients treated at the wound care center [23]. Interestingly, a recent animal study showed HBOT to have the greatest effect on time to healing in animals that were hyperglycemic, had ischemic wounds, or both [24]. It was hoped that the Does Applying More Oxygen (O2) Cure Lower Extremity Sores? (DAMO$_2$CLES) study with its multicenter prospective design would provide the best data to date on the

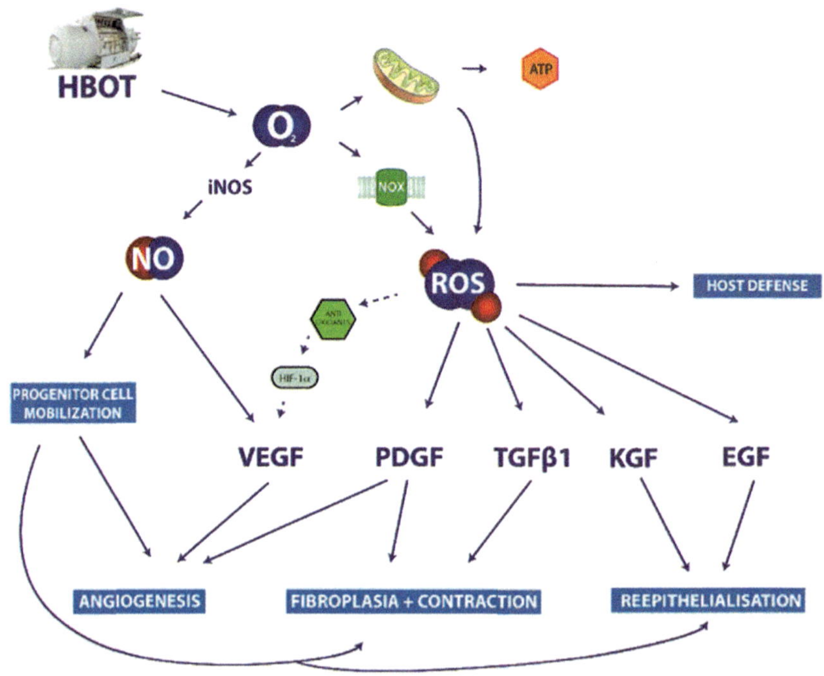

Fig. 4. Mechanisms of action for HBOT on chronic wounds. Solid arrows show direct interactions and dashed lines indirect actions. Increased oxygen availability leads to enhanced mitochondrial energy supply. ROS are produced in the presence of enhanced oxygen by nitric oxide enzymes. Key cytokines are also signaled that lead to increased fibroblast collagen production, through PDGF, angiogenesis through VEGF production, and epithelialization through keratinocyte growth factor (KGF). Progenitor cells are mobilized from the bone marrow. iNOS, inducible nitric oxide synthase. (*From* creative common version 4.0 license legend amended Andre-Levigne D, Modarressi A, Pepper MS and Pittet-Cuenod B. Reactive oxygen species and NOX enzymes are emerging as key players in cutaneous wound repair. International Journal of Molecular Sciences, 2017; 18: 2149. https://doi.org/10.3390/ijms18102149.)

utility of hyperbaric oxygen in the treatment of DFUs with associated ischemia. However, because of low patient accrual, the sample size was decreased from the originally calculated 226 to 120. In addition, 18% of the treatment group failed to complete the study. This study did not show improvement in either amputation or wound healing, but, given its flaws, these findings may not be generalizable [22]. A study analyzing big data from a multicenter wound database gave some more insights into the complexity of analyzing the effect of HBOT. They found that, of 5742 patients that received HBOT, only 2597 (or 45.2%) completed a full course. Furthermore, when comparing those receiving a full course with those receiving standard care, healing occurred in 75% versus 47% [25]. Given the heterogeneity and flaws in the design and reporting of the studies identified, the most recent Cochrane Review concluded that HBOT significantly improved short-term healing of DFUs but not the

Table 2
Prospective studies evaluating hyperbaric oxygen therapy for diabetic foot ulcer

Author, year	Study design	HBO	Standard care	Outcome
Doctor 1992[121] Chronic ulcers	Prospective randomized	15	15	Amputation HBO 13%; SC 47% ($P<.05$)
Faglia 1996[122] DFU Wagner grade 4>3 mo	Prospective randomized	36	34	Amputation HBO 8.6%; SC 33% ($P<.02$)
Kessler 2003[123] Wagner grade 1–3 >3 mo	Prospective randomized	14	13	Size reduction Week 2: HBO 42%; SC 22% ($P<.04$) Week 4: HBO 48%; SC 42% (NS)
Abidia 2003[124] • 6 wk • ABI<0.08 • HbA1c<8.5%	Prospective randomized	9	9	Ulcer healing HBO 63%; SC 0 ($P<.03$) Amputation HBO 13%; SC 13%
Duzgun 2008[125] >4 wk	Prospective randomized	50	50	Healing with no OR debridement at 1 y HBO 66%; SC 0
Londahl et al, [21] 2010 At least 2 mo good treatment Well vascularized	Prospective randomized	49	45	PP healing at 1 y HBO 61%; SC 27% ($P<.01$) Amputation HBO 3%; SC 3%

(*continued on next page*)

Table 2
(*continued*)

Author, year	Study design	HBO	Standard care	Outcome
Margolis et al, [23] 2013 Diabetes Foot wound Adequate arterial flow • 4 wk	Longitudinal observational database with propensity matching	793	5466	Healing at16 wk HBO 43% / SC 49% (*P*<.0001) Amputation at 16 wk HBO 6.7% / SC 2.1% (*P*<.0001)
Fedorka 2016[126] Wagner grade 2–4	Prospective randomized	54	49	Amputation HBO 23% / SC 24% (NS) Wound healing HBO 20% / SC 22%
Santema et al, [22] 2018 Diabetes Wagner grade 3–4 ABI<0.7	Multicenter prospective randomized	39	56	Amputation HBO 22% / SC 5% (NS) Complete healing HBO 55% / SC 48% (NS)

Abbreviations: ABI, ankle brachial index; HbA1c, hemoglobin A1c; HBO, hyperbaric oxygen; NS, not significant; PP, per protocol; SC, standard care.

long-term healing [26]. In addition, a recently published systematic review and meta-analysis of the controlled trials of HBOT in DFUs concluded that complete healing occurred more frequently and major amputation less frequently in patients undergoing HBOT. The investigators called for more trials with adequate power and design to minimize bias [27].

Venous ulcers are the most common lower extremity ulcer and account for 70% to 90% of leg wounds [15]. Chronic venous insufficiency leading to chronic venous hypertension is the underlying mechanism. Standard treatment involves the use of compression bandages and moist wound healing principles. It is estimated that more than 30% of venous ulcers fail to heal despite receiving adequate treatment [28]. HBOT has been used to augment healing in some patients with hard-to-heal venous ulcers. HBOT in this patient population has not been studied as extensively as in patients with DFUs. A randomized trial of patients with venous ulcers included patients that failed to show a 50% reduction of ulcer size (Percent Area Reduction [PAR]) after 4 weeks of standard care. Patients were further required to have adequate ankle brachial indices (ABIs) and evidence of a hypoxic wound responsive to an oxygen challenge. Thirty patients were randomized: 15 received HBOT and 15 received standard treatment. There was no difference in healing at 12 weeks between the groups. The patients receiving HBOT had a significantly greater PAR. There was also no difference between the groups regarding pain scores or quality-of-life assessments. The investigators suggest HBOT may be useful in indolent ulcers that have failed to reduce in size by 50% after 4 weeks of good ulcer treatment. However, this study was underpowered and the follow-up period of 12 weeks may have been too short to show relapses and delayed healing effects [28]. Venous ulcers are not currently an accepted indication for treatment with HBOT.

There are few data on the use of HBOT in ulcers of unusual causes, such as vasculitis, calcific uremic arteriolopathy, and pyoderma gangrenosum. Case reports and series have reported positive outcomes in selected cases [29].

TREATMENT

The standard protocol used for wounds is 2.0 to 2.4 ATA for 90 to 120 minutes 5 days weekly. Patients are prescribed 20 days of treatment to start with and closely monitored for improvement of the wound. If the wound is improving with HBOT, the number of treatments is increased until the wound is nearly healed.

OSTEOMYELITIS

Osteomyelitis is infection in the bone or bone marrow. Osteomyelitis is difficult to eradicate. It is estimated that 90% of patients with osteomyelitis are cured with their initial treatment [30]. There is a paucity of blood vessels in bone, and antimicrobial agents therefore do not reach the point of infection. Osteomyelitis is considered refractory when it does not respond to or recurs after appropriate treatment has been provided. Standard treatment is considered to be surgical debridement of nonviable bone, removal of foreign bodies and tissue, and antibiotics directed to cultures [31]. Cultures are ideally from bone at the site of infection. In some cases, excision of bone may be impossible because of the location or function.

In 1965, a case report was published in *Lancet* describing the successful use of HBOT to treat a case of refractory osteomyelitis [32]. Several animal series were subsequently published confirming the findings of success reported in the case studies. Experimental work has shown that infected bone has decreased oxygen content. This low oxygen level can be reversed while receiving HBOT [33].

There are 4 proposed mechanisms for the positive effect of HBOT in patients with chronic refractory osteomyelitis [34]:

1. Augmentation of host defenses against infection. Leukocyte killing mechanisms are enhanced in a high-oxygen-tension environment. A 1978 study in an animal model found HBOT alone to be as effective as cephalosporins in treating staphylococcal osteomyelitis [35].
2. HBOT enhances neovascularization, which can result in improved delivery of antibiotics and neutrophils to the area of infection [36].
3. HBOT increases osteoclastic activity, which removes dead and infected bone from the area, allowing the intrinsic immune responses to be more effective as well as improving the efficacy of antibiotics by improving their penetration to the site of infection [37].
4. HBOT affects anaerobes and facultative anaerobes directly [36].

Several retrospective reviews reported remission of chronic refractory osteomyelitis in 63% to 89% of patients treated with HBOT. Follow-up in these studies ranged from 17 to 84 months. There are no randomized studies to inform the efficacy of this therapy [38]. The Cierney-Mader classification system (Table 3) for osteomyelitis has been used to characterize the patients that are most likely to benefit from the addition of HBOT [39]. Patients with stage 3 or 4 infections that have systemic compromise of immune function or metabolism and/or local vascular compromise are considered most likely to have improvement [38]. Other investigators suggest that patients with recurrence of osteomyelitis after appropriate medical and surgical treatment should be eligible for HBOT.

TREATMENT

The treatment protocol delivers treatment daily for a total of 15 to 40 treatments at 2.0 to 2.5 ATA for 90 to 120 minutes. Markers of infection should be followed, and reimaging may also be performed to assess for evidence of improvement.

SUMMARY

There is a large volume of flawed data evaluating the use of HBOT in patients with chronic wounds. The most robust literature is in DFUs. A recently

Table 3
Cierney-Mader classification for osteomyelitis

Anatomic description			
Stage			Anatomy
1			Medullary osteomyelitis
2			Superficial osteomyelitis
3			Localized osteomyelitis
4			Diffuse osteomyelitis
Physiologic classification			
A Normal	B Compromised		C Poor clinical conditions
No comorbidities	Systemic Malnutrition Renal failure Liver failure DM Chronic hypoxia Immune deficiency Malignancy Extremes of age Immunosuppression Tobacco abuse	Local Chronic lymphedema Venous stasis Major vascular compromise Arteritis Extensive scarring Radiation fibrosis Small vessel disease Complete local sensory loss	Surgical treatment has higher risk than the osteomyelitis

Abbreviation: DM, diabetes mellitus.

Modified from Kaide CG and Khandelwal S. Hyperbaric Oxygen: Applications in Infectious Disease. Emergency Medicine Clinics of North America, 2008; 26(2):571-595.

published systematic review and meta-analysis concluded that HBOT was associated with decreased major amputation in patients with DFU and arterial vascular disease. However, there was no difference in minor amputation, percentage of ulcer healing, or mortality [40]. Matching wound characteristics and descriptions as well as patient factors offers one set of challenges in the design of a study to answer the question of efficacy in HBOT for chronic wounds. Appropriate end points with adequate power to determine real differences is another hurdle to overcome. In addition, treatment protocols vary from center to center and must be standardized to determine utility. Variations in the number of treatments, duration, and depth may affect whether the intervention is found useful. It is also likely that there is a population that is best suited for treatment based on chronicity of the wound, presence of ischemia or infection, and depth of the wound that has not been shown by the current body of literature. HBOT has been uniformly associated with few serious complications and is mechanistically appealing to augment healing in chronic wounds. Until better data become available, it seems reasonable to use it selectively to treat recalcitrant wounds. The evidence supporting use in osteomyelitis is scant and only retrospective. Using it to salvage cases that have failed debridement and antibiotics or where debridement is not possible seems reasonable.

GAS GANGRENE AND NECROTIZING SOFT TISSUE INFECTIONS

Gas gangrene or clostridial myonecrosis is a rapidly progressive clostridial infection that produces massive local tissue destruction of previously healthy tissue. It is an uncommon infection, with 3800 to 5800 cases reported annually in the United States [41]. Necrotizing soft tissue infections (NSTIs) represent a spectrum of severe soft tissue infections that may affect any part of the body. These infections can be difficult to diagnose, rapidly progressive, and are uncommon. They often present in advanced stages. A 2006 publication using an insurance database in the United States reported there to be 4 cases per 100,000 person years [42]. Group A *Streptococcus pyogenes* (GAS)–related NSTI was shown to range from 0.1 to 0.4 per 100,000 person years in a Canadian study [43]. More recently May and colleagues [44], using the 2018 National Inpatient Sample and Watson Health datasets, reported much higher incidences. They estimate 10.3 and 8.4 per 100,000 persons based on finding 33,600 and 28,500 cases of NSTI respectively in the datasets [44]. Gratifyingly the mortality has decreased over time. In studies published before 2000, the average mortality was more than 20%. In more recent publications, the reported mortality has decreased to 9% with timely operative intervention [44]. Morbidity remains substantial. Amputation is performed in 22% of extremity NSTIs [45]. Surgical treatment in the form of wide excisional debridement results in large wounds that may require advanced procedures for reconstruction. Patients frequently have long-term functional deficits leading to unemployment and a decreased quality of life. Interventions that potentially limit tissue loss and speed the control of infection may affect both mortality and morbidity.

Pathophysiology

NSTIs involve the superficial fascia and can involve deeper tissues. They are caused by diverse microbes, including fungi. Bacteria produce endotoxins and exotoxins that unleash an inflammatory response that amplifies tissue injury. Obliterating endarteritis, thrombosis, and tissue necrosis are hallmarks seen on microscopic evaluation [46]. Polymicrobial infections include aerobes and anaerobes. An average 4.4 organisms are cultured per patient in these infections [47]. Frequently cultured organisms are *Staphylococcus aureus*, *Streptococcus* species, *Escherichia coli*, and *Klebsiella* species. Monomicrobial infections feature *S pyogenes* (GAS), *S aureus*, *Aeromonas* species, *Vibrio* species, *Klebsiella pneumoniae*, *Pseudomonas aeruginosa*, and clostridial species [47].

Gas gangrene spreads through tissues rapidly. The speed of spread is caused by the elaboration of exotoxins by bacteria. These toxins produce local effects, including breakdown of connective tissue, lysis of blood components, and muscle death. Systemic effects can produce shock, myocardial depression, capillary leak, renal failure, and death [48]. Many patients affected with NSTIs are immunocompromised in some way and have at least 1 comorbidity [45]. The mainstays of treatment are prompt administration of broad-spectrum antibiotics and timely operative intervention.

WHY IT WORKS

The cornerstones of treating NSTIs include broad-spectrum antibiotic, resuscitation, and timely operative debridement. HBOT is used as an adjunct to this standard approach. The first reported treatment of an NSTI was reported by Brummelkamp and colleagues [49] when they treated 2 patients with gas gangrene in 1960. They logically assumed that increased tissue oxygen would kill the anaerobic clostridial species. Tissues damaged by NSTIs are edematous and are relatively hypoxic. Anaerobic organisms are often cultured, especially from polymicrobial NSTIs, and it is reasonable to posit that the provision of an environment with a high oxygen concentration could result in bacterial killing. Even facultative anaerobes would be affected in such an environment because they lack the ability to resist oxygen free radicals. In addition, toxin production by anaerobes is inversely proportional to the oxygen levels they are exposed to. Alpha toxin produced by clostridial species is completely halted at a tissue Po_2 of 250 mm Hg [50]. This degree of tissue oxygenation is easily reached at 3 ATA. The logic for the effectiveness in infections caused by aerobic organism is not as obvious. White blood cells exposed to oxygen-rich environments produce increased respiratory bursts and are thereby more efficient at killing both aerobic and anerobic organisms [36,50]. Certain antibiotics are less effective in hypoxic tissues, including aminoglycosides, some sulfonamides, and quinolones [51]. Tobramycin, trimethoprim-sulfamethoxazole, and ciprofloxacin have shown increased function in conditions of hyperoxia [51–53]. In addition, patients with diabetes may further benefit from continued treatments with HBOT to augment granulation tissue formation. Increased oxygen tension provides needed energy for protein synthesis and fibroblast activity. New capillary growth is encouraged in this oxygen-rich environment. Nutritive blood supply is thereby increased as the diffusion distance for oxygen to reach hypoxic tissues is decreased.

EVIDENCE FOR NECROTIZING SOFT TISSUE INFECTION AND GAS GANGRENE

Several animal studies have shown improved survival in animals treated with HBOT after being infected with *Clostridium perfringens.* The timing of HBOT was found to be important, with survival decreasing when treatment was initiated more than 18 hours from infection [54]. Other studies showed no improvement in survival. A sentinel article by Demello and colleagues [55] published in 1973 treated dogs with combinations of antibiotics, surgery, and HBOT and found the greatest survival in the group receiving all 3 modalities (Fig. 5). Hirn [56] reported enhanced wound healing and earlier wound closure when HBOT was used. Animals treated with both surgical debridement and hyperbaric oxygen had 94% wound healing, but only 20% of animals treated

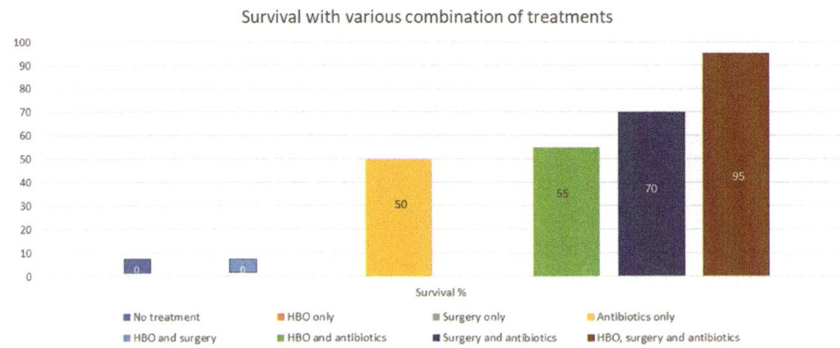

Fig. 5. Dogs inoculated with clostridia show best survival when treated with a combination of antibiotics, surgery, and HBOT. (*Data from* Demello FJ, Haglin JJ, and Hitchcock R. Comparative study of experimental Clostridium. perfringens infection in dogs treated with antibiotics, surgery, and hyperbaric oxygen Surgery, 1973; 73(6): 936-941.)

with surgery alone instead of only with surgery healed their wounds completely. Korhonen and colleagues [57] measured oxygen tensions in healthy volunteers and patients with NSTI. The arterial PO_2 increased to a maximum of 7 times higher than the starting value. Patients with NSTI had greater increase of PO_2 in the area of the wound than in healthy tissue, suggesting hyperbaric oxygen created an oxygen barrier to the further spread of infection. There have been no randomized controlled trials in humans comparing HBOT with standard therapy in patients with gas gangrene. Many researchers in the 1980s and 1990s considered HBOT to be standard in addition to antibiotics and surgery and thought that to compare modalities would not be ethical.

Several retrospective reviews have shown an association between HBOT use and improved survival from NSTI [58–62,64] (Table 4). Other retrospective reports have claimed earlier wound closure in patients receiving hyperbaric oxygen. Closure was achieved at 28 days in hyperbaric oxygen–treated patients but 48 days in those patients not receiving hyperbaric oxygen. There was also a corresponding decrease in hospital length of stay of 20 days [47]. Another retrospective review of the outcome in 42 patients receiving HBOT for NSTI found a mortality of 11.9% and that no patients with extremity NSTI required amputation [63]. Yet another retrospective review of 67 patients treated over 6 years compared outcomes of patients that received hyperbaric oxygen in addition to standard treatment with those that did not. There was no statistically significant difference in survival (17% vs 26%) or amputations (1 vs 6) in the treated and nontreated groups respectively. There was a statistically significant increase in the number of debridements required (4.15 ± 2.68 vs 2.65 ± 1.84 HBOT vs no HBOT; $P = .03$) [68]. A recent Cochrane Review failed to identify studies of sufficient quality to allow inclusion in a meta-analysis [69]. Thrane and Ovensen [70] also recently attempted a systematic analysis but failed to identify studies of adequate quality to allow inclusion in such a review. Hedetoft and

Table 4
Summary of hyperbaric oxygen therapy in necrotizing soft tissue infection

Author, year	Study type	N		Mortality (%)		Treatment	Operations (N)		Amputations (%)	
Riseman et al, [60] 1990	Retrospective	17	12	HBO 23[a]	No HBO 66[a]	90 min at 2.5 ATA Average 7.4 treatments	HBO 1.2[a]	No HBO 3.3[a]	Not described	
Brown et al, [67] 1994[b]	Retrospective	HBO 30	No HBO 24	HBO 30	No HBO 42	90 min at2.5–3.0 ATA 1- >5	HBO 3.2[a]	No HBO 1.7[a]	Not reported	
Shupak et al, [66] 1995[b]	Retrospective	HBO 25	No HBO 12	HBO 36	No HBO 25	45 min at 2.5 ATA No. of treatments not specified	HBO 3.3[a]	No HBO 1.5[a]	Not reported	
Mindrup et al, [58] 2005	Retrospective Fournier gangrene	HBO 26	No HBO 16	HBO 26.9	No HBO 12.5	Median 6 treatments at 2.4–3.0 ATA for 30–90 min	HBO 1	No HBO 1	Not applicable	
Wilkinson et al, [64] 2004	Retrospective	HBO 33	No HBO 11	HBO 6a	No HBO 36a	1–30	HBO 5	No HBO 1	HBO 0	No HBO 50[a]
Soh et al, [62] 2012	Retrospective National inpatient sample	HBO 405	No HBO 45,508	HBO 4.5[a]	No HBO 9.4[a]	Not described	Not described		HBO 14.1	No HBO 14.7
Massey et al, [65] 2012[b]	Retrospective	HBO 32	No HBO 48	HBO 15.6	No HBO 18.8	45 min at 2.8 ATA 1-8 treatments	HBO 7	No HBO 3.5	HBO 25	No HBO 16.7
Shaw et al, [59] 2014	Retrospective Consortium database	HBO 117	No HBO 1466	HBO 5a	HBO 12a	not described	not reported		no reported	
Devaney et al, [61] 2015	Retrospective	HBO 275	Not reported 66	Not reported 12[a]	No HBO 24.3[a]	2.8 ATA Average 6.1 treatments	HBO 4.8[a]	No HBO 3.0[a]	HBO 7.6[a]	No HBO 15.2[a]

[a]Statistically significant.
[b]Studies show no outcome improvement with HBOT.
Data from Refs. [58–62,64–67].

colleagues [71] performed a systematic review and meta-analysis that included data from 21 nonrandomized studies including 48,744 patients. They found lower odds of death during the sentinel hospitalization in patients receiving HBOT and determined that approximately 19 patients would need to be treated to prevent 1 death [71]. A recently published systematic review evaluated the use of HBOT in treating Fournier gangrene. They found a lower mortality in patients treated with HBOT, 16.6% compared with 25.9% in those not receiving treatment. They acknowledged a moderate to high risk of bias given the retrospective nature of the studies and differences in study design and reporting details [72]. A review of the Nationwide Inpatient Sample from 1988 to 2009 found a significant decreased in hospital mortality, from 9.4% in those not treated with HBOT to 4.5% in those treated with hyperbaric oxygen. This decrease was despite a higher cost of hospitalization and increased length of hospital stay [62]. A more recent evaluation of the same database from 1998 to 2010 showed HBOT was rarely used, occurring in 0.8% to 1.6% of the study population depending on the year, with no difference in mortality observed in those treated with HBOT [59].

Treatment

Some investigators recommend treatment of patients with gas gangrene with HBOT before surgical intervention [54]. They have even described improvement of patents considered too unstable to undergo aggressive operative intervention after receiving 1 session of HBOT. Patients with gas gangrene are treated at 3 ATA for 90 minutes 3 times in 24 hours followed by twice daily for the ensuing 2 to 5 days. Treatment is extended if patients remain toxic. Reevaluation for the need for ongoing treatments is performed after 10 treatments.

Treatment of patients with NSTI is started at 2 to 2.5 ATA for 90 to 120 minutes twice daily until the patient is stabilized. The treatments are then decreased to once daily. Treatment continuation is reviewed after 10 treatments. HBOT should not delay surgical treatment in the case of NSTI.

ACUTE TRAUMATIC PERIPHERAL ISCHEMIAS

Pathophysiology

Crush, compartment syndrome, and compromised flaps result from tissue injury and/or ischemia within a myofascial compartment. Injury and or ischemia produces swelling causing an increase in pressure within the compartmental space. The increase in pressure leads to compression of veins, nerves, and (if left untreated) arteries, leading to diminished perfusion of the tissues in the involved compartment. Injured muscle produces and releases inflammatory cytokines that cause increased vascular permeability, migration of neutrophils, and swelling. As the perfusion decreases, damaged muscles release histaminelike substances that further increase vascular permeability. The increased permeability causes plasma fluid leakage, leading to further diminution of tissue perfusion, causing more tissue hypoxia and ischemia. Muscle and

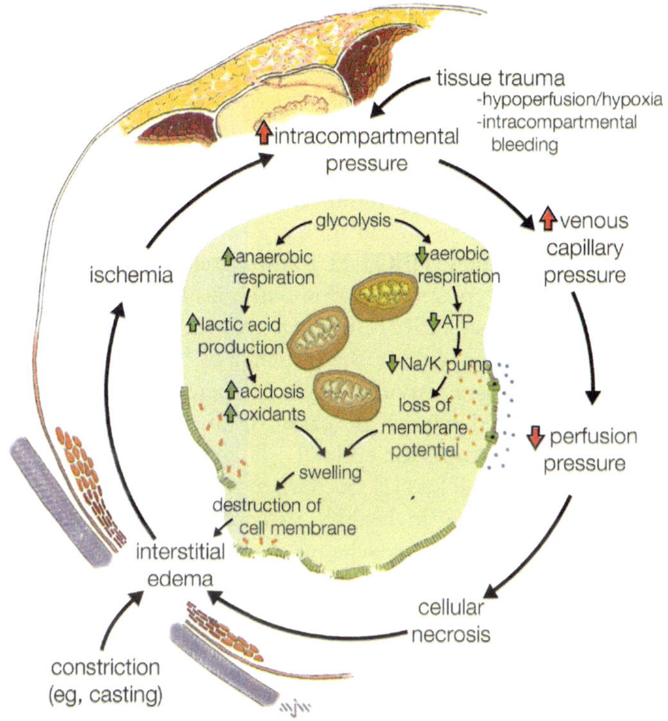

Fig. 6. Pathophysiology of acute traumatic peripheral ischemias. Constriction, tissue trauma, edema, or bleeding cause increased pressure within a myofascial or osteofascial compartment. As the intracompartmental pressure increases, the venous capillary pressure increases leading to hypoperfusion (*red arrows*). Intracellular metabolism converts from aerobic to anaerobic. The cell becomes acidotic and oxidants accumulate. The cell swells as the Na/K pump fails. The cell membrane is destroyed and intracellular contents enter the interstitium resulting in more edema. When perfusion is decreased below critical thresholds for an extended time, cell death and necrosis result. (*Reproduced from*: Henry S and Park H. Extremity Fasciotomies. In The Shock Trauma Manual of Operative Techniques ed Scalea T. 2nd edition, 2021 Springer Baltimore, Maryland pp. 521-588.)

nerve death ensue unless the cycle is broken (Fig. 6) [73]. Damaged muscle releases myoglobin into the systemic circulation, which can result in renal injury and profound electrolyte disturbances that can result in cardiac arrythmias.

Tissue at the point of injury is devitalized and nonviable and requires surgical debridement. Fracture stabilization, when required, remains an immediate priority using techniques that minimize further tissue injury. Tissue outside the zone injury is vulnerable, with varying degrees of damage leading to a susceptible zone outside the area of injury. Hyperbaric oxygen has the potential to affect this midzone by improving local conditions and perfusion [39,50]. In acute trauma, these tissue disorders often occur in association with fractures, further complicating wound healing and potential for infection.

Why it works

Oxygen is a universal requirement for cellular metabolic function. Tissue edema and increased compartmental pressure eliminate oxygen transfer across the capillary endothelium, worsening the hypoxic injury. Oxygen tensions less than 30 mm Hg inhibit cellular metabolic functions [39]. The hypoxic insult causes endothelium to be activated, causing the adhesion of neutrophils to it. Neutrophils release reactive oxygen radicals that cause tissue damage and vasoconstriction, resulting in reperfusion injury [74]. HBOT aids in these healing processes by multiple routes. HBOT at 2 atm increases the blood oxygen content by 125% [39]. Oxygen is increased in both plasma and tissue fluids by 10-fold [39]. While receiving HBOT, enough oxygen can be dissolved in the plasma to maintain tissues without the presence of hemoglobin-borne oxygen [75]. This dissolved oxygen provides ample compensation from the tissue hypoxia caused by increased oxygen diffusion distance from edema. Reversing acute tissue hypoxia interrupts the cycle of cellular ischemia leading to progressive edema and limits tissue loss [1]. Second, hyperoxygenation causes a reduction of blood flow by 20% in healthy vasculature, minimizing edema and interrupting the self-perpetuating ischemia cycle [39]. Fluid is resorbed at the capillary level while the vasoconstriction decreases the filtration of fluid from the capillary to the extracellular space. At the same time, vascular outflow is maintained and oxygen delivery improved. Hyperoxia of the plasma maintains delivery of oxygen to the tissues [76] In addition, HBOT can interrupt the reperfusion injury that accompanies crush and compartment syndromes. HBOT inhibits neutrophil sequestration and activation on the endothelium by inhibiting tumor necrosis factor alpha and intracellular adhesion molecule 1 (ICAM-1) production [74]. In addition, fibrinolysis is stimulated through activation of tissue plasminogen activator. When activated, neutrophils produce superoxide anions that interact with nitric oxide, producing a highly reactive peroxynitrite radical capable of producing further tissue injury. The highly oxygenated environment generates free oxygen radical scavengers such as superoxide dismutase, catalase, peroxidase, and glutathione [77]. These free oxygen radical scavengers decrease neutrophil-released ROS, which, in a hypoxic environment, are harder to clear [78].

Evidence for crush injury

The first described use of HBOT to treat crush injury was published in 1961 and involved a 16-year-old that sustained a Gustilo III C fracture dislocation of the ankle [79]. Complications arising from extensive crush injuries include osteomyelitis, amputations, failed flaps, and fracture nonunion. These complications in Gustilo type IIIB and IIIC injuries can be as high as 50% with standard techniques [1]. A double-blind, placebo-controlled clinical trial was done by Bouachour and colleagues [80] showing complete healing in 94% of patients after HBOT for crush injury treatment, as opposed to 55% in the control group (P<.01). In addition, only 6% required further surgery in the HBOT group compared with 33% of the control group (P<.05). The study was limited

Table 5
Gustilo classification of open fractures and risk of healing complications

Grade	Findings	Complications (infections, nonhealing, amputation)
I	Puncture type wound, usually from inside to out	Almost nil
II	Laceration associated with the open fracture	10%
III	Crush component to the injury	Vary with the subtype
A	Sufficient soft tissue to cover the bone	~10%
B	Exposed bone remains after debridement	~50%
C	Concomitant major vascular injury to the extremity	>50%

From Buettner M F and Wolkenhauer D. Hyperbaric Oxygen Therapy in the Treatment of Open Fractures and Crush Injuries. Emergency Medicine Clinics of North America, 2007; 25(1): 177-188 https://doi.org/10.1016/j.emc.2007.01.008.

to 36 patients (18 in each arm); however, the groups were matched for multiple potential confounders. It concluded that HBOT improved healing in Gustilo grade III soft tissue injuries in older adults [80]. A 2005 systematic review containing 150 patients suggested beneficial effects of adjunct HBOT in 8 of the 9 studies. The study concluded that adjunctive hyperbaric oxygen is not likely to be harmful and could be beneficial if administered early [81]. The Hyperbaric Oxygen in Lower Limb Trauma (HOLLT) study, a multicenter prospective randomized trial, is underway to evaluate the use of HBOT on the outcome of patients with acute open tibial fractures judged to be at high risk for injury-related complications based on the injury and or host status [82].

Which patients benefit?

Despite an understanding of the physiologic effects of HBOT, precise guidelines are lacking for its use. Gustilo's classification of open fractures (Table 5) was used in 2 studies reporting clinical outcomes with the use of HBOT [83]. Patients with crush injury who benefit most from early HBOT are those who have Gustilo type IIIB and IIIC injuries. Intuitively, other factors are likely to affect healing in patients with these injuries, including the severity of injury, age, and comorbidities. Strauss [39] has published guidelines using a 10-point assessment tool. He suggests patients deemed moderately and severely compromised with lower Gustilo grade fractures would also benefit from the addition of HBOT to their treatments [39]. Table 6 describes Strauss' tool.

TREATMENT

There is no standard treatment protocol for patients with acute traumatic peripheral ischemias. HBOT should not delay surgical intervention but should be provided as soon as logistically possible. Most protocols call for 12

Table 6
Strauss criteria for using hyperbaric oxygen therapy in patients with acute traumatic peripheral ischemias

	Findings			
Criteria	2 points[a]	1 point[a]	0 points[a]	Interpretation
Age (y)	< 40	40–60	>60	Healthy 8–10 points
Ambulation[b]	Community	Household	None	—
Cardiovascular/renal function[c]	Normal	Compensated with medication	Decompensated even under medication	Impaired 4-7 points
Smoking/steroid use[c]	None	> 5 years	Current	—
Neuropathy/deformity[c]	None	Mild to moderate	Severe	Severely compromised 3 or less points

[a]Use half-points if observations are between 2 findings.
[b]Subtract one-half point if walking aids required.
[c]Whichever gives the lower score.
From Strauss MB. Hyperbaric oxygen for crush injuries and compartment syndromes. In: Bakker DJ, Cramer FS, editors. Hyperbaric surgery perioperative care. Flagstaff (AZ): Best Publishing Company; 2002. p. 344.

treatments delivered at 2.0 to 2.4 ATA. Treatments are usually delivered twice daily, but some clinicians recommend 3 treatments per day for the first 2 days. Early initiation of treatment is preferred for crush injuries. The schedule is determined by the injury's specific pathophysiology, but most recommend 2 ATA in monoplace chambers or 2.4 ATA in multiplace chambers. For critical ischemia, 3 treatments within 24 hours are warranted. For resultant threatened flaps and wound healing, twice-daily treatment is suggested. In addition, daily or isolated treatments are considered for infections, resorption of calcified tissue, and reperfusion after thrombectomy/revascularization. The HOLLT study protocol calls for treatment to begin within 48 hours of injury for a total of 12 treatments. In this study, schedule variability is allowed based on the logistics of the center. The plan includes delivery of a dose with the bioequivalency of 90 minutes at 2.4 ATA [82].

Evidence for compartment syndrome

At present, there are no randomized controlled trials for the use of HBOT in compartment syndrome, but there are hundreds of case studies showing its benefit in practice [84–87]. If the American Heart Association's criteria for effectiveness are used, treatment with HBOT for compartment syndrome would fit into class I level C because of the inherent low risk of the therapy and its large potential benefit, especially in the impending stage of compartment syndrome. It is the only intervention with the potential to stop impending compartment syndrome from progressing to the established stage [39]. The groundwork for HBOT use in compartment syndrome derives from the study of canine injury models, which showed statistically significantly less skeletal muscle necrosis, defined by technetium 99m uptake, in HBOT-treated subjects compared with controls [88]. Bartlett and colleagues [89] performed electrophysiologic monitoring in a canine model of compartment injuries. HBOT-treated animals showed significantly better muscle function than those animals treated with fasciotomy alone [1,89].

HBOT is an adjunct treatment and does not replace fasciotomy. Compartment syndrome can generally be divided into 3 stages: suspected, impending, and established. Suspected compartment syndrome in this staging system occurs when the injury sustained was severe enough to risk progression to compartment syndrome. In these cases, HBOT is not warranted [39]. Frequent neurovascular evaluations are performed to recognize progression. With impending compartment syndrome, signs such as increased pain, hyperesthesias, muscle weakness, compartment tenseness, and discomfort with passive stretch are observed, but criteria for fasciotomy are not met. Initiating HBOT at this stage potentially prevents progression to the next stage. Established compartment syndrome by this definition occurs when 3 or more findings associated with impending compartment syndrome are present or serial compartment pressure measurements reach the threshold that warrants fasciotomy. Surgical decompression is the priority; however, postoperative HBOT is warranted if there is ischemic muscle, unclear demarcation between viable and nonviable tissue, massive swelling, threatened skin flap/graft, residual neuropathy, or continued decompensation [1,39].

TREATMENT

Impending stage treatment involves HBOT at 2.0 to 2.4 ATA for 90 to 120 minutes twice over the first 24 hours. Clinical observation is needed to decide when treatments should be stopped thereafter. When used after fasciotomy, HBOT should be used twice a day for 7 to 10 days at the same ATA and treatment duration listed earlier [1,39].

EVIDENCE FOR COMPROMISED FLAPS

The standard treatment of compromised flaps is surgical debridement, local wound care, and when possible revisional reconstruction. HBOT has been included as an adjunct to this standard treatment. Evidence supporting the use of HBOT to salvage compromised flaps came from animal experiments. Exposure to HBOT resulted in significantly improved tissue survival [88]. The human data supporting HBOT use are small retrospective reviews. Variable outcomes have been reported, from complete healing in 36% in 1 study to improvement or significant improvement in 64% [90]. A systematic review included 10 case series or case reports, all with positive outcomes. Patients in these studies received, on average, 30 treatments. Nine of the 10 studies had low strength, leading the investigators to conclude that there was a low to moderate level of evidence supporting the use of HBOT for compromised grafts and flaps [12].

THERMAL BURNS

Thermal injuries are classified according to their cause and depth. In general, 3 zones are found at the injury site. The zone of coagulation represents the area of irreversible injury. The zone of stasis neighbors the zone of coagulation and has been subjected to injury but has the potential to survive or necrose. Last, there is the zone of hyperemia. This tissue is uninjured but affected by vasodilation induced by inflammation [91].The goal of burn care is to preserve the viable tissue in the zone of stasis along the margins of the thermal injury. Minimizing major complications that can follow thermal injuries, such as cellulitis, pneumonia, urinary tract infections, and sepsis, by decreasing the recovery time are other objectives of burn treatment. Both obstruction and destruction of the microvasculature occurs at the initial burn injury site. A cascade of events leads to depression of humoral and cellular immunity [92]. This compromised immunity is the most critical in the first 12 to 24 hours after the injury, resulting from the rapid development of ischemic necrosis in these wounds [92]. Thermal burns additionally cause extensive edema because of increased capillary permeability and eventual hypoproteinemia with resultant decreased intravascular oncotic pressure. A multitude of animal studies have shown that HBOT can aid in preserving tissues along the zone of stasis by numerous potential mechanisms. These mechanisms include reducing edema at the site of injury [93] , attenuating dermal ischemia [94], prevention of partial to full thickness tissue injury [95], preservation of both cellular and microcirculation integrity [96], enhancing neutrophil killing [36], and maintaining ATP levels for normal endothelial physiology [96,97]. Newer studies also suggest that HBOT can reduce the mechanical allodynia of burn injuries by upregulating opioid and melatonin receptors at multiple sites, further enhancing recovery [98].

Evidence for thermal injury

In the 1960s, HBOT was first observed to aid in the healing of burns when coal miners undergoing treatment of CO poisoning showed concurrent improvement of their thermal injuries after HBOT use [1,99]. Cianci and colleagues [100] then showed that HBOT can significantly reduce ($P<.012$) the length of hospital stays in patients with burns over 18% to 39% of their total body surface area (TBSA). A study in 1987 then compared 226 patients receiving HBOT with 609 historic controls with 35% TBSA. There was a significant reduction in fluid loss as well as earlier reepithelialization in the HBOT-treated patients, but there was only a reduction in mortality for high-risk groups [101,102]. In a 2018 study, 18 patients with 25% TBSA burns were compared with 17 historic controls. Patients treated with HBOT had a statistically significant improvement in pain and satisfaction scores [103]. In a 2021 systemic review of the use of HBOT in burn injuries, 47 publications met inclusion criteria with more than 3000 animal models, 58 human volunteers, and 2208 clinical study patients accounted for [102].

This study, which contained 3 prospective randomized trials, concluded that 29 out of 32 experimental and 10 out of 11 clinical studies showed positive effects of HBOT on healing, with a generally unanimous finding of decreased edema and fluid requirements in the HBOT-treated groups [102]. Future randomized controlled trials will be necessary to make a definitive assessment of the clinical value of HBOT in thermal burn injuries.

WHICH PATIENTS BENEFIT?

HBOT has been found to be the most clinically useful as an adjunctive treatment in patients with deep second-degree burns [103]. HBOT should be used in combination with standard-of-care burn treatment, including excision and grafting, dressing changes, nutritional support, and judicious use of antibiotics [1]. In addition, HBOT should be strongly considered when second-degree burns involve 20% or greater of the TBSA. It should also be considered when burns are located within areas where surgical debridement is difficult and imprecise, including hands, fingers, perineum, face, and ears [104]. Anecdotal evidence of ocular burn injuries improving at a more rapid rate with hyperbaric oxygen has been reported.

Treatment

Patients with no contraindications to HBOT and deemed fit should ideally have 3 treatments in the first 24 hours, with the first treatment being within 6 to 8 hours of the incident. For the following days, treatment should continue twice daily at the burn surgeon's discretion. Usually, 10 to 14 days of treatment are used for larger burns (TBSA 40%). All treatments should be at 2.0 or 2.4 ATA for 90 minutes each [1]. It is extremely important in these patients to monitor fluid status because HBOT may mask hypovolemia. Patients should only be treated with HBOT if the facility has both a hyperbaric chamber and a burn unit, as well as staff who are comfortable monitoring the patient and delivering therapy in a critical care setting [1,104].

SOFT TISSUE RADIONECROSIS AND DELAYED EFFECTS OF RADIATION

Radiation is successfully used to kill cancer cells through DNA damage but also affects surrounding normal cells. The DNA damage to normal cells occurs in rapidly dividing cells that are present in the gastrointestinal tract as well as the genitourinary tract. Damage that persists beyond a few months after initial radiation can be improved with HBOT. Radiation has been observed to lead to apoptosis and chronic fibrosis from fibrogenic cytokines triggered by remote radiation exposure [105]. HBOT enhances angiogenesis, reduces fibrosis, and mobilizes stem cells [106].

Hyperbaric oxygen has been used for treatment of mandibular radiation necrosis and patients that have had radiation doses greater than 6000 cGy.

Although most patients with osteoradionecrosis resolve well with conservative management, those with exposed bone benefit from HBOT. Like chronic osteomyelitis, the treatment of osteoradionecrosis requires surgical debridement. The Marx protocol is commonly used when treating osteoradionecrosis. Thirty HBOT treatments are administered before surgical debridement, followed by 10 treatments after [107]. The success of hyperbaric hyperoxia combined with surgery also depends on surgical technique. Several studies with negative or equivocal results of HBOT for osteoradionecrosis did not use the prescribed Marx protocol and cannot be compared with earlier studies showing remarkably positive effects. Nonadjunctive HBOT can be used in patients before and after mandibular tooth extraction. In addition, management of osteoradionecrosis of the jaw needs to occur with a surgical plan in mind, with frequent and direct communication between head and neck or oral surgeon and hyperbaric physician [107].

HBOT has a role in other areas with radiation injury, including patients with head and neck cancer where curative doses of radiation were used beyond the effect on the mandible. These patients have esophageal and tracheal lesions related to radiation [108,109]. Chest wall wounds are also seen in patients with breast cancer who have received radiation that stalled wound healing or who progress to necrotic wounds after extensive reconstructive breast surgery [110,111]. Hyperbaric oxygen has been used for nipple-sparing surgery with and without prior radiation.

In patients who receive pelvic radiation with resultant radiation cystitis, proctitis, and other rectal lesions, multiple studies have shown significant improvement in bleeding, pain, and frequency with HBOT [112–114]. Radiation cystitis is one of the most common indications for hyperbaric oxygen. Patients are treated until hematuria and other related symptoms resolve or improve. In multiplace chambers, very ill patients admitted to the hospital and on continuous bladder irrigation can be treated.

HBOT has also been successfully used for radiation proctitis and enteritis. Many studies report improvement in symptoms of both enteritis and proctitis when HBOT is used [115].

HBOT has been used in patients with neurologic radiation injuries such as radiation myelitis, brain necrosis, optic neuritis, and plexopathies [116]. These rare conditions require further documentation of efficacy. This goal is difficult, with few cases sent for hyperbaric consultation.

Some physicians hesitate to consider HBOT as a treatment modality in patients with cancer because of the incorrect belief that HBOT promotes cancer growth. There are numerous studies in both animals and humans that conclude that cancer growth is not potentiated by hyperbaric hyperoxia [117].

Patient selection for each of these indications requires in-depth review of the patient's prior radiation therapy as well as other treatments used for the resultant radiation damage. Most patients with delayed effects of radiation can be treated 6 months after the last dose of radiation or when they have evidence of delayed radiation effects.

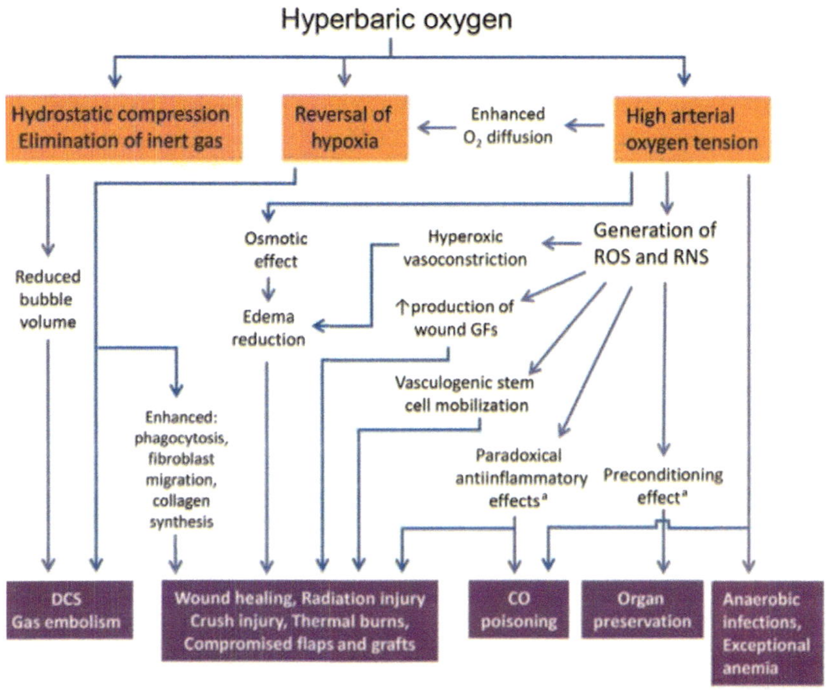

Fig. 7. Three principal therapeutic mechanisms of HBOT with linkage to some common indications. [a]Includes induction of multiple reactive species, including heat shock proteins and hemoxygenase-1. DCS, decompression sickness; GF, growth factors; RNS, reactive nitrogen species. (*Reproduced from* Bennett MH and Mitchell SJ. Emerging indications for hyperbaric oxygen, Curr Opin Anesthesiol 2019: 32(6): 792-798.)

Treatment

Standard dose and treatment of radiation injury requires 40 treatments at 2.0 to 2.4 ATA for 90 to 120 minutes. If patients have persistent symptoms, the number of treatments is increased incrementally until symptoms resolve or plateau.

For osteoradionecrosis of the jaw, the Marx protocol is typically used. That is, 30 treatments before surgical debridement and 10 treatments postoperatively. Nonadjunctive hyperbaric oxygen treatments before dental extraction of mandibular teeth typically involve 20 treatments before the procedure and 10 treatments after extraction.

OTHER AREAS OF INTEREST

Indications that are not yet approved but may be in the next few years include inflammatory bowel disease and severe traumatic brain injury (TBI). Both are current areas of research. The Hyperbaric Oxygen Brain Injury Trial (HOBIT) is an ongoing National Institutes of Health (NIH)–funded, phase 2, interventional, multicenter study evaluating the dose and duration of hyperbaric oxygen treatments for patients with initial Glasgow Coma Scale score of 3 to 8 following TBI [118]. This adaptive trial's results are not yet available.

Both Crohn disease and ulcerative colitis are areas of interest where HBOT shows promise. A recent phase 2B multicenter, randomized controlled trail showed lower rates of colectomy in HBOT-responsive patients at 3 months compared with controls [,[119,120]]. A larger phase 3 study is planned. Patients are treated for 5 days at 2.4 ATA for 90 minutes.

Severe complications such as fistula formation caused by Crohn disease have been treated with HBOT with promising results [120]. Optimal dosing is based on individual response and typically exceeds 20 treatments. Rigorous trials for Crohn disease are needed.

SUMMARY

HBOT is an acceptable treatment modality and should be considered for appropriate surgical patients. Although treatment with HBOT has been available and extensively studied for 80 years, it is not maximally used because of mixed clinical data caused by a variety of methodological constraints. Hyperbaric oxygen treatment is associated with a variety of physiologic responses that could intuitively reverse the pathophysiology of several conditions. Fig. 7 shows some of these. HBOT is also not universally readily available as an emergent or urgent treatment; however, knowledge of HBOT can allow informed use to assist surgeons in optimizing patient outcomes in a variety of conditions.

CLINICS CARE POINTS

- Timing of hyperbaric oxygen is important for most indications. Clinicians should consult hyperbaric medicine specialists at the earliest opportunity. This recommendation is especially important for NSTIs and acute peripheral ischemia, including crush and compartment syndrome.
- Patients with graft failure need emergent hyperbaric oxygen treatments.
- Patients with at-risk flaps can use hyperbaric oxygen if surgical or interventional options are not available.
- Pretreatment with hyperbaric oxygen when performing a procedure on previously irradiated areas should be considered. Postoperative wound healing complications in these areas may require hyperbaric oxygen for resolution.

Disclosure

The authors have nothing to disclose.

References

[1] Moon RE. UHMS hyperbaric oxygen therapy indication. 14th edition. North Palm Beach (FL): Best Publishing Company; 2019.

[2] Available at: https://www.medicare.gov/coverage/hyperbaric-oxygen-therapy. Accessed November 28, 2021.
[3] Hardy K. Physics of hyperbaric oxygen therapy in physiology and medicine of hyperbaric oxygen therapy E-Book. Neuman TS, Thom SR, editors. Philadelphia: Elsevier Health Sciences, 2008;57–64.
[4] Tibbles PM, Edelsberg JS. Hyperbaric-oxygen therapy. N Engl J Med 1996;334:1642–8.
[5] Rollins MD, Gibson JJ, Hunt TK, et al. Wound oxygen levels during hyperbaric oxygen treatment in healing wounds. Undersea Hyperb Med 2006;33(1):17–25.
[6] Londahl M, Fagher K, Katzman P. What is the role of hyperbaric oxygen in the management of diabetic foot disease? Curr Diab Rep 2011;11:285–93.
[7] Hart GB, Strauss MB. Gas gangrene-clostridial myonecrosis: a reveiw. J Hyperb Med 1990;5:125–44.
[8] Jokinen-Gordon H, Barry RC, Watson B, et al. A retrospective analysis of adverse events in hyperbaric oxygen therapy (2012-2015): lessons learned from 1.5 million treatments. Adv Skin Wound Care 2017;20(3):125–9.
[9] Lam G, Fontaine R, Ross FL, et al. Hyperbaric oxygen therapy: exploring the clinical evidence. Adv Skin Wound Care 2017;30(4):181–90.
[10] Goldstein LJ. Hyperbaric oxygen for chronic wounds. Dermatol Ther 2013;26(3): 207–14.
[11] Londahl M. Hyperbaric oxygen therapy as treatment of diabetic foot ulcers. Diabetes Metab Res Rev 2012;28(Supp 1):78–84.
[12] Goldman RJ. Hyperbaric oxygen therapy for wound healing and limb salvage: a systematic review. Am Acad Phys Med Rehabil 2009;1(5):471–88.
[13] Thackham JA, McElwain S, Long RJ. The use of hyperbaric oxygen therapy to treat chronic wounds: a review. Wound Regen Repair 2008;16:321–30.
[14] Amsler F, Willenberg T, Blattler W. In search of optimal compression therapy for venous leg ulcers: a meta-analysis of studies comparing divers' bandages with specifically designed stockings. J Vasc Surg 2009;50:668–74.
[15] Sen CK, Gordillo GM, Roy S, et al. Human skin wounds: a major and snowballing threat to public health and the economy. Wound Repair Regen 2009;17:763–71.
[16] Demidova-Rice TN, Hamblin MR, Herman IM. Acute and impaired wound healing: pathophysiology and current methods for drug delivery, part 1: normal and chronic wounds: biology, causes, and approaches to care. Adv Skin Wound Care 2012;25(7):304–14.
[17] Thom SR. Hyperbaric oxygen- its mechanisms and efficacy. Plast Reconstr Surg 2011;127(11):131S–41S.
[18] Hajhosseinin B, Kuehlmann BA, Bonham CA, et al. Hyperbaric oxygen therapy: descriptive review of the technology and current application in chronic wounds. Plast Reconstr Surg Glob Open 2020;8:e3136.
[19] Tiaka EK, Papanas N, Manolakis AC, et al. The role of hyperbaric oxygen in the treatment of diabetic foot ulcers. Angiology 2012;63:302–14.
[20] Baroni G, Porro T, Faglia E, et al. Hyperbaric oxygen in diabetic gangrene treatment. Diabetes Care 1987;10:81–6.
[21] Londahl M, Katzman P, Nilsson A, et al. Hyperbaric oxygen therapy facilitates healing of chronic foot ulcers in patients with diabetes. Diabetes care 2010;33:998–1003.
[22] Santema KTB, Stoekenbroek RM, Koelemay MJW, et al. Hyperbaric oxygen therapy in the treatment of ischemic lower-extremity ulcers in patients with diabetes: results of the DAMO2CLES multicenter randomized clinical trial. Diabetes Care 2018;41:112–9.
[23] Margolis DJ, Gupta J, Hoffstad O, et al. Lack of effectiveness of hyperbaric oxygen therapy for the treatment of diabetic foot ulcer and the prevention of amputation: a cohort study. Diabetes care 2013;36:1961–6.
[24] Andre-Levigne D, Modarressi A, Pignel R, et al. Hyperbaric oxygen therapy promotes wound repair in ischemic and hyperglycemic conditions, increasing tissue perfusion and collagen deposition. Wound Repair Regen 2016;24:954–65.

[25] Ennis WJ, Huang ET, Gordon H. Impact of Hyperbaric Oxygen on More Advanced Wagner Grades 3 and 4 diabetic foot ulcers: matching therapy to specific wound conditions. Adv Wound Care 2018;7(12):397–407.
[26] Kranke P, Bennet MH, Marty-St, et al. Hyperbaric oxygen therapy for chronic wounds. Cochrane Database Syst Rev 2015;6; https://doi.org/10.1002/14651858.CD004123.pub4:Art. No.: CD004123.
[27] Sharma R, Sharma SK, Mudgal SK, et al. Efficacy of hyperbaric oxygen therapy for diabetic foot ulcer, a systematic review and meta-analysis of controlled clinical trials. Sci Rep 2021;11:2189.
[28] Thistlethwaite KR, Finlayson KJ, Cooper PD, et al. The effectiveness of hyperbaric oxygen therapy for healing chronic venous leg ulcers: a randomized, double-blind placebo-controlled trial. Wound Repair Regen 2018;26:324–31.
[29] Huang E, Heyboer M, Savaser DJ. Hyperbaric oxygen therapy for the management of chronic wounds: patient selection and perspectives. Chronic Wound Care Management Research 2019;6:27–37.
[30] Cierny G. Surgical treatment of osteomyelitis. Plast Reconstr Surg 2011;127:190S–204S.
[31] Hatzenbuehler J, Pulling TJ. Diagnosis and management of osteomyelitis. Am Fam Physician 2011;84(9):1027–33.
[32] Calhoun JH, Cobos JA, Mader JT. Does Hyperbaric Oxygen have a Place in the treatment of osteomyelitis? Orthop Clin North Am 1991;22(3):467–71.
[33] Mader JT, Brown GL, Guckian JC, et al. A Mechanism for the amelioration by hyperbaric oxygen of experimental staphylococcal osteomyelitis in rabbits. J Infect Dis 1980;142: 915–20.
[34] Wang J, Li F, Calhoun JH. The role and effectiveness of adjunctive hyperbaric oxygen therapy in the management of musculoskeletal disorder. J Postgrad Med 2002;48(3):226–31.
[35] Mader JT, Guckian JC, Glass DL, et al. Therapy with hyperbaric oxygen for experimental osteomyelitis due to Staphylococcus aureus in rabbits. J Infect Dis 1978;138(3):312–8.
[36] Memar MY, Yekai M, Alizadeh N, et al. Hyperbaric oxygen therapy; antimicrobial mechanisms and clinical application for infections. Biomed Pharmacother 2019;109:440–7.
[37] Eltorai I, Hart GB, Strauss MB. Osteomyelitis in the spinal cord injured: A review and a preliminary report on the use of hyperbaric oxygen therapy. Paraplegia 1984;22:19–24.
[38] Kaide CG, Khandelwal S. Hyperbaric Oxygen: Applications in Infectious Disease. Emerg Med Clin North Am 2008;26:571–95.
[39] Strauss MB. Hyperbaric oxygen for crush injuries and compartment syndromes. In: Bakker DJ, Cramer FS, editors. Hyperbaric surgery perioperative care. Flagstaff (AZ): Best Publishing Company; 2002. p. 344.
[40] Brouwer RJ, Lalieu C, Hoencamp R, et al. A systematic review and meta-analysis of hyperbaric oxygen therapy for diabetic foot ulcers with arterial insufficiency. J Vasc Surg 2020;71:682–92.
[41] Psoinos CM, Flahive JM, Shaw JJ, et al. Contemporary trends in necrotizing soft-tissue infections in the United States. Surgery 2013;153:819–27.
[42] Simonsen SME, van Orman ER, Hatch BE, et al. Cellulitis incidence in a defined population. Epidemiol Infect 2006;134(2):293–9.
[43] Ontario Group A Streptococcal Study, Kaul R, McGeer A, Low DE, et al. Population based surveillance for group A streptococcal necrotizing fasciitis: Clinical features, prognostic indicators, and microbiologic analysis of seventy-seven cases. Ontario Group A Streptococcal Study. Am J Med 1997;103:18–24.
[44] May AK, Talisa VB, Wilfret DA, et al. Estimating the impact of necrotizing soft tissue infections in the United States: incidence and re-admissions. Surg Infections 2021;22(5): 509–15.
[45] Dworkin MS, Westercamp MD, Park L, et al. The epidemiology of necrotizing fasciitis including associated with death and amputation. Epidemiol Infect 2009;137:1609–14.
[46] Stevens DL, Bryant AE. Necrotizing Soft tissue infection. NEJM 2017;337:2263–5.

[47] Elliott DC, Kufera JA, Myers RAM. Necrotizing soft tissue infections risk factors for mortality and strategies for management. Ann Surg 1996;224(5):672–83.
[48] Henry S. Surgical Infections of skin and soft tissue. In: Britt LD, Peitzman AB, Barie PS, et al, editors. Acute care surgery. 2nd edition. New York: Wolters Kluwer; 2019. p. 706–22.
[49] Brummelkamp WH, Hogendijk J, Boerema I. Treatment of anerobic infections (clostridial myositis) by drenching the tissues with oxygen under high atmospheric pressure. Surgery 1961;49:299–302.
[50] William STB. The role of hyperbaric oxygen therapy in trauma. Trauma 2010;12:13–20.
[51] Marzella L, Vezzani G. Effect of Hyperbaric Oxygen on Activity of Antibacterial Agents. In: Oriani G, Marroni A, Wattel F, editors. Handbook on hyperbaric medicine. Milano (Italy): Springer; 1996; https://doi.org/10.1007/978-88-470-2198-3_24.
[52] Lerche CJ, Christophersen LJ, Kolpen M, et al. Hyperbaric oxygen therapy augments tobramycin efficacy in experimental Staphylococcus aureus endocarditis. Int J Antimicrob Agents 2017;50:406–12.
[53] Kolpen M, Mousavi N, Sams T, et al. Reinforcement of the bactericidal effect of ciprofloxacin on Pseudomonas aeruginosa biofilm by hyperbaric oxygen treatment. Int J Antimicrob Agents 2016;47:163–7.
[54] Hart GB, Lamb RC, Strauss MB. Gas Gangrene. J Trauma Inj Infect Crit Care 1983;23(11): 991–1000.
[55] Demello FJ, Haglin JJ, Hitchcock R. Comparative study of experimental Clostridium. perfringens infection in dogs treated with antibiotics, surgery. Hyperb oxygen Surg 1973;73(6): 936–41.
[56] Hirn M. Hyperbaric oxygen in the treatment of gas gangrene and perineal necrotizing fasciitis. A clinical and experimental study. Eur J Surg Suppl 1993;570:1–36.
[57] Korhonen K, Kuttila K, Niinikoski J. Tissue gas tensions in patients with necrotising fasciitis and healthy controls during treatment with hyperbaric oxygen: a clinical study. Eur J Surg 2000;166(7):530–4.
[58] Mindrup SR, Kealey P, Fallon B. Hyperbaric oxygen for the treatment of Fournier's gangrene. J Urol 2005;173:1975–7.
[59] Shaw JJ, Psoinos C, Emhoff TA, et al. Not just full of hot air: hyperbaric oxygen therapy increases survival in cases of necrotizing soft tissue infections. Surg Infections 2014;15(3): 328–35.
[60] Riseman JA, Zamboni WA, Graham DR, et al. Hyperbaric oxygen therapy for necrotizing fasciitis reduces mortality and the need for debridements. Surgery 1990;108(5):847–50.
[61] Devaney B, Frawley G, Frawley L, et al. Necrotising soft tissue infections: the effect of hyperbaric oxygen on mortality. Anaesth Intensive Care 2015;43:685–92.
[62] Soh CR, Pietrobon R, Freiberger JJ, et al. Hyperbaric oxygen therapy in necrotising soft tissue infections: a study of patients in the United States Nationwide Inpatient Sample. Intensive Care Med 2012;38(7):1143–51.
[63] Escobar SJ, Slade JB, Hunt TK, et al. Adjuvant Hyperbaric oxygen therapy (HB02) for treatment of necrotizing fasciitis reduces mortality and amputation rate. UHM 2005;32(6): 437–43.
[64] Wilkinson D, Doolette D. Hyperbaric oxygen treatment and survival from necrotizing soft tissue infection. Arch Surg 2004;139:1239–345.
[65] Massey PR, Sakran JV, Mills AM, et al. Hyperbaric oxygen therapy in necrotizing soft tissue infections. JSR 2012;177:146–51.
[66] Shupak A, Shoshani O, Goldenberg I, et al. Necrotizing fasciitis: an indication for hyperbaric oxygenation therapy? Surgery 1995;118:873–8.
[67] Brown DR, Davis NL, Lepawsky M, et al. A multicenter review of the treatment of major truncal necrotizing infections with and without hyperbaric oxygen therapy. Am J Surg 1994;167(5):485–9.
[68] Hassan Z, Mullins RF, Friedman BC, et al. Treating necrotizing fasciitis with or without hyperbaric oxygen therapy. Undersea Hyperb Med 2010;37(2):115–23.

[69] Levett D, Bennett MH, Millar I. Adjunctive hyperbaric oxygen for necrotizing fasciitis. Cochrane Database Syst Rev 2015;1; https://doi.org/10.1002/14651858.CD007937.pub2:Art. No.: CD007937.
[70] Thrane JF, Ovensen T. Scarce evidence of efficacy of hyperbaric oxygen therapy in necrotizing soft tissue infection: a systematic review. Infect Dis 2019;51(7):485–92.
[71] Hedetoft M, Bennett MH, Hyldegaard O. Adjunctive hyperbaric oxygen treatment for necrotising soft-tissue infections: a systematic review and meta-analysis. Diving Hyperb Med 2021;51(1):34–43.
[72] Schneidewind L, Anheuser P, Schönburg S, et al. Hyperbaric Oxygenation in the Treatment of Fournier's Gangrene: A Systematic Review. Urol Int 2021;105(3–4):247–56.
[73] Henry S, Park H. Extremity Fasciotomies. In: The shock trauma manual of operative techniques ed Scalea T. 2nd edition. Maryland (MD): Springer Baltimore; 2021. p. 521–88.
[74] Francis A, Baynosa R. Ischaemia-reperfusion injury and hyperbaric oxygen pathways: a review of cellular mechanisms. Diving Hyperb Med 2017;47(2):110–7.
[75] Greensmith JE. Hyperbaric oxygen reverses organ dysfunction in severe anemia. Anesthesiology 2000;93:1149–52.
[76] Gill AL, Bell CNA. Hyperbaric oxygen: its uses mechanisms of action and outcomes. Q J Med 2004;97:385–95.
[77] Camporesi EM. Side effects of hyperbaric oxygen therapy. Undersea Hyperb Med 2014;41:253–7.
[78] Ferrari R, Ceconi C, Curello S, et al. Oxygen-mediated myocardial damage during ischaemia and reperfusion: role of the cellular defenses against oxygen toxicity. J Mol Cell Cardiol 1985;17(10):937–45.
[79] Smith G, Stevens J, Griffiths JC, et al. Near-avulsion of foot treated by replacement and subsequent prolonged exposure of patients to oxygen at two atmospheres pressure. Lancet 1961;2:1122–3.
[80] Bouachour G, Cronier P, Gouello JP, et al. Hyperbaric oxygen therapy in the management of crush injuries: a randomized double-blind placebo-controlled clinical trial. J Trauma 1996;41(2):333–9.
[81] Garcia-Covarrubias L, McSwain NE Jr, Van Meter K, et al. Adjuvant hyperbaric oxygen therapy in the management of crush injury and traumatic ischemia: an evidence-based approach. Am Surg 2005;71(2):144–51.
[82] Millar IL, McGinnes RA, Williamson O, et al. Hyperbaric Oxygen in Lower Limb Trauma (HOLLT); Protocol for a randomised controlled trial. BMJ Open 2015;5:e008381.
[83] Yamada N, Toyoda I, Doi T, et al. Hyperbaric oxygenation therapy for crush injuries reduces the risk of complications: research report. UHM 2014;41(4):283–9.
[84] Hoy G, Hasenkam C, Fock A, et al. Hyperbaric oxygen as an adjunctive therapy post fasciotomy for unilateral supraspinatus rhabdomyolysis and compartment syndrome. Case Rep Orthop 2018;5485767; https://doi.org/10.1155/2018/5485767.
[85] Karam MD, Amendola A, Mendoza-Lattes S. Case report: successful treatment of acute exertional paraspinal compartment syndrome with hyperbaric oxygen therapy. Iowa Orthop J 2010;30:188–90.
[86] Fitzpatrick DT, Murphy PT, Bryce M. Adjunctive treatment of compartment syndrome with hyperbaric oxygen. Mil Med 1998;163(8):577–9.
[87] Malerba F, Oriani G, Farnetti A. HBO in orthopedic disorders. In: Oriani G, Marroni A, Watterl F, editors. Handbook on hyperbaric medicine. Milan (Italy): Springer; 1996. p. 409–27.
[88] Strauss MB, Hargens AR, Gershuni DH, et al. Reduction of skeletal muscle necrosis using intermittent hyperbaric oxygen in a model compartment syndrome. J Bone Joint Surg Am 1983;65(5):656–62.
[89] Bartlett RL, Stroman RT, Nickels M, et al. Rabbit model of the use of fasciotomy and hyperbaric oxygen in the treatment of compartment syndrome. Undersea Hyperb Med 1998;25(Suppl):29.

[90] Larson JV, Steensma EA, Flikkema RM, et al. The application of hyperbaric oxygen therapy in the management of compromised flaps. Undersea Hyperb Med 2013;40:499–504.
[91] Arturson G. Pathophysiology of the burn wound and pharmacological treatment. The Rudi Hermans Lecture, 1995. Burns 1996;22(4):255–74.
[92] Edwards M, Singh M, Selesny S, et al. Hyperbaric treatment of thermal burns. In: StatPearls. Treasure Island (FL): StatPearls Publishing; 2021.
[93] Oley MH, Oley M, Aling DMR, et al. Effects of hyperbaric oxygen therapy on the healing of thermal burns and its relationship with ICAM-1: A case-control study. Ann Med Surg (Lond) 2020;61:104–9.
[94] Türkaslan T, Yogun N, Cimşit M, et al. Is HBOT treatment effective in recovering zone of stasis? An experimental immunohistochemical study. Burn 2010;36(4):539–44.
[95] Stewart RJ, Yamaguchi KT, Cianci PE etc. Burn wound levels of ATP after exposure to elevated levels of oxygen. In: Proceedings of the American burn association, New Orleans (LA); 1989. p. 67.
[96] Zamboni WA, Roth AC, Russell RC, et al. Morphologic analysis of the microcirculation during reperfusion of ischemic skeletal muscle and the effect of hyperbaric oxygen. Plast Reconstr Surg 1993;91(6):1110–23.
[97] Wu ZS, Wu SH, Lee SS, et al. Dose-Dependent Effect of Hyperbaric Oxygen Treatment on Burn-Induced Neuropathic Pain in Rats. Int J Mol Sci 2019;20(8):1951.
[98] Wada J, Ikeda T, Kamata K, et al. Oxygen hyperbaric treatment for carbon monoxide poisoning and severe burn in coal mine (hokutanyubari) gas explosion. Igakkunoaymi (Japan) 1965;5:53.
[99] Cianci P, Lueders HW, Lee H, et al. Adjunctive hyperbaric oxygen therapy reduces length of hospitalization in thermal burns. J Burn Care Rehabil 1989;10(5):432–5.
[100] Niu AKC, Yang C, Lee HC. Burns treated with adjunctive hyperbaric oxygen therapy: A comparative study in humans. J Hyperb Med 1987;2:75–85.
[101] Smolle C, Lindenmann J, Kamolz L, et al. The History and Development of Hyperbaric Oxygenation (HBO) in Thermal Burn Injury. Medicina (Kaunas) 2021;57(1):49.
[102] Chen K-L, Wu C-J, Tseng W-S, et al. Improvement of satisfaction in burn patients receiving adjuvant hyperbaric oxygen therapy. Formos J Surg 2018;51:184–92.
[103] Mathieu D, Marroni A, Kot J. Tenth European Consensus Conference on Hyperbaric Medicine: recommendations for accepted and non-accepted clinical indications and practice of hyperbaric oxygen treatment. Diving Hyperb Med 2017;47(1):24–32 [Erratum appears in Diving Hyperb Med 2017;47(2):131-132].
[104] Delanian S, Lefaix JL. The radiation-induced fibroatrophic process: therapeutic perspective via the antioxidant pathway. Radiother Oncol 2004;73(2):119–31.
[105] Fleckenstein K, Gauter-Fleckenstein B, Jackson IL, et al. Using biological markers to predict risk of radiation injury. Semin Radiat Oncol 2007;17(2):89–98.
[106] Feldmeier JJ, Gesell LB. Delayed Radiation Injuries (Soft tissue and bony necrosis) and Potential for Future Research. In: Moon R, editor. Hyperbaric oxygen therapy indications. 14th edition. North Palm Beach (FL): Best Publishing Company; 2019. p. 163–202.
[107] Ariza-Prota M, Morales A, Grajeda J, et al. Successful Healing of Tracheal Radionecrosis: Role of Hyperbaric Oxygen Therapy. Chest 2016;150(6):e147–50.
[108] Ajayi OD, Leggett CL, Myburgh SJ, et al. Esophageal stricture following radiation, concurrent immunochemotherapy, treated with hyperbaric oxygen and dilation. Mayo Clin Proc Innov Qual Outcomes 2019;3(2):241–5.
[109] Rajpal N, Walters ET, Elmarsafi T, et al. Use of hyperbaric oxygen therapy for tissue ischemia after breast reconstruction. Undersea Hyperb Med 2019;46(4):461–5.
[110] Carl UM, Feldmeier JJ, Schmitt G, et al. Hyperbaric oxygen therapy for late sequelae in women receiving radiation after breast-conserving surgery. Int J Radiat Oncol Biol Phys 2001;49(4):1029–31.

[111] Oscarsson N, Müller B, Rosén A, et al. Radiation-induced cystitis treated with hyperbaric oxygen therapy (RICH-ART): a randomised, controlled, phase 2-3 trial. Lancet Oncol 2019;20(11):1602–14.

[112] Cooper JS, Hanley ME. Hyperbaric Treatment of Radiation Proctitis. In: StatPearls. Treasure Island (FL: StatPearls Publishing; 2021.

[113] Yuan JH, Song LM, Liu Y, et al. The effects of hyperbaric oxygen therapy on pelvic radiation induced gastrointestinal complications (rectal bleeding, diarrhea, and pain): a meta-analysis. Front Oncol 2020;10:390.

[114] Hampson NB, Holm JR, Wreford-Brown CE, et al. Prospective assessment of outcomes in 411 patients treated with hyperbaric oxygen for chronic radiation tissue injury. Cancer 2012;118(15):3860–8.

[115] Stowe HB, Mullins BT, Chera BS. Hyperbaric oxygen therapy for radiation-induced brachial plexopathy, a case report and literature review. Rep Pract Oncol Radiother 2020;25(1):23–7.

[116] Moen I, Stuhr LE. Hyperbaric oxygen therapy and cancer–a review. Target Oncol 2012;(4):233–42.

[117] Available at: https://clinicaltrials.gov/ct2/show/NCT02407028?term=NCT02407028&rank=1. Accessed November 28, 2021.

[118] Dulai PS, Raffals LE, Hudesman D, et al. A phase 2B randomised trial of hyperbaric oxygen therapy for ulcerative colitis patients hospitalised for moderate to severe flares. Aliment Pharmacol Ther 2020;52(6):955–63.

[119] Dulai PS, Buckey JC Jr, Raffals LE, et al. Hyperbaric oxygen therapy is well tolerated and effective for ulcerative colitis patients hospitalized for moderate-severe flares: a phase 2A pilot multi-center, randomized, double-blind, sham-controlled trial. Am J Gastroenterol 2018;113(10):1516–23.

[120] Lansdorp CA, Gecse KB, Buskens CJ, et al. Hyperbaric oxygen therapy for the treatment of perianal fistulas in 20 patients with Crohn's disease. Aliment Pharmacol Ther 2021;53(5): 587–97.

[121] Doctor N, Pandya S, Supe A. Hyperbaric oxygen therapy in diabetic foot. J Postgrad Med 1992;38(3):112–4, 1303408.

[122] Faglia E, Favales F, Aldeghi A, Calia P, Quarantiello A, Oriani G, et al. Adjunctive systemic hyperbaric oxygen therapy in treatment of severe prevalently ischemic diabetic foot ulcer. A randomized study. Diabetes Care 1996;19(12):1338–43.

[123] Kessler L, Bilbault P, Ortega F, Grasso C, Passemard R, Stephan D, Pinget M, Schneider F. Hyperbaric oxygenation accelerates the healing rate of nonischemic chronic diabetic foot ulcers: a prospective randomized study. Diabetes Care 2003;26(8):2378–82; https://doi.org/10.2337/diacare.26.8.2378, 12882865.

[124] Abidia A, Laden G, Kuhan G, Johnson BF, Wilkinson AR, Renwick PM, et al. The role of hyperbaric oxygen therapy in ischaemic diabetic lower extremity ulcers: a double-blind randomised-controlled trial. European Journal of Vascular and Endovascular Surgery 2003;25:513–8.

[125] Duzgun AP, Satir HZ, Ozozan O, Saylam B, Kulah B, Coskun F. Effect of hyperbaric oxygen therapy on healing of diabetic foot ulcers. Journal of Foot and Ankle Surgery 2008;47(6):515–9.

[126] Fedorko L, Bowen JM, Oreopoulos G, Goeree R, Hopkins RB, O'Reilly DJ. Hyperbaric Oxygen Therapy Does Not Reduce Indications for Amputation in Patients with Diabetes with Nonhealing Ulcers of the Lower Limb: A Prospective, Double-Blind, Randomized Controlled Clinical Trial. Diabetes Care 2016;39(3):392–9; https://doi.org/10.2337/dc15-2001, 26740639.

Advances in Surgery 56 (2022) 205–227

ADVANCES IN SURGERY

Endoscopic Treatment of Gastroesophageal Reflux Disease

William S. Richardson, MD[a,b,*],
Jessica Koller Gorham, MD, DABOM[a], Nicole Neal, MD[a],
Robert D. Fanelli, MD, MHA[c,d]

[a]Ochsner Clinic, 1514 Jefferson Highway, New Orleans, LA 70121, USA; [b]University of Queensland, Brisbane, Australia; [c]Department of Surgery, The Guthrie Clinic, One Guthrie Square, Sayre, PA 18840, USA; [d]Geisinger Commonwealth School of Medicine, Sayre, PA, USA

Keywords

• Endoscopic antireflux surgery • Antireflux operation
• Transoral incisionless fundoplication • TIF Stretta • Antireflux mucosectomy

Key points

- Stretta and TIF are relatively easy to learn although endoscopic suturing is a very new skill. Mucosectomy will require more training for surgeons not already doing the techniques involved.
- Stretta and TIF both have very good outcomes in appropriate patients. Complications of these procedures seem less than laparoscopic fundoplication.
- Mucosectomy is a newer procedure but seems promising.

Video content accompanies this article at http://www.advancessurgery.com.

RADIOFREQUENCY ENERGY

Introduction

The only FDA approved device for GERD treatment in this area is Stretta (Restech, Houston, TX, USA) which was approved in 2000 (Fig. 1). Stretta is indicated for patients with reflux and hiatal hernias less than 2 cm. Increased

*Corresponding author. *E-mail address:* wrichardson@ochsner.org

https://doi.org/10.1016/j.yasu.2022.04.001

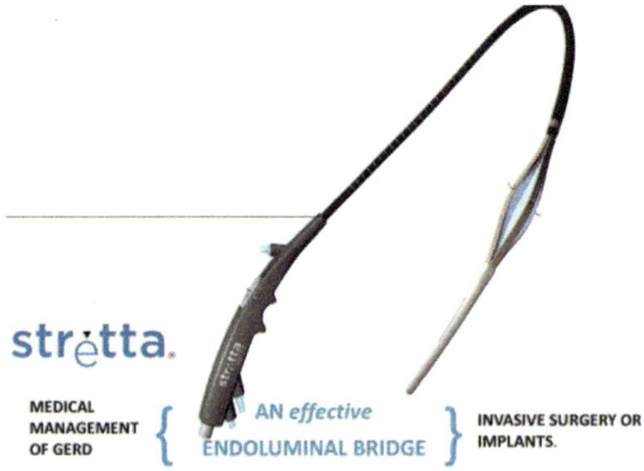

Fig. 1. Stretta. (*Courtesy* Restech, Houston, Texas).

complication rates are seen with larger hiatal hernias. In addition, patients with hiatal hernias may have difficulty with the device deploying well enough to cause the desired effect. Typically, the patient's reflux improves immediately after the procedure for a few days then worsens and finally improves again. Therefore, the full effect of the device is not known for approximately 3 months. Interestingly as this does not require any suturing to recreate a fundoplication this device can be used in patients who have had their fundus removed such as after bariatric surgery. It can also be used with patients who developed reflux after laparoscopic fundoplication.

Indications and contraindications

Workup is similar for any other reflux procedure and includes endoscopy, motility study and pH probe and/or gastric emptying study as indicated. Radiofrequency energy is indicated for all patients with significant reflux symptoms and workup showing reflux. Patients should have tried PPI with at least some improvement in symptoms, have side effects requiring stopping PPI, be allergic to PPI or are not compliant with taking PPI. Extraesophageal symptoms are an indication. Patients with prior surgery such as gastric bypass, sleeve edge, prior fundoplication, post lung transplant can also be treated with this modality. Patients under the age of 18, pregnant, with achalasia or LES obstruction and poor surgical candidates are not candidates for this therapy. Contraindications include hiatal hernia over 2 cm and dilated esophagus, and this is since the needles used with this device are unlikely to penetrate deep enough to be affective. Significant esophageal stricture would also be a contraindication but the device itself was not very wide. Also, erosive esophagitis is a contraindication. As this device uses radiofrequency, devices that could pick this up need to be turned off such as pacemakers and stimulators during use. This procedure avoids the implantation of any foreign body.

Mechanism of action

Stretta delivers radiofrequency energy to the lower esophageal sphincter muscle and gastric cardia. Studies are conflicting over how the procedure works. Radiofrequency application directly effects the muscle by decreasing compliance and increasing thickness, yield pressure and TLSRs in animal studies [1–3]. In humans, Stretta has been shown to decrease acid exposure [4]. In a double blind sham-controlled study, Stretta improved GERD symptoms and was shown to decrease GEJ compliance [5]. There are analyses that show no increase in LES pressure and will be discussed in the outcomes section. At the very least it seems that Stretta decreases LES compliance.

Procedure

The procedure can be performed under moderate sedation or general anesthesia (Stretta Incisionless Procedure to Treat Reflux, GERD - YouTube). Continuous pulse oximetry and blood pressure monitoring should be used throughout the procedure. Supplemental oxygen should be applied. The case can be conducted either in the left lateral decubitus position or with the patient prone and takes about 25 minutes. Endoscopy is performed with the evaluation of the esophagus, stomach and duodenum. Assessing the lower esophageal sphincter, size of hiatal hernia or esophageal dilation should be notas the procedure may be contraindicated. The z line should be measured twice from a fixed point such as the incisors and a wire is placed into the stomach and the endoscope removed. The radiofrequency procedure is performed in a standard technique with 8 antegrade treatments on the esophagus and 6 pullback treatments on the cardia (Fig. 2). The catheter is placed over the wire into the stomach and positioned above the z line. The balloon is inflated, and needles deployed. The needles are 5.5 mm and once deployed radiofrequency energy is delivered for approximately 60 seconds to achieve a tissue temperature of 80° Celsius. Additional treatments are conducted by deflating the balloon, retracting the needles and twisting the device 45°, balloon inflation, redeployment of needles and retreatment and repeating this several times along the distal esophagus and proximal stomach. There are a are a total of 56 administrations and it should be noted how many of them have note reached target temperature although it is common to have a few failures. Radiofrequency administration will stop once target temperature is reached or if impedance becomes elevated. After treatment the device and wire are removed, and endoscopy is performed which will show successful treatment and any complications (see Fig. 2).

Outcomes

There are 6 randomized studies and the 2 most recent give conflicting results on Stretta's efficacy on GERD symptoms [5–10]. All except the one of the most recent randomized studies have been included in some of the 4 meta-analyses on Stretta.

Perry and colleagues 2012 meta-analysis identified 22 publications with Stretta as primary treatment of gerd with at least 3-month follow-up [11]. This study

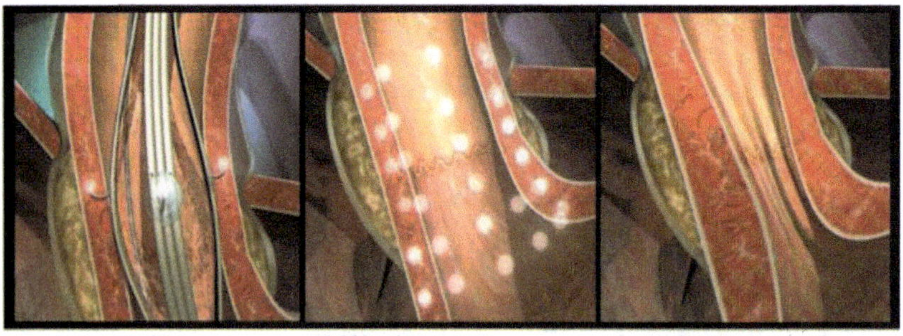

Fig. 2. LES and stretta. (*Courtesy* Restech, Houston, Texas).

included 2 rtcs on Stretta. This study showed a significant decrease in heartburn scores, acid exposure and LES pressure. Lipka and colleagues in their meta-analysis analyzed the randomized studies in 2015 and a total of 4 studies were included [12]. The overall quality of the evidence was considered very low but the outcomes showed no beneficial effect of Stretta. Fass and colleagues in a later meta-analysis which included at least 3-month follow-up, controlled trials and cohort studies included 28 studies with a total of 2468 patients and this study included 4 randomized studies and pooled and unpooled results of these studies [13]. Eleven of 12 studies that had heartburn score outcomes showed significant heartburn improvement, ph improvement (although not to normalization), Demeester score improvement with Stretta with pooled data. The LES pressure was significantly increased by Stretta in the pooled data but not significantly increased from the sham group. Adverse event reporting was available for 26 studies and showed an incidence of 0.93% in the Stretta group (vs 7.18% in the laparoscopic fundoplication group). The most frequent events were erosions and mucosal lacerations. Xie and colleagues in their 2021 meta-analysis included 5 randomized controlled trials [14]. This study identified 2 Stretta studies that had outcomes on quality of life and showed improvement, but the quality was graded as low. These studies compared with TIF (transoral incisionless fundoplication) which was not significantly different. 4 studies reported heartburn results and TIF and Stretta had significant improvement but were not significantly different from each other. 5 rcts reported on LES pressure and TIF was more significant at raising LES pressure than Stretta. 3 rcts reported on acid exposure using Stretta and this showed 89.1% improvement. 4 rcts reported on esophagitis rate and Stretta showed 57.3% improvement (TIF showed better improvement). Reduction or withdrawal of PPI was shown in 4 rcts and there was no significant difference in rate between TIF and Stretta but the overall change in rate was 92.1% for TIF, 56.5 for Stretta and 1.4% for ppi. The quality of evidence for the outcomes was low to moderate. Overall, most of the analyses show effectiveness for Stretta with low risk and relative cost to fundoplication.

Overall risks appear low. From the Maude database from 2006 to 2020 with 35,000 Stretta cases the adverse event rate was 0.0001% (3 events). The cost seems relatively low as well. From the manufacturer the cost is $3500 to 6000. This is likely less than TIF and certainly less than transabdominal procedures.

Durability

In Dughera's 8 year study on 26 patients Stretta showed improved Gerd hrql scores and Qol scores and 76.9% or patients were off PPI [15]. Motility showed no increase in LES pressure. Ph probes showed improvement at 4 years but returned to baseline at 8 years. The only adverse event was gastroparesis that was limited to 3 weeks.

In Noar's 10 year study 217 patients were prospectively followed [16]. Normalization of gerd-hrql was found in 72% of patients. 50% or greater reduction of ppi use was found in 64% of patients (41% off ppi). Regarding harms they noted occasional short-term chest pain following the procedure and 2 cases of bleeding requiring no treatment. They also noted regression of Barrett's in 85% of patients. They had a median procedure time of 25 minutes.

Reymunde and colleagues reported 4-year and 15-year follow-up but the 15 year is an abstract [17,18]. At 4 years there was significant improvement in QoL, GERD symptom scores significantly improved from 2.7 (baseline) to 0.6. PPI was reduced from 100% of patients to 13.75%. At 15 years with 35 patients followed up the QoL continued to be significantly improved, GERD symptom score significantly improved 2.7 to 1.1, ppi use for 100% to on demand ppi use for less than 25% of patients.

Radiofrequency energy for gerd after other operations

In patients with GERD and with reoperative fields or when the fundus has been removed with prior surgery Stretta is still effective and low risk if there are no contraindications to Stretta. Recurrent gerd after fundoplication or bariatric surgery are examples (Fig. 3). There is not as much literature to make strong recommendations in this area but there seems to be little risk to the procedure in the available literature. For example, in Noar's study of 18 patients after failed fundoplication and followed over 10 years showed continued improvement following Stretta (gerd-hrql scores) [19]. There were no adverse events reported.

TRANSORAL INCISIONLESS FUNDOPLICATION (TIF)

Introduction

Transoral Incisionless Fundoplication (TIF) is an endoluminal procedure for gastroesophageal reflux disease (GERD) that is performed using the EsophyX device manufactured by EndoGastric Solutions, Inc. to deploy proprietary SerosaFuse fasteners in the construction of a 270° to 300° partial fundoplication. The device launched in 2006, and was cleared for use by the Food and Drug Administration (FDA) in 2007, and both the device and procedure have undergone several important evolutionary steps [20]. The device currently used in

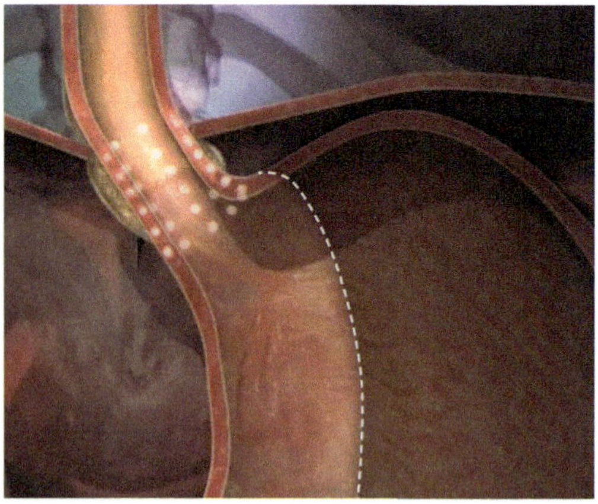

Fig. 3. LES post-Stretta. (*Courtesy* Restech, Houston, Texas).

the TIF 2.0 procedure, the EsophyX Z+, accommodates a standard adult gastroscope through its central channel, with the endoscope providing visual guidance during device insertion, fundoplication configuration, fastener deployment, and removal of the device. TIF 2.0 has been evaluated in more than 100 published articles. It provides effective symptom relief for appropriately selected patients, enabling more than 82% of treated patients to stop using daily pharmacologic therapy for GERD, and objectively healing GERD-related esophagitis in about 84% of patients [21–23]. In clinical practices that include the management of a significant number of patients with GERD, TIF represents an option worthy of consideration for those patients who meet the inclusion criteria for this minimally invasive endoluminal approach.

The first iteration of TIF used a device that while revolutionary at the time, would be seen as rudimentary at present, to perform a procedure known then as EndoLuminal Fundoplication (ELF). This gastro-gastric apposition was created by deploying fasteners below the esophagogastric junction (EGJ), attempting to remedy GERD by decreasing compliance in this region. Although this approach was not successful in eliminating GERD, it served as the foundation for later advancements that ultimately led to the creation of the well-studied EsophyX Z+ device. At the time that ELF was launched, there was great apprehension about the deployment of SerosaFuse fasteners across the esophageal wall, limiting that initial fundoplication to a gastro-gastric configuration. The fasteners were loaded individually for each firing of the device, making the process tedious, cumbersome, and time consuming. Understandably, adoption was limited [24,25]. Approximately 190 patients in total were treated using ELF.

TIF 1.0 incorporated numerous lessons learned from ELF, and was designed to allow the placement of fasteners 1 cm above the EGJ, creating an esophagogastric plication, although still falling short of creating a traditional fundoplication that mimicked those performed surgically. The device was bulky and required a nonstandard slim endoscope for guidance. Approximately 670 patients in total were treated using TIF 1.0 [25].

TIF 2.0, the current iteration of this procedure, benefits from preloaded cartridges that hold 20 fasteners each, enough for a typical TIF procedure. The EsophyX Z+ channel accepts a widely available standard adult gastroscope, and creates an esophagogastric fundoplication that exceeds 270°, that is fashioned by the placement of SerosaFuse fasteners ranging 1 cm to 4 cm above the EGJ, with enhanced length on the greater curvature aspect of the fundoplication. The wrap fashioned during this latest iteration adheres to many of the principles established for successful performance of antireflux surgery [26,27]. To date, TIF 2.0 has been performed in more than 22,000 patients. Fig. 4 illustrates the configuration of the anatomic reconstruction associated with each progression through TIF development, compared with Nissen, and native anatomy in patients with and without GERD.

Patient selection

In general, endoluminal therapies for GERD have accepted that no matter the approach, the basic construct is limited by the underlying patient anatomy. Therefore, patient selection for all endoluminal therapies has been limited to patients with documented GERD who have intact anatomy. Those without Barrett esophagus, a hiatus hernia smaller than 2 cm, or a Hill esophagogastric valve configuration I or II are generally considered candidates for endoluminal GERD therapy. These are the same criteria used to select most patients for consideration for TIF [28,29].

In our practice, we apply the same patient selection criteria to everyone being considered for antireflux therapy, whether operative or endoluminal. In general, these guidelines are as follows:

- Trial of behavioral modifications such as diminished food and fluid intake before recumbency, eliminating carbonated beverages and limiting caffeine, and if tolerated, elevating the head while lying down or sleeping.
- Free of nicotine addiction, or willing to become free of this addiction.
- Body Mass Index no greater than 35 Kg/M^2, or committed to losing weight to meet and maintain this threshold.
- Glycosylated hemoglobin less than 8%.
- No significant delay in gastric emptying, or one that cannot be addressed through other means.
- Secure diagnosis of GERD, either through biopsy proven esophagitis or significant esophageal acid exposure and symptom correlation during esophageal pH analysis.
- Esophageal manometry absent evidence of EGJ outflow obstruction, adequate esophageal body peristaltic function, no findings that contraindicate intervention.
- Response to pharmacologic therapy for GERD, even if partial.
- Endoscopic documentation of EGJ anatomy that includes the assessment of any hiatus hernia, type and size, and Hill configuration.

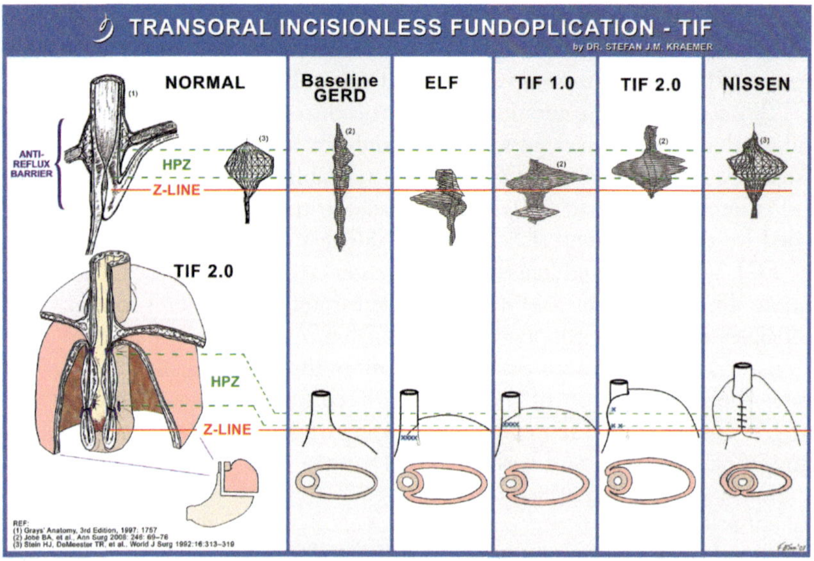

Fig. 4. Tif evolution.

We require the cessation of nicotine addiction for obvious reasons and as an important part of an overall esophageal health program, as well as our concern for its negative impact on healing. Our requirements for a controlled BMI and reasonable diabetic control are based on similar widely shared concerns for healing, health, and outcomes superiority. The remaining items listed are standard parts of a tailored physiologic evaluation for GERD, and help inform our counseling as patients are advised toward their menu of therapeutic options. All patients are asked to have engaged in a trial of behavioral modifications, and we identify at least partial responsiveness to pharmacologic agents an important indicator for treatment success.

Patients considered for TIF are those who meet the above criteria, have a Hill configuration I or II, no larger than a 2 cm Type I hiatus hernia, and who do not have Barrett esophagus. Most patients who are considered candidates for TIF, or any primary endoluminal therapy for GERD, also would be candidates for antireflux surgery, and such patients are provided with decision-making support through education and outcomes comparatives, and are asked to choose their therapy with input from our team. TIF fills an increasingly important role in our GERD practice as we see increasing numbers of patients with relatively intact anatomy who enjoy excellent symptom control on proton pump inhibitor (PPI) therapy but choose to end their use of those medications due to safety and side effect concerns.

Because TIF on its own has no capability to repair a hiatus hernia, patients with more than a slight anatomic defect will not realize optimal benefit from

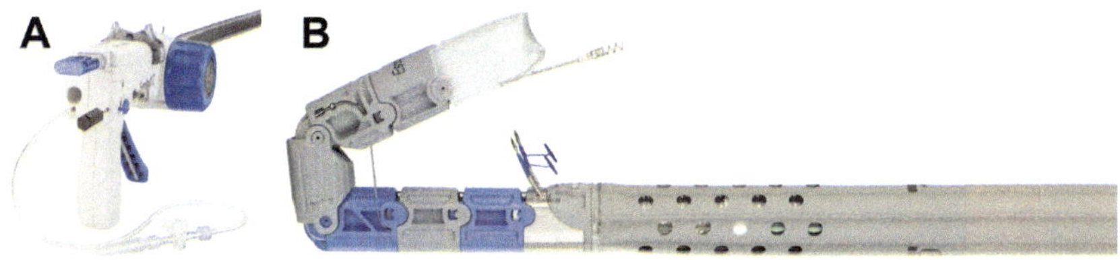

Fig. 5. (*A*) Rear handle view. (*B*) View of the distal working end.

TIF as traditionally performed. Similarly, concerns over the cancer risks associated with Barrett esophagus limit TIF application in those patients.

In our practice, aftercare is the same for patients undergoing TIF as for our patients undergoing laparoscopic fundoplication. We are intentional about this so that patients who interact with each other will support a single protocol, and to ensure that all staff members maintain expert level knowledge of postprocedure protocols in place regardless of the procedure that had been performed. The single difference is that patients with TIF typically are discharged within 90 minutes of their procedure, whereas laparoscopic fundoplication patients are discharged about 16 hours following the completion of their procedure.

The TIF procedure

- We use general endotracheal anesthesia, and position patients on their left side using a bean bag, padding, and securements to maintain a safe left lateral recumbent position throughout the procedure.
- We then perform diagnostic esophagogastroduodenoscopy (EGD) to ensure that there has been no change in anatomic configuration as conclusion of their workup, noting the depth of the EGJ, size of any hiatus hernia, and Hill configuration.
- Once satisfied that there are no contraindications to proceeding, the endoscope is removed and its shaft wiped down with an appropriate grade of mineral oil and sprayed with medical grade silicon spray, taking care to avoid contaminating the work area and floor with overspray.
- The Esophyx Z+ is removed from its packaging onto a covered worktable, and the 2 included SerosaFuse fastener cartridges are firmly tapped on the table several times each per manufacturer's guidance. Fig. 5 illustrate the working portions of the Esophyx Z+ device.
- The Esophyx Z+ is then lubricated by infusing mineral oil into the channels of the device, its hinged portions, and its loading wires before they are reseated. The external portion of the device is treated with a water-soluble lubricant.
- A SerosaFuse fastener cartridge then is attached to the Esophyx Z+, the device is dry fired several times, and the fasteners then are loaded. The fasteners will be seen in the observation window as they travel to the deployment zone. This is an important observation, especially on initial loading of the device.
- Mineral oil is dripped through the central channel before introducing the endoscope, and an alcohol pad is used to cleanse the endoscope lens, ensuring a clearer view.

- The combined platform is introduced gently into the esophagus and stomach under constant direct vision. A jaw thrust chin lift maneuver often is helpful in the initial advancement of the device.
- Once positioned within the stomach, the EsophyX Z+ tissue mold is closed, and the endoscope advanced about 15 cm and retroflexed to provide the visualization of the EGJ throughout the procedure.
- The stomach is maximally insufflated during tissue mold positioning, but slight decompression is useful in achieving fundoplication length just before the deployment of the fasteners, enabling the device to be nudged into optimal position.
- Carbon dioxide insufflation is used, and sometimes, having a laparoscopic insufflator with tubing attached through the instrument channel of the endoscope will be helpful in distending the stomach more expeditiously.
- The first set of fasteners is deployed at the 11 o'clock position. The retroflexed endoscope is advanced and withdrawn as needed, repositioned accordingly throughout the procedure to provide excellent visualization of all steps.
- With the Esophyx Z+ in position, the jaws are opened slightly, the helical retractor is engaged with tissues just distal to the Z-line, and the tissue mold is used to guide the fundus circumferentially around the distal esophagus. Once optimally positioned, the device components are locked.
- The integrated suction device is activated, allowing slight advancement of the device to lengthen the intraabdominal esophagus, resulting in a deeper fundoplication length.
- The device is tightened maximally, tension is allowed to be released from the shaft, the location markers are checked for reference to the EGJ location, and the fasteners are deployed by slowly and securely squeezing the handle.
- Each time the device is deployed, 2 nonabsorbable H-shaped fasteners are delivered through the layered walls of the distal esophagus and gastric fundus, securing the fundoplication.
- The invaginator suction is disconnected, the device reloaded, and it is readied for each subsequent deployment.
- Ultimately, 6 fasteners, 3 deployments, will be used in the corners at the 11 o'clock and 1 o'clock positions, whereby the gastric fundus approximates the lesser curvature anteriorly and posteriorly.
- Four fasteners will be deployed, 2 deployments, at each of the 5 o'clock and 7 o'clock positions, the deepest portion of the fund.
- In between each deployment at each location, the stomach is insufflated maximally, the device loosened, repositioned, the stomach decompressed slightly as the device is optimally positioned, and then the deployment sequence is followed.
- The underlying principle in creating the fundoplication is to place anchors at particular anatomic locations but to avoid deploying new fasteners directly onto the previous ones. This avoids damage to the previously placed fasteners and spreads the tissue apposition forces for optimal configuration and durability.
- Twenty fasteners are placed during the typical procedure, creating the Omega shaped fundoplication of at least 270° as demonstrated in the animated video of the TIF procedure (Video 1).

The cTIF procedure

One of the greatest impediments to the adoption of TIF has been the relatively small number of patients with GERD with pristine intact anatomy. Although there are many patients suffering GERD and its symptoms, most of these may not meet the stringent anatomic requirements of having a Hill configuration I or II, and at maximum, a 2 cm Type I hiatus hernia. As TIF literature evolved, it was observed that patients with a Hill II configuration enjoyed success, but those with a Hill III configuration were more likely to experience recurrent symptoms. It was determined that TIF 2.0 outcomes were adversely impacted when the hiatus was dilated to greater than 2.0 cm in transverse dimension 10 to 13 [30–34]. This and similar observations led to improved patient selection for TIF 2.0 procedures, which may explain the improved outcomes in the TEMPO and RESPECT trials compared with those from the 2012 TIF registry analysis. It was suggested that outcomes for TIF 2.0 likely would be improved if a hiatus hernia repair was undertaken before the TIF procedure [33].

Enter cTIF (concomittetent hiatal hernia with TIF), also referred to as HH-TIF, an approach that pairs a concomitant laparoscopic hiatus hernia repair with the TIF 2.0 procedure during a single session intervention. Although controversial, early outcomes suggest that the combination of a hiatus hernia repair and creation of the Omega fundoplication that characterizes TIF may offer effective GERD therapy with fewer side effects such as gas bloating and dysphagia [34]. In 2017, the FDA acted favorably on a request to amend the Instructions for Use for the EsophyX Z+ to include performance of TIF 2.0 immediately after hiatus hernia repair. It remains too early to tell if this combined intervention will offer sustainable benefit, and if its cost structure will be justified, but the concept has influenced research investigating the laparoscopic creation of a similarly configured Omega fundoplication. This type of innovation may not have come to the forefront without the influence of TIF and its evolution throughout the 15 years since its introduction.

Outcomes

TIF is a well-studied endoluminal therapy for patients with GERD. A recent PubMed search confirmed that 118 reports exist in the English-language medical literature as of November 2021. The analysis of results sometimes has been confounded by combining data sets from the different phases of procedural evolution. TIF 2.0 is quite different from TIF 1.0 and ELF, and combining these data does not accurately reflect the outcomes expected from the current approach. There have been several important trials that inform the current placement of TIF 2.0 within the GERD treatment armamentarium.

Important clinical trials

TIF versus Medical Proton Pump Inhibitor Management of Refractory GERD Symptoms: The TEMPO Trial [16]. ClinicalTrials.gov ID: NCT016437958.

Publications [35–38]:

SUMMARY

The TEMPO Trial was undertaken to assess the durability of TIF-related benefits. Sixty-three patients with chronic GERD symptoms refractory to proton pump inhibitor therapy and abnormal esophageal acid exposure were randomized to TIF or continued PPI use. All patients had no hiatus hernia or one that was 2 cm maximum if present. After the 6-month evaluation, all patients in the initial PPI group elected to crossover to TIF, meaning that all 63 enrolled patients who underwent eventually were treated using the TIF 2.0 procedure. Primary outcomes included the durable elimination of daily regurgitation and documented atypical symptoms, assessed at the 5-year follow-up. Secondary outcomes included improvements in GERD-HRQL symptom scores, PPI use, need for repeat intervention, and overall patient satisfaction. A cost comparison was conducted.

The results were based on the following enrolled patients long-term. Of the initial 63 patients, 60 were available for follow-up at 1 year, 52 available at 3 years, and 44 available at 5 years. Regurgitation was eliminated in 88% of patients at 1 year, 90% at 3 years, and 86% at 5 years, and atypical symptoms were resolved in 82%, 88%, and 80% of patients at these time intervals. No serious adverse events occurred in the performance of the 63 TIF 2.0 procedures. At 5 years, 66% of patients no longer used daily PPIs and overall GERD-HRQL scores improved from 22.2 to 6.8 ($P < .001$). Costs were estimated to be reduced by 27% over a 5 year period in patients treated with TIF as compared with those treated with continued PPI therapy.

Transoral Incisionless Fundoplication Registry Study for Treatment of Gastroesophageal Reflux Disease: The TIF Registry [39]. ClinicalTrials.gov ID: NCT01118585.

Publications [21,39–41]:

Summary: The TIF Registry Trial was created to prospectively assess 2-year outcomes after TIF 2.0 in a multicenter setting. This US-based registry enrolled more than 100 patients from 14 centers performing the TIF 2.0 procedure for chronic GERD. The primary outcome was symptom assessment and control, and the secondary outcomes changed in PPI use, healing or persistence of esophagitis, procedural safety, and changes in esophageal acid exposure.

During the enrollment period, January 2010 to April 2011, 127 patients were treated using TIF 2.0 for GERD; 15% were unavailable for complete follow-up. No serious adverse events were associated with performing TIF 2.0 in this study. GERD-HRQL scores improved by 50% or more in 66% of enrolled patients, and regurgitation scores improved in 70% of patients. The Reflux Symptom Index (RSI) score normalized in 65% of patients treated. Daily PPI use declined from 91% to 29% after treatment using TIF, and esophagitis was healed in 75% of those with pretreatment esophagitis. Esophageal acid exposure was normalized in 57% of patients after TIF 2.0 was performed. Eighty percent of patients were completely off pharmacologic therapy 2 years after undergoing TIF compared with 92% of patients found dependent on antisecretory medications before intervention. TIF was demonstrated as safe and effective for medically refractory GERD in a variety of community settings with 6-month follow-up.

Randomized EsophyX versus Sham/Placebo-Controlled TIF Trial: The RESPECT Study [42]. ClinicalTrials.gov I D: NCT01136980.

Publication [42]:

Summary: This prospective sham-controlled clinical trial was undertaken in patients with established refractory GERD on PPIs to assess the response of regurgitation and related symptoms to TIF. A group of 696 patients with refractory GERD despite daily PPI use was screened on and off PPIs using validated GERD assessments. Patients with GERD, and a hiatus hernia less than 2 cm, if one was present, were randomized to groups that either underwent TIF followed by 6 months of placebo substitution for PPIs (n = 87), or a sham procedure followed by 6 months of omeprazole prescribed either once or twice (n = 42) daily. All patients were blinded to therapy during the study and follow-up periods, and assessments were conducted at 2, 12, and 26 weeks. Endoscopic visualization and 48-hour pH probe monitoring were performed at 6 months. Cross-over was offered after unblinding at 6 months.

Regurgitation was eliminated in 67% of patients after TIF compared with 45% in patients treated using daily or twice daily PPIs ($P = .05$) at 6 months. Esophageal pH was improved in the TIF group and was unaffected in the sham group ($P < .001$) at 6 months. Seventy-six percent of sham-treated patients elected to crossover to TIF. At 12 month analysis, 72% of crossover patients had controlled regurgitation; 72% remained completely off pharmacologic therapy.

Transoral Incisionless Fundoplication versus Sham for Treatment of Gastroesophageal Reflux Disease: the TIF versus Sham Study [43]. ClinicalTrials.gov ID: NCT01110811.

Publication [43]:

Summary: Patients treated with TIF 2.0 were able to discontinue pharmacologic therapy 59% of the time compared with 9% of patients in the sham arm. Esophageal acid exposure time was significantly normalized after TIF; 8.89% preprocedure to 3.73% postprocedure. Acid exposure time was not improved in patients in the sham group. This randomized controlled study demonstrates that TIF 2.0 reduces the need for pharmacologic therapy and effectively controls GERD symptoms.

Safety of TIF 2.0 has been demonstrated to be at least equivalent to that of laparoscopic fundoplication. Industry-based registry data sets indicate the significant adverse event rate for TIF 2.0 is 0.41%, with 91 events reported in 22,000 procedures. The TEMPO trial concluded durability of TIF at 5 years, while additional European analyses have identified no significant changes in the rate of symptom relief at 5 and 10 years after TIF was performed.

SUMMARY

When a new procedure known as ELF was introduced in 2006, it was cumbersome and tedious, not particularly similar to laparoscopic fundoplication, and was associated with limited successes. It had all the hallmark features predicting that it would be another failed endoluminal therapy for GERD. What differed was a platform that would be modified as safety and efficacy data emerged, that would allow the endoluminal approach to fundoplication to evolve into an approach that now is associated with solid clinical outcomes, reliably demonstrated patient benefit, and a remarkable safety profile. While bulking agents, injectables, implants, and other suture and fastener-based approaches have failed, the team at EndoGastric Solutions, Inc. continued to coax better design and performance from their initial device. What once seemed to me, a 30-year veteran foregut surgeon, an interesting device no doubt destined for failure, now has emerged into an important tool in the treatment of the full spectrum of GERD symptoms and anatomic concerns that affect many patients along the reflux continuum.

The resolution of classical GERD symptoms, heartburn, and regurgitation, is critical to patient acceptance and the positive outcome of TIF 2.0 seems to have longevity as demonstrated in numerous studies. RSI scores are reported to be normalized after TIF 2.0 at 73% after 6 months and at 65% at 2 years. The TEMPO trial, a crossover study comparing TIF 2.0 treatment in medically refractory patients with GERD, reported complete eradication of regurgitation in 86% of patients at 5 years. TEMPO looked at atypical symptoms as well and revealed durable improvement in atypical GERD symptoms such as cough, hoarseness, dysphagia, mucus, and throat clearing in 80% of study patients at 5 years. The RESPECT trial, which compared TIF 2.0 against a sham procedure with PPI therapy, reported resolution of regurgitation in 67% of patients at 6 months and complete symptom elimination in 72% of patients at 12 months [21,35,40,43]

Pooled patient data presented in numerous meta-analyses demonstrate significant improvement in GERD-HRQL scores, reporting improvements with 95% confidence. Huang et all reported decreased reflux episodes and an absence of gas bloat symptoms after TIF 2.0 in a meta-analysis incorporating 13 prospective studies and 5 randomized trials [44]. Other reports have followed TIF 2.0 for 10 years, demonstrating the persistence of these benefits.

Another measure critical to patient acceptance of GERD interventions is the ability to end reliance on pharmacologic agents. The TEMPO trial reported PPI cessation rates of 71% and 46% at 3 years and 5 years after TIF 2.0, while RESPECT reported that 60% of patients with TIF were off antisecretory therapy at 6 months as compared with patients in the sham treatment arm. Ten-year rates of reduced antisecretory use are 91.7%, indicating through pooled data analysis that even if some medication still is required occasionally, pharmacologic dependance is dramatically reduced in most of the patients. As has been seen with other GERD interventions, data collected suggest that there is at best a loose correlation between esophageal pH normalization and symptom control. TIF 2.0 studies report esophageal pH normalization in 57% to 69% of treated patients. Despite these disappointing observations, esophagitis was resolved in 77% to 100% of patients after TIF 2.0, perhaps indicating that a critical threshold of acid reduction had been reached to allow tissue recovery in most treated patients even without complete normalization [21,35,42,43].

When evaluating TIF data in the assessment of durability and treatment failure, it is important to evaluate data sets pertaining only to TIF 2.0, the current procedure that is offered. As an example of the influence of earlier data sets, the combined failure rate of ELF and TIF 1.0 approached 40%. Overall evaluation of the literature indicates a TIF failure rate of 5% to 18%, but the TEMPO trial reported a 5% failure rate at 5 years after the index TIF 2.0 procedure among study participants. This compares favorably with the 5% to 6% failure rate typically reported with laparoscopic fundoplication.

There is an assumption that surgical revision after failed TIF is less complex than revision of a prior surgical fundoplication. Surgical fundoplication following failed TIF is a complex undertaking that requires division of the SerosaFuse fasteners and the scar tissue that develops along their pathways and adjacent to opposed surfaces. Increased rates of esophagogastric perforation, bleeding, and abscess formation have been reported during surgical revision after TIF, 27%, as compared with operative revision of prior surgical fundoplication, 13%, and initial surgical fundoplication, 2% [45–47]. Some studies have suggested a higher rate of dysphagia in patients undergoing surgical revision for failed TIF [21,22].

Some TIF failures are mitigated through careful adherence to selection criteria when considering patients for TIF 2.0, eliminating those with greater than a 2.0 cm wide hiatus. Others have reported that deploying an increased number of fasteners during TIF is associated with improved outcomes and durability [20,21,48].

The most commonly reported adverse events associated with TIF are perforation, bleeding, pleural effusion, and dysphagia, with an overall reported complication rate of 2.4% [49]. Mortality related directly to the TIF procedure remains exceptionally low. While the most common untoward outcomes after surgical fundoplication are reported to be dysphagia, bloating, and increased flatulence, these are reported to occur less frequently after TIF, and patients with preprocedural bloating and flatulence often report improvement after TIF. The most common issues reported by patients after TIF are transient nausea and abdominal discomfort.

The Centers for Medicare and Medicaid Services (CMS) instituted payment coverage for TIF 2.0 using the EsophyX Z+ device effective 1 January 2018. Some commercial insurers have followed suit and TIF is now an option for an increasing number of appropriately evaluated and selected patients with GERD. The TIF 2.0 procedure is a well-studied treatment of patients with refractory GERD and intact anatomy, who also meet other established inclusion criteria for intervention, with symptoms most appropriately addressed by a treatment positioned between continued pharmacologic therapy and laparoscopic fundoplication [50].

ANTIREFLUX MUCOSECTOMY

Introduction

Gastroesophageal reflux is a normal physiologic process that occurs during brief episodes of transient lower esophageal sphincter relaxation and usually without symptoms, esophageal injury, or complications. Gastroesophageal reflux becomes a pathologic disorder when it causes symptoms (eg, heartburn, regurgitation) or injury to the esophagus (eg, erosive esophagitis) and is thought to be due to a poorly functioning esophagogastric junction (EGJ), the antireflux barrier. Gastroesophageal reflux disease (GERD) is one of the most common gastrointestinal disorders with a significant impact on quality of life and an increasing burden on the health care system [51]. Medical management with acid-reducing medications (most commonly with PPIs) and lifestyle modifications have become first-line treatment. However, many patients remain symptomatic despite optimal medical therapy and there are increasing concerns about the safety of long-term PPI use [52]. The gold-standard therapy for refractory GERD is laparoscopic fundoplication with or without hiatal hernia repair. As alternatives to surgery, less invasive, endoscopic procedures have been described. These include endoscopic EGJ plication, radiofrequency ablation, and transoral incisionless fundoplication. However, the lack of efficacy, high cost, need for special equipment and implantation of foreign devices make these procedures less favored.

Antireflux mucosectomy (ARMS) is a novel endoscopic approach that uses endoscopic mucosal resection (EMR) techniques to promote contraction and scarring at the gastric cardia resulting in tightening of the EGJ and restoration of the acid reflux barrier. This procedure was formally described in 2014 by Inoue and colleagues when a patient-reported improved GERD symptoms after undergoing EMR for Barrett's esophagus with high-grade dysplasia [53]. Several studies have been published describing its' feasibility and safety. The short-term outcomes have been encouraging with improved GERD symptoms, including the discontinuation of PPIs and normalized DeMeester score [54–58]. Continued observation and long-term data may further prove its efficacy.

Patient selection

ARMS should be considered for patients with typical reflux symptoms who are refractory to PPIs or do not wish to continue long-term PPI therapy and those who are not candidates for antireflux surgery or refuse it. One study demonstrated ARMS as a feasible therapeutic option for a patient with refractory GERD after sleeve gastrectomy who otherwise would have been recommended to undergo a Roux-en-Y gastric bypass [59].

Patients with a hiatal hernia greater than 2 cm or esophageal dysmotility are not candidates for this procedure because current therapies do not fix the hiatus or enhance esophageal motility or LES competence.

Procedure

Several techniques have been described for the ARMS procedure. Initially performed by endoscopic submucosal dissection and later using cap- or banded-assisted mucosal resection. The later techniques were found to be faster and easier to perform with the same effectiveness.

Preop workup should include upper GI endoscopy (assess for hiatal hernia and evaluate gastric flap valve), high-resolution manometry (rule out esophageal motility disorders), and pH testing.

CAP ASSISTED (ARMS-C)

There is not yet a standardized technique. Most studies describe using a regular endoscope equipped with a medium-sized hard cap and a thin diameter crescent snare. A thorough inspection of the esophagus, stomach, and duodenum is performed with scope advancement. One study describes performing the procedure anteriorly, otherwise, the procedure is performed in retroflexion. An argon plasma coagulation (APC) is used to mark out a 270° to 320° area for resection. 1–2 cm (or 1–2 cap lengths) of the greater and lesser curves are spared (butterfly technique). Compared with preserving the greater curve only, the butterfly technique has been shown to decrease postoperative stenosis. A mixture of normal saline, epinephrine, and indigo carmine (or methylene blue) is injected into the submucosa along the markings with a 25-gauge needle. The snare is prelooped on the internal ridge of the cap. The mucosa is suctioned into the cap and resected with electrosurgical current. This is repeated until the marked mucosa is completely resected. Bleeding is controlled with APC.

The procedure is similar to the banded technique except for a band is placed after the mucosa is suctioned into the cap and before the tissue is resected. The banded technique allows for improved visualization before resection and decreased bleeding [55].

Antireflux mucosal ablation

In 2020 Inoue and colleagues introduced a second technique, antireflux mucosal ablation (ARMA). This was initially performed on a post-ARMS patient who had poor results. Repeating the ARMS procedure was believed to be too technically challenging which led to the development of ARMA. Twelve total patients were included in the study using the ablation technique. Two patients had previously undergone ARMS. The preoperative workup and inclusion criteria were similar in ARMS. The procedure is like ARMS but rather than resecting the mucosa, argon plasma coagulation or endoknife coagulation is used to ablate the mucosa. Saline with indigo carmine is injected into the submucosal to provide a marker for adequate ablation and to reduce thermal injury. The results showed similar scarring and tightening effects as ARMS as well as a decrease in DeMeester score, discontinuation of PPI, and improvement in symptom scoring. This simplified technique has a lower risk of perforation and the advantage of allowing for repeat procedures [60].

Outcome

A 2021 meta-analysis by Rodriquez de Santiago evaluated 15 nonrandomized studies (12 on ARMS and 3 on ARMA) including over 400 patients that have been conducted to evaluate the safety and effectiveness of the techniques. Follow-up ranged from 2 months to 3 years. Dysphagia is the most common adverse outcome, occurring in 5% to 10% of patients, all treated successfully with endoscopic balloon dilation. The most feared compilation, perforation, occurred in 4 patients undergoing ARMS and none undergoing ARMA. Outcomes were measured using a combination of patient-reported symptom scoring (including the discontinuation of PPI or decrease in dosage), DeMeester scores, and/or flap valve grade. Clinical success ranged from 58% to 100% at 2 to 6 months and 26% to 76% at 3 years. Additional studies and long-term data are needed to further evaluate the outcomes; however, currently, the results are promising as a less-invasive alternative to laparoscopic fundoplication for patients with refractory GERD [54].

Wong, et all compared ARMS to fundoplication, matching 33 patients with ARMS to 67 laparoscopic Nissen fundoplication patients. This found a higher

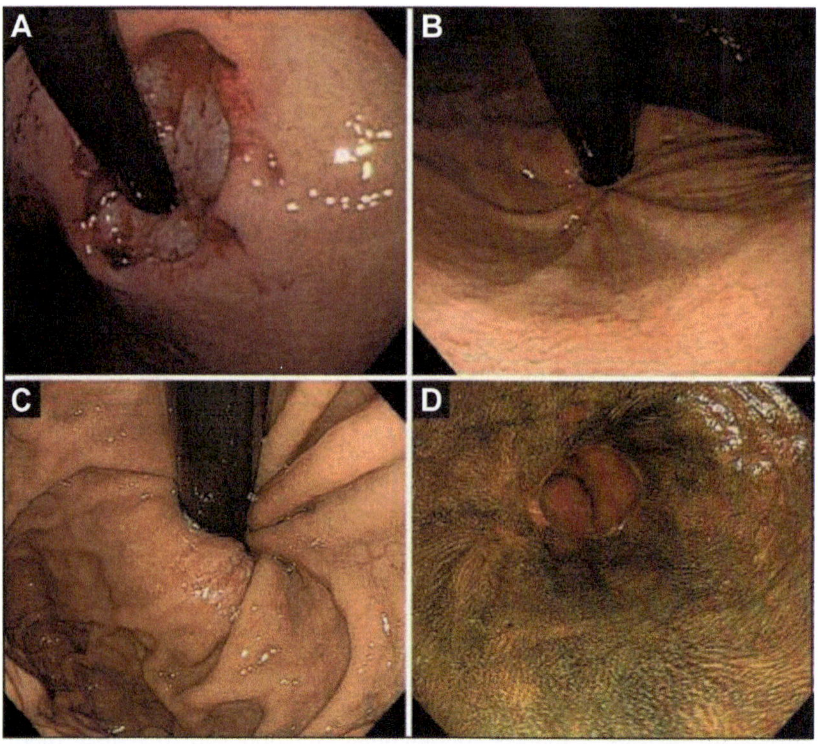

Fig. 6. Reproduced with permission from Annals of Gastroenterology. Endoscopic follow up of circumferential anti-reflux mucosectomy (ARMS) (retroflexed views). (*A*) Immediately after circumferential ARMS. Approximately 2 cm-wide gastric cardia mucosa was circumferentially resected by cap-endoscopic mucosal resection method. (*B*) Appearance at 3 years. A tight gastro-esophageal junction. Convergence of three gastric folds was observed along the lesser curve of the stomach. (*C*) More than 10 years after circumferential ARMS. Appearance is similar to B. (*D*) More than 10 years after circumferential ARMS (forward view). Chromoendoscopy with Lugol's solution demonstrated well-stained squamous epithelium with neither recurrence of esophagitis nor Barrett's esophagus.

rate of esophagitis in the fundoplication group as well as hiatal hernia size compared with the ARMs group (2 cm vs 1 cm). ARMS had shorter OR time, less blood loss, shorter length of hospital stay (same-day discharge), less pain at discharge, earlier discontinuation of narcotics for pain, and sooner return to normal daily activities compared to fundoplication. One ARMS patient postop bleeding was managed conservatively. There was no difference in 30-day complication rates, hospital visits, or readmissions. GERD-HRQL and dysphagia scores were similar between the 2 groups. In the ARMS group, 90.9% of patients discontinued PPI therapy and 9.1% required dilation. 10 patients (30.3%) progressed to require future antireflux procedures including laparoscopic fundoplication, LINX, or bypass [61]. Fig. 6 and 7 show patient results up to 10 years with good valve integrety.

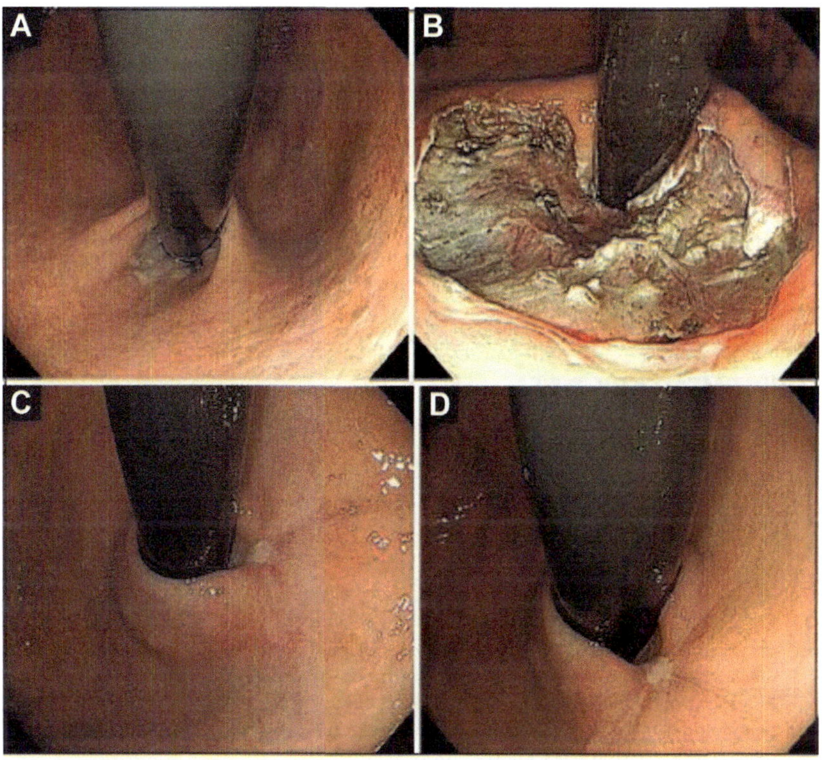

Fig. 7. Reproduced with permission from Annals of Gastroenterology. Endoscopic follow up of crescentic anti-reflux mucosectomy (ARMS). (*A*) Before ARMS. Endoscopy in retroflexion demonstrated significant hiatal hernia (Flap valve score 3) but no sliding component. Chest pain and regurgitation were prominent in this case (DeMeester score 5) and symptoms were not controlled by double dose proton pump inhibitor. (*B*) Immediately after procedure. Endoscopy in retroflexion showed two-thirds circumferential artificial ulcer. ARMS was centered at lesser curve and the mucosal flap valve at greater curve was preserved. (*C*) Appearance at 2 months. Mucosal valve was re-shaped and well-defined (Mucosal flap valve Grade 1). (*D*) Alternative endoscopic view at 2 months. Mucosal valve as appeared as though "stitched" at the lesser curve of gastric cardia.

SUMMARY

Antireflux mucosectomy or mucosal resection is an effective and safe technique for managing patients with GERD and may be considered in the armamentarium of antireflux procedural interventions with appropriate patient selection. It avoids the use of foreign bodies and does not complicate future antireflux operations if required.

CLINICS CARE POINTS

- Appropriate work up is necessary to get the best results.
- Attention to detail with the techniques is important to outcomes so obtain appropriate preprocedure training and consider having a case mentor until you feel comfortable.
- These cases have rare complications. Be very careful IF a patient doesn't seem to be doing well as this could be a warning sign.

DISCLOSURE

The authors have nothing to disclose. There were no grants or funding sources for this chapter.

SUPPLEMENTARY DATA

Supplementary data related to this article can be found online at https://doi.org/10.1016/j.yasu.2022.04.001.

References

[1] Herman RM, Berho M, Murawski M, et al. Defining the histopathological changes induced by nonablative radiofrequency treatment of faecal incontinence—a blinded assessment in an animal model. Colorectal Dis 2015;17:433–40.

[2] Utley DS, Kim M, Vierra MA, et al. Augmentation of lower esophageal sphincter pressure and gastric yield pressure after radiofrequency energy delivery to the gastroesophageal junction: a procine model. Gastrointest Endosc 2000;52:81–6.

[3] Kim MS, Holloway RH, Dent J, et al. Radiofrequency energy delivery to the gastric cardia inhibits triggering of transient lower esophageal sphincter relaxation and gastroesophageal reflux in dogs. Gastrointest Endosc 2003;57:17–22.

[4] Triadafilopoulos G. Changes in gerd symptom scores correlate with improvement in esophageal acid exposure after the Stretta procedure. Surg Endosc 2004;18:1038–44.

[5] Arts J, Bisschops R, Blondeau K, et al. A double -blind sham-controlled study of the effect of radiofrequency energy on symptoms and distensibility of the gastro-esophageal junction in GERD. Am J Gastroenerol 2012;107:222–30.

[6] Corley DA, Katz P, Wo JM, et al. Improvement of gastroesophageal reflux symptoms after radiofrequency energy: a randomized, sham controlled trial. Gastroenerology 2003;125:668–76.

[7] Coron E, Sebille V, Cadiot G, et al. Clinical trial: radiofrequency energy delivery in proton pump inhibitor dependent gastro-oesopheal reflux disease patients. Aliment Pharmacol Ther 2008;28:1147–58.

[8] Abdel Aziz AM, El-Khayat HR, Sadek A, et al. A prospective randomized trial of sham, single-dose stretta, and double-dose Stretta for the treatment of gastroesopheal reflux disease. Surg Endosc 2010;24:818–25.
[9] Kalapala R, Shah H, Nabi Z, et al. Treatment of gastroesophageal reflux disease using radiofrequency ablation (stretta procedure): an interim analysis of a randomized trial. Indian J Gastroenterol 2017;36:337–42.
[10] Zerbib F, Sacher-Huvelin S, Coron E, et al. Randomized clinical trial: oesophageal radiofrequencey energy delivery versus sham for PPI-refractory heartburn. Aliment Pharmacol Ther 2020;52:637–45.
[11] Perry KA, Banerjee A, Melvin WS. Radiofrequency energy delivery to the lower esophageal sphincter reduces esophageal acid exposure and improves GERD symptoms: a systematic review and meta-analysis. Surg Laparosc Endosc Percutan Tech 2012;22:283–8.
[12] Lipka S, Kumar A, Richter JE. No evidence for efficacy of radiofrequency ablation for treatment of gastroesophageal reflux disease: a systematic review and meta-analysis. Clin Gastroenterol Hepatol 2015;13:1058–67.
[13] Fass R, Cahn F, Scotti D, et al. Systematic review and meta-analysis of controlled and prospective cohort efficacy studies of endoscopic radiofrequency for treatment of gastroesophageal reflux disease. Surg Endosc 2017;31:4865–82.
[14] Xie P, Yan J, Ye L, et al. Efficacy of different endoscopic treatments in patients with gastroesophageal reflux disease: a systematic review and network meta-analysis. Surg Endosc 2012;35:1500–10.
[15] Dughera I, Rotondano G, De Cento M, et al. Durability of Stretta Radiofrequency treatment for GERD: results of an 8-year follow-up. Gastroenterol Res Pract 2014;2014:531907.
[16] Noar M, Squires P, Noar E, et al. Long-term maintenance effect of radiofrequency energy delivery for refractory GERD: a decade later. Surg Endosc 2014;28:2323–33.
[17] Reymunde A, Santiago N. Long-term results of radiofrequency energy delivery for the treatmtn of GERD: sustained improvement in symptoms, quality of life and drug use at 4-year follow-up. Gastrointest Endosc 2007;65:361–6.
[18] Reymunde A Santiago N. Fifteen plus years after stretta antireflux endoscopy procedure: quality of life and ppi requirements. Am J Gastroenterol 2017;112:ps459–60.
[19] Noar M, Squires P, Khan S. Radiofrequency energy delivery to the lower esophageal sphincter improves gastroesophageal reflux patient-reported outcomes in failed laparoscopic Nissen fundoplication cohort. Surg Endosc 2017;31:2854–62.
[20] Ihde GM. The evolution of TIF: transoral incisionless fundoplication. Therap Adv Gastroenterol 2020;13:1756284820924206.
[21] Bell RC, Barnes WE, Carter BJ, et al. Transoral incisionless fundoplication: 2-year results from the prospective multicenter U.S. study. Am Surg 2014;80(11):1093–105.
[22] Chimukangara M, Jalilvand AD, Melvin WS, et al. Long-term reported outcomes of transoral incisionless fundoplication: an 8-year cohort study. Surg Endosc 2019;33(4):1304–9.
[23] Testoni PA, Testoni S, Mazzoleni G, et al. Long-term efficacy of transoral incisionless fundoplication with Esophyx (Tif 2.0) and factors affecting outcomes in GERD patients followed for up to 6 years: a prospective single-center study. Surg Endosc 2015;29(9):2770–80.
[24] Repici A, Fumagalli U, Malesci A, et al. Endoluminal fundoplication (ELF) for GERD using EsophyX: a 12-month follow-up in a single-center experience. J Gastrointest Surg 2010;14(1):1–6.
[25] Velanovich V. Endoscopic, endoluminal fundoplication for gastroesophageal reflux disease: initial experience and lessons learned. Surgery 2010;148(4):646–51 [discussion: 651-643].
[26] DeMeester TR, Wernly JA, Bryant GH, et al. Clinical and in vitro analysis of determinants of gastroesophageal competence. A study of the principles of antireflux surgery. Am J Surg 1979;137(1):39–46.
[27] Patti MG, Allaix ME, Fisichella PM. Analysis of the causes of failed antireflux surgery and the principles of treatment: a review. JAMA Surg 2015;150(6):585–90.

[28] Barnes WE, Hoddinott KM, Mundy S, et al. Transoral incisionless fundoplication offers high patient satisfaction and relief of therapy-resistant typical and atypical symptoms of GERD in community practice. Surg Innov 2011;18(2):119–29.
[29] Demyttenaere SV, Bergman S, Pham T, et al. Transoral incisionless fundoplication for gastroesophageal reflux disease in an unselected patient population. Surg Endosc 2010;24(4): 854–8.
[30] Reavis KM, Perry KA. Transoral incisionless fundoplication for the treatment of gastroesophageal reflux disease. Expert Rev Med Devices 2014;11(4):341–50.
[31] Horgan S, Pellegrini CA. Surgical treatment of gastroesophageal reflux disease. Surg Clin North Am 1997;77(5):1063–82.
[32] Testoni PA, Corsetti M, Di Pietro S, et al. Effect of transoral incisionless fundoplication on symptoms, PPI use, and ph-impedance refluxes of GERD patients. World J Surg 2010;34(4):750–7.
[33] Ihde GM, Besancon K, Deljkich E. Short-term safety and symptomatic outcomes of transoral incisionless fundoplication with or without hiatal hernia repair in patients with chronic gastroesophageal reflux disease. Am J Surg 2011;202(6):740–6 [discussion: 746-747].
[34] Janu P, Shughoury AB, Venkat K, et al. Laparoscopic hiatal hernia repair followed by transoral incisionless fundoplication with EsophyX Device (HH + TIF): Efficacy and Safety in Two Community Hospitals. Surg Innov 2019;26(6):675–86.
[35] Trad KS, Barnes WE, Prevou ER, et al. The TEMPO Trial at 5 Years: Transoral Fundoplication (TIF 2.0) Is Safe, Durable, and Cost-effective. Surg Innov 2018;25(2):149–57.
[36] Trad KS, Simoni G, Barnes WE, et al. Transoral Fundoplication offers durable symptom control for chronic GERD: 3-year report from the TEMPO randomized trial with crossover arm. Surg Endosc 2017;31(6):2498–508.
[37] Trad KS, Simoni G, Barnes WE, et al. PG Mavrelis Efficacy of transoral fundoplication for treatment of chronic gastroesophageal reflux disease incompletely controlled with high-dose proton-pump inhibitors therapy: a randomized, multicenter, open-label, crossover study. BMC Gastroenterol 2014;14:174.
[38] Trad KS, Barnes WE, Simoni G, et al. Transoral incisionless fundoplication effective in eliminating GERD symptoms in partial responders to proton pump inhibitor therapy at 6 months: the TEMPO randomized clinical trial. Surg Innov 2015;22(1):26–40.
[39] Bell RC, Mavrelis PG, Barnes WE, et al. A prospective multicenter registry of patients with chronic gastroesophageal reflux disease receiving transoral incisionless fundoplication. J Am Coll Surg 2012;215(6):794–809.
[40] Bell RC, Fox MA, Barnes WE, et al. Univariate and multivariate analyses of preoperative factors influencing symptomatic outcomes of transoral fundoplication. Surg Endosc 2014;28(10):2949–58.
[41] Wilson EB, Barnes WE, Mavrelis PG, et al. The Effects of Transoral Incisionless Fundoplication on Chronic GERD Patients: 12-Month Prospective Multicenter Experience. Surg Laparosc Endosc Percutan Tech 2014;24(1):36–46.
[42] Hunter JG, Kahrilas PJ, Bell RC, et al. Efficacy of transoral fundoplication vs omeprazole for treatment of regurgitation in a randomized controlled trial. Gastroenterology 2015;148(2): 324–33.e5.
[43] Hakansson B, Montgomery M, Cadiere GB, et al. Randomised clinical trial: transoral incisionless fundoplication vs. sham intervention to control chronic GERD. Aliment Pharmacol Ther 2015;42(11–12):1261–70.
[44] Huang X, Chen S, Zhao H, et al. Efficacy of transoral incisionless fundoplication (TIF) for the treatment of GERD: a systematic review with meta-analysis. Surg Endosc 2017;31(3): 1032–44.
[45] Furnee EJ, Broeders JA, Draaisma WA, et al. Laparoscopic Nissen fundoplication after failed EsophyX fundoplication. Br J Surg 2010;97(7):1051–5.
[46] Bell RC, Kurian AA, Freeman KD. Laparoscopic anti-reflux revision surgery after transoral incisionless fundoplication is safe and effective. Surg Endosc 2015;29(7):1746–52.

[47] Puri R, Smith CD, Bowers SP. The spectrum of surgical remediation of transoral incisionless fundoplication-related failures. J Laparoendosc Adv Surg Tech A 2018;28(9):1089–93.
[48] Chang KJ, Bell R. Transoral incisionless fundoplication. Gastrointest Endosc Clin N Am 2020;30(2):267–89.
[49] Ramai D, Shapiro A, Barakat M, et al. Adverse events associated with transoral incisionless fundoplication (TIF) for chronic gastroesophageal reflux disease: a MAUDE database analysis. Surg Endosc 2021.
[50] Rabach L, Saad AR, Velanovich V. How to choose among fundoplication, magnetic sphincter augmentation or transoral incisionless fundoplication. Curr Opin Gastroenterol 2019;35(4):371–8.
[51] Yamasaki T, Hemond C, Eisa M, et al. The changing epidemiology of gastroesophageal reflux disease: are patients getting younger? J Neurogastroenterology Motil 2018;24: 559–69.
[52] Katz P, Dunbar K, Schnoll-Sussman F, et al. ACG clinical guideline for the diagnosis and management of gastroesophageal reflux disease. Am J Gastroenterol 2022;117:27–56.
[53] Sumi K, Inoue H, Kobayashi Y, et al. Endoscopic treatment of proton pump inhibitor-refractory gastroesophageal reflux disease with anti-reflux mucosectomy: Experience of 109 cases. Dig Endosc 2021;33:347–54.
[54] Rodriguez de Santiago E, Albeniz E, Estremera-Arevalo F, et al. Endoscopic anti-reflux therapy for gastroesophageal reflux disease. World J Gastroenterol 2021;27:6601–15.
[55] Monino L, Gonzalez JM, Vitton V, et al. Antireflux mucosectomy band in treatment of refractory gastroesophageal reflux disease: a pilot study for safety, feasibility and symptom control. Endosc Int Open 2020;8:E147–54.
[56] Hedberg H, Kuchta K, Ujiki M. First experience with banded anti-reflux mucosectomy (arms) for gerd: feasibility, safety, and technique. J Gastrointest Surg 2019;23:1274–8.
[57] Yoo I, Ko W, Kim H, et al. Anti-reflux mucosectomy using a cap-assisted endoscopic mucosal resection method for refractory gastroesophageal disease: a prospective feasibility study. Surg Endosc 2020;34:1124–31.
[58] Yang X, Tan J, Liu Y, et al. Comparison of 180° anti-reflux mucosectomy versus 270° anti-reflux mucosectomy for treatment of refractory gastroesophageal reflux disease: a retrospective study. Surg Endosc 2021; https://doi.org/10.1007/s00464-021-08857-5.
[59] Debourdeau A, Vitton V, Monino L, et al. Antireflux Mucosectomy Band (ARM-b) in treatment of refractory gastroesophageal reflux disease after bariatric surgery. Obes Surg 2020;30: 4654–8.
[60] Inouel H, Tanabe M, de Santiago ER, et al. Anti-reflux mucosal ablation (ARMS) as a new treatment for gastroesophageal reflux refractory to proton pump inhibitors: a pilot study. Endosc Int Open 2020;8:133–8.
[61] Wong H, Su B, Attaar M, et al. Anti-reflux mucosectomy (ARMS) results in improved recovery and similar reflux quality of life outcomes compared to laparoscopic Nissen fundoplication. Surg Endosc 2020; https://doi.org/10.1007/s00464-020-08144-9.

Advances in Surgery 56 (2022) 229–245

ADVANCES IN SURGERY

Direct Peritoneal Resuscitation for Trauma

Samuel J. Pera, MD, Jessica Schucht, MD, PhD,
Jason W. Smith, MD, PhD, MBA*

Hiram C. Polk Jr. Department of Surgery, University of Louisville, 550 South Jackson Street, Louisville, KY 40202, USA

Keywords

• Direct peritoneal resuscitation • Damage Control Surgery • Trauma

Key points

- Direct peritoneal resuscitation (DPR) has been found to be a useful adjunct for severely injured trauma patients requiring damage control surgery.
- DPR can be performed using items commonly found in most operating rooms—temporary abdominal closure, surgical drain, and peritoneal dialysis solution.
- DPR has been found to decrease the time to definitive fascial closure, increased likelihood of primary fascial closure, and fewer abdominal complications following damage control surgery.
- Clinical scenarios where DPR has been found beneficial include traumatically injured patients, emergency general surgery patients, and organ donors.

INTRODUCTION

Severely injured patients present unique challenges to the receiving center and treating physicians. These patients require rapid assessment, quick thinking, and a well-functioning team to determine the source of the problem and necessary treatment quickly. Hemorrhagic shock is most commonly the source of instability in the trauma patient with many associated consequences and physiologic changes [1–3]. The 1993 seminal article by Rotondo and colleagues described damage control surgery and instantly changed the management of these patients [4]. Surgical practice shifted from attempting a definitive repair

*Corresponding author. *E-mail address:* Jasonw.smith@louisville.edu
Twitter: @DrJtrauma (J.W.S.)

https://doi.org/10.1016/j.yasu.2022.03.003

Abbreviations

DPR	Direct Peritoneal Resuscitation
PD	Peritoneal Dialysis
IRI	Injury Reperfusion Injury
FFP	Fresh Frozen Plasma
CR	Conventional Resuscitation
MODS	Multiorgan Dysfunction Syndrome
ICU	Intensive Care Unit
ISS	Injury Severity Score

on the index operation to controlling the immediate threats to life with subsequent open abdomen, Intensive Care Unit (ICU) resuscitation, and further surgery once stabilized [5]. This strategy was effective in keeping patients alive. However, this resulted in more open abdomens, thus creating further questions on the proper management. This change, along with the resuscitation strategies of the 1990s focusing on large volume crystalloid infusion, resulted in abdominal cavities that could not achieve primary fascial closure, high rates of intra-abdominal complications, and long-term hernia formation [6,7]. During the next 2 decades, surgeons investigated ways to better care for these critically ill patients requiring damage control laparotomies. Techniques ranging from specialized abdominal closure devices, scheduled takebacks with sequential closure, or hypertonic saline have been studied as adjuncts to the closure of the open abdomen [8–10]. This article will discuss an alternative technique called direct peritoneal resuscitation (DPR).

DIRECT PERITONEAL RESUSCITATION PATHOPHYSIOLOGY

Before discussing the clinical applications, it is essential to discuss the underlying pathophysiology and cellular changes associated with DPR. DPR is a validated resuscitative method that augments visceral microcirculatory flow. Following the initial hemorrhagic shock insult, significant morbidity and mortality occur due to an ischemia reperfusion injury (IRI) that restored blood flow to the visceral organs [11]. Despite restoring central hemodynamics, studies have shown that the visceral microvascular experiences persistent and progressive vasoconstriction, prolonging the ischemic insult. The duration of this ischemia has been shown to directly correlate with the extent of the injury on visceral organs and dysfunction [12]. The IRI damages endothelial and epithelial barriers, activating an aberrant inflammatory cascade that leads to multisystem organ dysfunction.

DPR augmented resuscitation is a way to combat IRI-mediated vasoconstriction. This vasoconstriction results from an overall imbalance of vasoconstrictors and vasodilators, decreased responsiveness to humoral vasodilators and disruption of endothelial-mediated vasodilation [13]. Put simply, although the vascular smooth muscle capability to dilate remains intact, the endothelium loses the ability to respond to mediators that initiate vasodilation adequately [14,15]. Glucose-based peritoneal dialysis (PD) solution, most frequently used for DPR, contains glucose and glucose degradation products that lead to visceral vasodilation due to adenosine and nitric oxide release. The release of these mediators shifts the balance toward vasodilation, therefore, augmenting visceral blood flow. This solution's hypertonicity also decreases transcellular diffusion of water through aquaporin channels following ischemia. This reverses the vasoconstriction and causes a significant sustained and instantaneous vasodilation and subsequent hyperperfusion of the visceral organs [11,14–17]. The augmented flow limits the duration of the IRI, decreasing the release of inflammatory mediators and limiting cellular swelling and apoptosis.

Initial laboratory studies focused on DPR augmented resuscitation in hemorrhagic shock and its ability to augment intestinal microcirculation and hepatic blood flow relative to crystalloid resuscitation alone. Compared with crystalloid resuscitation alone, DPR decreases tissue necrosis, attenuates the release of damage-associated molecular proteins, decreases organ edema, and improves mortality [18–21]. Because hemostatic resuscitation has become the standard of care for hemorrhagic shock, more recent studies have focused on using DPR in conjunction with fresh frozen plasma resuscitation (FFP). The combination of DPR and FFP has been shown to improve intestinal microcirculatory flow, decrease intestinal barrier breakdown and glycocalyx degradation, and decrease end-organ injury relative to either method of resuscitation alone [11,12].

Augmenting visceral blood flow, attenuating IRI, and blunting the resultant aberrant immune response are 3 main qualities that make DPR valuable in not only hemorrhagic shock but other disease pathologies with a significant component of microvascular and immune system dysfunction. Brain death is another phenomenon known to cause the release of significant inflammatory mediators resulting in organ damage. Laboratory studies show that DPR dampens this response, decreasing cellular and functional damage to the lungs, kidneys, and intestinal barrier [18,22–25]. Through similar mechanisms, DPR has also been shown to be beneficial in intra-abdominal sepsis, ischemia-reperfusion injury to the spinal cord, necrotizing enterocolitis in neonates, and improved survival following crush injuries and hemorrhagic shock/burn injury [26–30].

DIRECT PERITONEAL RESUSCITATION IN ABDOMINAL TRAUMA

Initial study

In 2010, Smith and colleagues published the first series using DPR in a clinical setting [31]. The study focused on severely injured trauma patients who required damage control surgery between 2004 and 2008. A retrospective case-control study was performed with 2:1 matching. The treatment group consisted of 20 patients who were found to be in hemorrhagic shock requiring surgical intervention. Each of these patients was found to have substantial tissue edema, hemodynamic instability, or both at the time of laparotomy. The decision was made to follow damage control principles–abbreviate the initial operation and proceed expeditiously to the ICU for further resuscitation. For the treatment group, each patient received adjunctive DPR in addition to conventional resuscitation (CR). The treatment group was then matched to 40 controls based on Injury Severity Score (ISS), age, gender, mechanism of action, initial systolic blood pressure, and presenting pH. The decision was made to exclude patients with severe head injuries.

In the DPR treatment group, each patient had a 19F Blake drain (Ethicon) placed through the left upper lateral quadrant and directed to the root of the mesentery. The abdomen was then temporarily closed with a vacuum device. The institutional practice used an improvised vacuum-assisted closure device (Barker type), which included an underlay sterile radiograph cassette fashioned to cover the abdominal viscera completely. A sterile operating room towel was then placed over the sterile cassette, 2 large 28F chests placed on top of the towel, and finally an adherent dressing such as Ioban (3M) to form a seal. The chest tubes were then connected to continuous low wall suction. The chest tubes must not contact the viscera, resulting in injury or fistula. Further, an adequate seal must be maintained.

Once in the ICU, DPR would be started by infusing dialysate through the 19F Blake drain. The 2.5% glucose-based PD solution (Delflex; Fresenius USA) was selected. The 2.5% glucose-based PD solution was more effective than the hypertonic solution with a lower likelihood of tissue desiccation and intravascular fluid shifts [32,33]. In the initial study, 500 mL of Delflex fluid was initially infused, followed by an hourly rate of 1.5 mL/kg after that. The flow rate has now been updated to be 800 mL in the first hour, followed by an hourly rate of 5 mL/kg or 400 mL/h until the weight was verified. In this initial study, crystalloid infusion and blood transfusions were left to the treating physician's discretion with the overall goal of restoring hemodynamic stability.

A wide range of variables was evaluated, comparing the DPR treatment group to the matched controls. There were no significant differences between the 2 groups in comparing baseline characteristics. Both groups had similar operative times and initial injuries. Major hepatic injuries were typical for patients suffering blunt force injury, whereas great vessel or pelvic vessel injuries were more common after penetrating trauma. ISS scores were similar in each group, with an average ISS of 36 for DPR patients and 34 for control patients. Further, both groups required more than 20 units of blood products in the first 24 hours. Mortality, hospital length of stay, ICU length of stay (ICU LOS), and ventilator days were also similar in both groups.

There were several significant differences between the 2 groups. The time to definitive fascial closure was significantly shorter in the DPR group than in the control group (4.4 ± 1.7 days vs 7.0 ± 3.4 days). Furthermore, patients in the treatment group had a higher likelihood of achieving primary fascial closure with a significant odds ratio of 10.7:1. These results are shown in Fig. 1.

The overall complication rate was similar between the 2 groups. However, the number of abdominal complications was considerably less in the DPR

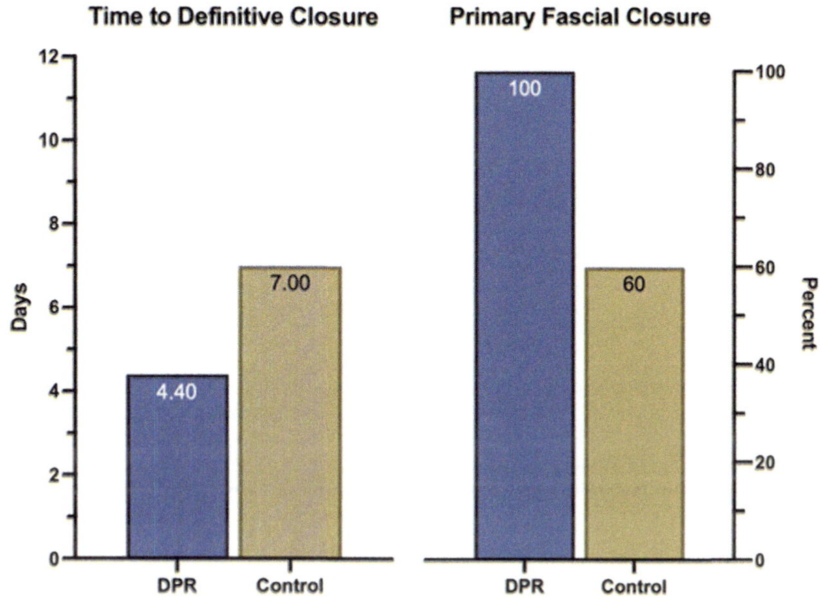

Fig. 1. Time to definitive closure and ability to achieve primary fascial closure in the control group versus DPR treatment group, both statistically significant.

group, with an odds ratio for intra-abdominal complications of 5:1 in favor of DPR over controls ($P = .05$). Further, 6 patients developed enterocutaneous fistula in the control group versus zero in the DPR group. The patients were followed for 6 months from the point of discharge. There were significantly fewer hernias seen in the DPR group than in the control (6% vs 34%, $P = .034$), with an odds ratio for hernia development of 8.5:1 in favor of the treatment group ($P = .04$). These results are seen in Fig. 2.

Finally, hepatocellular enzymes were measured in both the control and treatment groups to proxy visceral blood flow. At presentation and at 24 hours postinjury, both the aspartate transaminase (AST) and alanine transaminase (ALT) levels were found to be equal between the 2 groups. At 24 hours postresuscitation, there was a substantial difference in the rate of improvement of AST/ALT levels in favor of the DPR group. The normalization of these levels would imply improved splanchnic perfusion in the DPR treatment group despite equivalent intravenous resuscitation. These changes can be seen in Fig. 3.

There were a few weaknesses associated with this study. For starters, the study was retrospective in nature, had a small sample size, and the patients selected for DPR could not be randomized or controlled. Further resuscitation was not directly controlled and was at the discretion of the attending surgeon. The study was a case-control design, and the controls were selected to match the treatment group in terms of ISS, resuscitation volume, mortality, and base deficit on arrival. Based on this study design, it is possible the groups

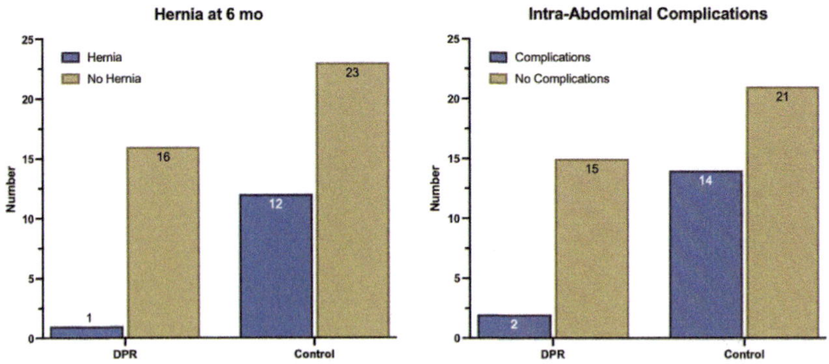

Fig. 2. Hernia development and intra-abdominal complications in the control group versus DPR treatment group with hernia development at 6 months reaching significance. The decreased hernia rate and fewer intra-abdominal complications reached statistical significance in favor of the DPR treatment group.

were not comparable, which would increase the possibility of a type 1 error. However, it is worth noting that the primary fascial closure rate in the control group was comparable to other published studies, indicating that the accelerated closure rate for the DPR group was indeed significant [34–36]. Despite some limitations, this study formed the foundation for future studies using DPR.

Randomized controlled clinical trial

In 2016, a randomized controlled trial was performed evaluating the efficacy of DPR for severely injured trauma patients [37]. The study's goal was to elucidate better if DPR could reduce systemic inflammation, improve abdominal closure rates, and reduce morbidity following damage control laparotomy. The study was performed as a single-center, nonblinded, block randomized prospective study at an American College of Surgeons-verified Level 1 trauma center. The study was conducted from January 2011 to December 2015. Patients were included if they presented in hemorrhagic shock requiring abdominal exploration. Hemorrhagic shock was defined as occurring within 4 hours of admission and 3 of the following variables:

- Tachycardia (HR > 120 beats/min)
- Hypotension (SBP < 90 mm Hg or initiation of vasopressor
- Global hypoperfusion (pH < 7.32, base deficit < −4, serum lactate > 3.0 mmol/L, or SvO_2 < 60%)
- Oliguria (urine output < 0.5 mL/kg/h for 2 hours)
- Blood transfusion requirement of >4u in initial 2 hours

Patients were excluded if they were younger than 18 years, pregnant, incarcerated at the time of presentation, not expected to survive beyond 24 hours after the initial operation, or if next of kin was unavailable or declined to enroll

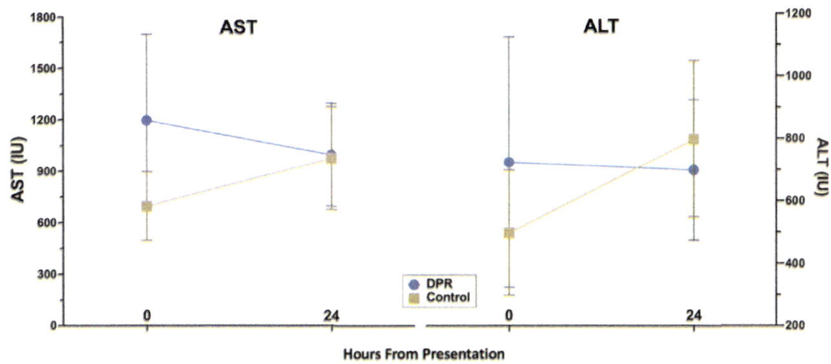

Fig. 3. Changes in liver enzymes between the control and DPR treatment groups show a trend toward improvement in the DPR group compared with worsening AST and ALT levels in the control group.

in the study. During these 5 years, 162 patients met inclusion criteria, with 110 patients being randomized. Randomization was done following a blinded individual randomization scheme, with 1:1 allocation into the conventional and peritoneal resuscitation groups. The final analysis included 51 patients in the CR group and 52 in the DPR group. This can be seen in Fig. 4.

The temporary abdominal closure device was standardized for all patients and was the Barker type improvised vacuum-assisted closure. DPR patients

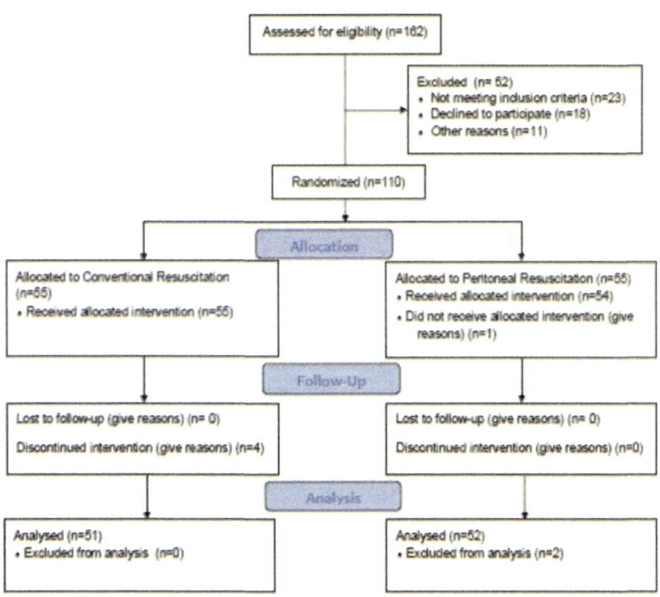

Fig. 4. Consort diagram for peritoneal resuscitation study enrollment.

had a 19F Blake drain (Ethicon) inserted into the abdomen directed around the root of the mesentery. Once stable in the ICU, continuous lavage consisting of 2.5% glucose-based PD solution (Delflex, Fresenius USA) was infused into the abdominal cavity. The initial flow rate was 800 mL for the first hour, followed by an hourly 5 mL/kg. DPR was continued until definitive abdominal closure. Patients were resuscitated using both crystalloid and blood products at the discretion of the treating physician in order to restore stable hemodynamics.

Many variables were collected with many typical of a critical care study, including basic demographics, mechanism of injury, organ injury scores, ISS, initial vitals, presenting pH, the volume of resuscitation for both crystalloid and blood products, and mortality. Unique to this study included time to definitive fascial closure, rate of primary fascial closure, and intra-abdominal complications. Additional variables such as volume removed from the open abdomen, multiorgan dysfunction syndrome (MODS) score, and various cytokines and inflammatory markers were sampled. These were accomplished as follows. For the treatment DPR group, the amount of dialysate instilled was subtracted from the volume removed from the midline vacuum device to estimate the volume of fluid lost. The control group volume was found from the total volume removed from the midline vacuum device. These were sampled for cytokines and inflammatory markers at the time of operation and then every 6 hours for the first 48 hours to assess for any differences over that initial, critical time frame.

There were several important takeaways and conclusions from this study. For starters, the 2 comparison groups were well matched after randomization. There was no notable difference in either ISS, abdominal Abbreviated Injury Scale (AIS), or head AIS. Both groups had an average ISS greater than 25, representing a severely injured patient population. Further, there was no difference in the volume of either crystalloid or blood products during the first 24 hours of resuscitation. There were some significant findings worth mentioning. The time to definitive fascial closure was found to be significantly faster in the DPR group as compared with the CR group (4.1 ± 2.2 days vs 5.9 ± 3.5 days, $P \leq .002$) and requiring significantly fewer operations in order to do so (2.4 ± 1.4 vs 3.1 ± 1.3, $P = .01$). Moreover, the primary fascial closure rate was higher in the DPR group than in the CR group (83% vs 66%, $P \leq .05$). Speed to fascial closure is a crucial variable, particularly when considering the significant intra-abdominal complications that can occur if the abdomen is left open for a prolonged period. Other studies have found significant complications in patients whose abdomen were left open for significant periods, reaffirming the importance of early closure [6,38–40]. In this study, the early closure rate likely contributed to the overall decrease for intra-abdominal complications (8% vs 18% in DPR and CR groups, respectively) and significantly reduced the likelihood of intra-abdominal abscess in the DPR group (3% vs 14%, $P < .05$). Finally, although not reaching significance, there was also a trend toward reduced mortality in the treatment group,

Table 1
Comparison of fluid removed via vacuum-assisted closure dressing in open abdomen

	Conventional Resuscitation, mean ± SD (n = 51)		Peritoneal Resuscitation, mean ± SD (n = 52)			
Hours	Total removed	Instilled	Total removed	Instilled	Difference	*P* value
12	1135 ± 498	0	5600 ± 604	4320 ± 333	1280 ± 271	0.08
24	746 ± 222	0	5625 ± 701	4641 ± 252	624 ± 449	0.08
48	908 ± 397	0	9100 ± 896	7784 ± 564	1316 ± 432	0.001
72	1101 ± 366	0	9665 ± 821	8462 ± 487	1233 ± 334	0.06
96	752 ± 279	0	8805 ± 908	7694 ± 501	1111 ± 407	0.001
120	566 ± 332	0	9368 ± 755	8321 ± 422	1407 ± 333	0.001

with a DPR 30-day mortality rate of 13% versus 28% ($P = .06$) in the CR group.

One theory supporting why the treatment group had a significant early abdominal closure and high primary fascial closure rates was based on the net removal of fluid from the abdomen, which was thought to be a proxy for reducing visceral edema. In the control group, this was monitored and recorded daily. The amount of instilled dialysate was subtracted from the output giving the net removal for the DPR group. In comparing each group per time interval and considering the instilled dialysate, the DPR group has a consistently higher output, frequently reaching statistical significance. This can be seen in Table 1.

Multiple different variables were evaluated when comparing the degree of systemic inflammation and cellular injury. They included the MODS score, cytokines, and inflammatory markers. For the 16 cytokines and inflammatory markers that were sampled, 4 (interleukin-6, tumor necrosis factor-α, high mobility group box one protein, and intestinal fatty acid-binding protein) demonstrated trends of possible clinical significance. These markers have previously been associated with improved outcomes after trauma [41–43]. Each of these markers was decreased in the treatment DPR group versus the control group. This decrease was typically seen 12 hours after exploration and did reach clinical significance for each marker. This finding may signify a reduction in visceral and systemic inflammation initiated by peritoneal resuscitation. Further clinical research will be necessary to make more definitive conclusions.

The MODS score was the other marker comparing the degree of systemic inflammation and cellular injury. The MODS score is a validated scoring system used to stratify clinical outcomes in the critically ill. Input variables include the partial pressure of oxygen (PaO_2), fraction of inspired oxygen (FiO_2), central venous pressure, mean arterial pressure (MAP), heart rate, platelets, bilirubin, creatinine, and the Glasgow Coma Scale. The scoring system will predict ICU mortality, ICU length of stay, and in-hospital mortality with the lower the score, the more favorable the outcome [44]. The MODS score was tracked over time and compared between the 2 groups. Although being an imprecise measure, the MODS score for the DPR group was consistently lower than the CR group, frequently reaching statistical levels. These results can be seen in Table 2.

Table 2
MODS score changes between the conventional and peritoneal resuscitation groups

Time, h	Conventional resuscitation, mean ± SD (n = 51)	Peritoneal resuscitation, mean ± SD (n = 52)	*P* value
Initial	4.3 ± 0.6	3.5 ± 0.9	0.001
12	6 ± 3.6	6.6 ± 2.9	0.35
24	9.4 ± 4	7.9 ± 3.2	0.04
48	8.7 ± 4.1	6.1 ± 4.6	0.003
72	8.8 ± 3.7	6.9 ± 2.5	0.003
96	6.7 ± 3	5.5 ± 2.7	0.04
120	6 ± 3.3	4 ± 2.1	0.004
144	4.4 ± 2.5	3.3 ± 1.9	0.02
168	4 ± 2	3.3 ± 1.8	0.06

Finally, multivariate analysis was performed to determine predictors of mortality concerning CR versus DPR. Several predictors were identified, each associated with increased mortality in either treatment group, and they included increasing ISS, age, head AIS, low Systolic Blood Pressure (SBP), and pH on arrival. The analysis identified control group patients as 2.4 times more likely to die after damage control surgery than treatment group patients; however, this was not statistically significant (odds ratio = 2.4, 95% CI 0.88–6.653, $P = .06$). Power analysis demonstrated that a sample size of approximately 350 patients would be required to find a significant difference.

There were weaknesses associated with the study that are important to acknowledge. Although this was a randomized controlled trial, it was a single institution. Randomization was completed; however, blinding the treating physicians was not possible due to the nature of the study and could have increased the risk of bias. This study was performed over 5 years, and during that time frame, fundamental shifts occurred regarding resuscitation methodology. Specifically, as the study progressed, far less crystalloid was administered with a greater focus on blood products and focused resuscitation with discernible endpoints. Further, resuscitation practices were left to the treating physician's discretion and were not explicitly controlled in the study.

Other applications for direct peritoneal resuscitation

As DPR has evolved, so have the indications for using the therapy and patient populations who may benefit from the intervention. The first patient population for whom DPR may benefit were emergency general surgery (EGS) patients undergoing emergency laparotomy, typically due to abdominal sepsis. The second population was individuals who met the brain death criteria and became organ donors. Each will be discussed further.

Direct peritoneal resuscitation for emergency general surgery patients

In 2014, Smith and colleagues investigated the utility of DPR for EGS patients as the next logical step of implementation as many of these patients required damage control surgery due to intra-abdominal sepsis [45,46]. Similar to trauma patients in hemorrhagic shock, EGS patients in septic shock were prone to developing acidosis, hypothermia, and coagulopathy with resultant poor clinical outcomes [47]. DPR has already been shown an effective adjunct for trauma patients due to its ability to improve microvascular perfusion and reduce tissue injury [14,33]. In trials involving trauma patients, DPR had been shown to increase primary fascial closure rates, decrease time to fascial closure, and have an improved profile regarding intra-abdominal infection [31,37]. The investigators hypothesized a similar benefit for EGS patients.

The study was performed from January 2008 to December 2012 at an American College of Surgeons Level 1 academic institution. Patients were enrolled in a sequential cohort manner, first enrolling the control arm from 2008 to 2010, followed sequentially by the DPR arm from 2010 to 2012. All patients older than 18 years, up to 80 year old, were included. After the first operation, all patients underwent damage control surgery with an open abdomen. The temporary abdominal closure was standardized for all patients and described in the prior sections. DPR was performed as previously described. The indications for surgery included necrotizing pancreatitis, perforated viscous, small bowel obstruction, anastomotic leak, and bowel ischemia.

A total of 118 patients enrolled in the study. Due to the sequential enrollment, 67 patients were enrolled in the control, CR group, and 51 patients in the DPR treatment group. In comparing the 2 groups, there were several significant differences, including age, heart rate and respiratory rate on arrival, platelet counts, the partial pressure of CO_2, and multiple electrolytes. The study investigators performed propensity matching to control for some of these variables and create 2 comparable groups. The matching process was done following the GMATCH algorithm developed by the Mayo Clinic [48,49]. In short, the process matched a DPR patient to a control patient with prespecified parameters to create a good match; further, each patient was matched only once. Once this was complete, there were 44 matched pairings, and there were no longer statistically significant differences between the 2 groups. The remainder of the study analysis was performed on these matched pairings.

The most common indications for surgery in the matched pairs were perforated viscous, small bowel obstruction, and intestinal ischemia. The most common indications for damage control surgery were bowel viability, contamination, and hemodynamic instability. Both indications were similar between the 2 groups. Measured variables including blood product administration in the first 24 and 48 hours were not significantly different. There was a significant difference in the volume of crystalloid received at both 24 and 48 hours, with the control group receiving significantly higher volumes as compared with the DPR treatment group (IVF @ 24 hours, 10, 840 $\pm$ 1740 vs 9870 $\pm$ 1600 $P = .01$ and IVF @ 48 hours, 18,300 $\pm$ 2650 vs 15,900 $\pm$ 3100 $P < .001$).

Multiple critical care scoring systems were calculated, including the Acute Physiology and Chronic Health Evaluation II, Sequential Organ Failure Assessment score, and Simplified Acute Physiology Score, in order to compare the physiologic response to illness in the 2 groups [50–55]. Initially, the scoring systems were equal between groups as the matching process used many independent variables to create the cohorts. However, at 48 hours after laparotomy, the DPR group was found to have significantly lower scores than the control group. DPR seemed to have a significant impact in improving the underlying physiology in these critically ill patients.

Next, several outcome variables were measured and compared between the 2 groups. The variables measured include time to definitive abdominal closure, rate of primary fascial closure, intra-abdominal complications, ventilator days and ICU LOS, and mortality, to name a few. These findings are summarized in Table 3.

As seen in the table, many of these variables reached statistical significance. However, neither total LOS nor mortality was significant in this matched cohort. To rule out a type II error, the necessary power required for a study of that type would require nearly double the sample size. It is noteworthy that many of the same significant findings in the DPR group used in abdominal trauma (no. of trips to the operating room, time to definitive abdominal closure, achieving primary fascial closure, and abdominal complications) were also significant in the EGS population. Thus, DPR played a positive role in managing the open abdomen.

There are several limitations in this study that deserve mention. First, again, this was a single institution, prospective cohort study. Due to the mismatch in the natural accrual of patients, the comparison groups required propensity score matching to have 2 homogenous groups. Further, the matching process mitigates the variability and natural discrepancy between 2 groups to have similar baseline demographics. Second, as this study was unable to be blinded, investigator bias is possible. Finally, the study was completed between 2008 and 2012. During this time frame, many advances in resuscitation were made, particularly in using blood products instead of crystalloid [56,57]. The total volumes of crystalloid given to both treatment and control groups would be exceedingly uncommon in practice today.

Direct peritoneal lavage to human cadaver organ donor improves organ procurement

The final article to mention was written in 2015. This study specifically evaluated the role of DPR in brain dead (BD) organ donors [58]. DPR was a helpful

Table 3
Propensity-matched cohort outcome variables

	Controls (n = 44)	DPR (n = 44)	*P* value
No. trips to the operating room	4(2)	3(2)	0.02
Time to definitive abdominal closure, d	7.7(4.1)	5.9(3.2)	0.02
Primary fascial closure, n%	19(43)	29(68)	0.03
No. abdominal complications	21(47%)	12(27%)	0.04
Ventilators days	14(6)	10(5)	0.01
ICU LOS, d	24(11)	17(9)	0.002
Total LOS, d	41(13)	34(16)	0.06
ICU-free days	26(11)	31(13)	0.05
Mortality, n%	12(27)	7(16)	0.15

adjunct because BD organ donors have several physiologic derangements that decrease organ function. These donors have altered central hemodynamics, impaired hormone physiology, exaggerated systemic inflammatory response, end-organ microcirculatory dysfunction, and tissue hypoxia. These derangements have explicitly been evaluated in prior animal models that showed improvement after undergoing DPR [18,22–25].

The study's goal was to see if DPR increased the organs transplanted per donor [59]. Patients were prospectively enrolled from January 2012 to August 2014. Those in the control group underwent the standard organ donor resuscitation. This resuscitation is based on donor management goals set by the local organ procurement organizations [60–63]. The patients in the treatment group had the same donor management goals for resuscitation, and DPR was performed. DPR therapy was performed by placing a peritoneal lavage catheter into the abdomen via the open technique. Once done, peritoneal dialysate was instilled via passive infusion. The dialysate remained in the abdomen for 2 hours before being siphoned off for an hour. This process was repeated a second time with the dialysate left in the abdomen until the time of organ removal.

The 2 groups were compared with one another with a few significant findings. For starters, the DPR group was found to require significantly less IV crystalloid and reduced use of IV vasopressor agents during the initial resuscitation. There were no adverse effect on UOP, MAP, or specific donor management goals. Next, effective hepatic blood flow was measured by infusing galactose at a steady state and assessing clearance [25]. The DPR treatment group was found to have significantly increased effective hepatic blood flow compared with the control. This effect was seen to taper down over time; however, the DPR group always had a significantly higher flow over the first 12 hours. Finally, the number of organs donated per treatment group was compared against the expected number of organs to be donated. The expected number of organs was calculated using the Scientific Registry of Transplant Recipient (SRTR) organ yield per donor calculator [64]. The calculator takes baseline clinical information about the donor and estimates an expected yield for each organ in each donor. There was no significant difference when comparing the donors SRTR between the treatment and control groups. However, when calculating the actual number of organs donated per donor in each group, there was a statistical difference in favor of the DPR group.

There were a few limitations associated with this study. For starters, the donors could not be randomized at the time of enrollment due to the availability of a surgeon to place the catheter. Even though the physician managing the resuscitation was blinded to the treatment group, bias cannot be excluded entirely. Further, the sample size was small, and the patient population was from one region, potentially limiting the generalizability of the study. Finally, the data included in this study were entirely about the donor; no information was available regarding the recipient. This information would be vital in determining the effect DPR had on the transplanted organs.

FUTURE DIRECTIONS FOR DIRECT PERITONEAL RESUSCITATION

DPR has shown promising results across a broad spectrum of patient populations. The limitations of the studies listed have been small sample sizes, lack of randomization, and the studies performed at one institution. Therefore, to definitively determine the utility of DPR, large randomized multicenter trials will need to be performed. Further, more extensive trials involving abdominal sepsis should be performed to determine DPR's effect on outcomes. Different patient populations should also be studied, including burn patients and vascular patients requiring an open abdomen approach. Finally, patients in fulminant sepsis could be considered a target population, mainly when a significant IRI occurs. Disease processes such as clostridium difficile colitis, pneumonia, and urinary tract infections could be potential targets.

SUMMARY

DPR has shown to be effective in both animal models and small-scale human trials. There is good evidence to suggest that DPR helps minimize the effect of shock by reducing organ edema, improving hepatic blood flow, and reducing serum levels of inflammatory cytokines. In the patient trials, DPR has been shown to increase the rate of primary fascial closure, decrease the time to definitive closure, and decrease the incidence of intra-abdominal complications. Further studies are needed to validate these findings.

CRITICAL CARE POINTS

- Damage control surgery is the mainstay of treatment of patients who present in extremis, whether from hemorrhagic or septic shock.
- Damage control surgery involves an expedited surgical exploration, hemorrhage or source control, temporary abdominal closure, and further resuscitation in the intensive care unit. Definitive surgical care would proceed once the patient has been physiologically corrected.
- DPR should be considered whenever a damage control laparotomy is being performed.

Disclosure

The authors have nothing to disclose.

References

[1] Feliciano DV, Mattox KL, Jordan GL Jr. Intra-abdominal packing for control of hepatic hemorrhage: a reappraisal. J Trauma 1981;21(4):285–90.
[2] Stone HH, Strom PR, Mullins RJ. Management of the major coagulopathy with onset during laparotomy. Ann Surg 1983;197(5):532–5.
[3] Wilson RF, Dulchavsky SA, Soullier G, et al. Problems with 20 or more blood transfusions in 24 hours. Am Surg 1987;53(7):410–7.

[4] Rotondo MF, Schwab CW, McGonigal MD, et al. Damage control': an approach for improved survival in exsanguinating penetrating abdominal injury. J Trauma 1993;35(3):375–82.
[5] Rotondo MF, Zonies DH. The damage control sequence and underlying logic. Surg Clin North Am 1997;77(4):761–77.
[6] Miller RS, Morris JA Jr, Diaz JJ Jr, et al. Complications after 344 damage-control open celiotomies. J Trauma 2005;59(6):1365–71.
[7] Bradley MJ, Dubose JJ, Scalea TM, et al. Independent predictors of enteric fistula and abdominal sepsis after damage control laparotomy: results from the prospective AAST Open Abdomen registry. JAMA Surg 2013;148(10):947–54.
[8] Burlew CC, Moore EE, Biffl WL, et al. One hundred percent fascial approximation can be achieved in the postinjury open abdomen with a sequential closure protocol. J Trauma Acute Care Surg 2012;72(1):235–41.
[9] Dennis A, Vizinas TA, Joseph K, et al. Not so fast to skin graft: transabdominal wall traction closes most "domain loss" abdomens in the acute setting. J Trauma Acute Care Surg 2013;74(6):1486–92.
[10] Harvin JA, Mims MM, Duchesne JC, et al. Chasing 100%: the use of hypertonic saline to improve early, primary fascial closure after damage control laparotomy. J Trauma Acute Care Surg 2013;74(2):426–30.
[11] Schucht JE, Matheson PJ, Harbrecht BG, et al. Plasma resuscitation with adjunctive peritoneal resuscitation reduces ischemic intestinal injury following hemorrhagic shock. J Trauma Acute Care Surg 2020;89(4):649–57.
[12] Schucht JE, Matheson PJ, Harbrecht BG, et al. Plasma resuscitation with adjunctive peritoneal resuscitation reduces ischemia-induced intestinal barrier breakdown following hemorrhagic shock. J Trauma Acute Care Surg 2021;90(1):27–34.
[13] Torres Filho I. Hemorrhagic Shock and the Microvasculature. Compr Physiol 2017;8(1):61–101.
[14] Zakaria el R, Li N, Garrison RN. Mechanisms of direct peritoneal resuscitation-mediated splanchnic hyperperfusion following hemorrhagic shock. Shock 2007;27(4):436–42.
[15] Garrison RN. Zakaria el R. Peritoneal resuscitation. Am J Surg 2005;190(2):181–5.
[16] Khaneki S, Jensen AR, Drucker NA, et al. Direct peritoneal resuscitation improves mesenteric perfusion by nitric oxide dependent pathways. J Surg Res 2017;213:274–80.
[17] Weaver JL, Smith JW. Direct Peritoneal Resuscitation: A review. Int J Surg 2016;33(Pt B):237–41.
[18] Weaver JL, Matheson PJ, Hurt RT, et al. Direct Peritoneal Resuscitation Alters Hepatic miRNA Expression after Hemorrhagic Shock. J Am Coll Surg 2016;223(1):68–75.
[19] Crafts TD, Hunsberger EB, Jensen AR, et al. Direct peritoneal resuscitation improves survival and decreases inflammation after intestinal ischemia and reperfusion injury. J Surg Res 2015;199(2):428–34.
[20] Hurt RT, Matheson PJ, Smith JW, et al. Preservation of hepatic blood flow by direct peritoneal resuscitation improves survival and prevents hepatic inflammation following hemorrhagic shock. Am J Physiol Gastrointest Liver Physiol 2012;303(10):G1144–52.
[21] Matheson PJ, Mays CJ, Hurt RT, et al. Modulation of mesenteric lymph flow and composition by direct peritoneal resuscitation from hemorrhagic shock. Arch Surg 2009;144(7):625–34.
[22] Weaver JL, Schucht JE, Matheson PJ, et al. Direct Peritoneal Resuscitation Reduces Lung Injury and Caspase 8 Activity in Brain Death. J Invest Surg 2020;33(9):803–12.
[23] Weaver JL, Matheson PJ, Matheson A, et al. Direct peritoneal resuscitation reduces inflammation in the kidney after acute brain death. Am J Physiol Ren Physiol 2018;315(2):F406–12.
[24] Weaver JL, Matheson PJ, Matheson A, et al. Direct Peritoneal Resuscitation Alters Leukocyte Infiltration in the Lung After Acute Brain Death. Shock 2018;50(5):565–71.
[25] Smith JW, Ghazi CA, Cain BC, et al. Direct peritoneal resuscitation improves inflammation, liver blood flow, and pulmonary edema in a rat model of acute brain death. J Am Coll Surg 2014;219(1):79–87.

[26] Xiong Y, Xia Y, Deng J, et al. Direct Peritoneal Resuscitation with Pyruvate Protects the Spinal Cord and Induces Autophagy via Regulating PHD2 in a Rat Model of Spinal Cord Ischemia-Reperfusion Injury. Oxid Med Cell Longev 2020;2020:4909103; https://doi.org/10.1155/2020/4909103.

[27] Jung AD, Friend LA, Stevens-Topie S, et al. Direct Peritoneal Resuscitation Improves Survival in a Murine Model of Combined Hemorrhage and Burn Injury. Mil Med 2020;185(9–10):e1528–35.

[28] Zhou XL, Ni SZ, Xiong D, et al. Fluid resuscitation with preventive peritoneal dialysis attenuates crush injury-related acute kidney injury and improves survival outcome. Scand J Trauma Resusc Emerg Med 2019;27(1):68.

[29] Maki AC, Matheson PJ, Shepherd JA, et al. Intestinal microcirculatory flow alterations in necrotizing enterocolitis are improved by direct peritoneal resuscitation. Am Surg 2012;78(7):803–7.

[30] Luo X, Jian D, Lv Z. The beneficial effect of direct peritoneal resuscitation on septic shock in rats. J Biomed Biotechnol 2011;2011:743763.

[31] Smith JW, Garrison RN, Matheson PJ, et al. Direct peritoneal resuscitation accelerates primary abdominal wall closure after damage control surgery. J Am Coll Surg 2010;210(5):658–64.

[32] Zakaria el R, Patel AA, Li N, et al. Vasoactive components of dialysis solution. Perit Dial Int 2008;28(3):283–95.

[33] Zakaria el R, Spain DA, Harris PD, et al. Generalized dilation of the visceral microvasculature by peritoneal dialysis solutions. Perit Dial Int 2002;22(5):593–601.

[34] Bee TK, Croce MA, Magnotti LJ, et al. Temporary abdominal closure techniques: a prospective randomized trial comparing polyglactin 910 mesh and vacuum-assisted closure. J Trauma 2008;65(2):337–42.

[35] Barker DE, Green JM, Maxwell RA, et al. Experience with vacuum-pack temporary abdominal wound closure in 258 trauma and general and vascular surgical patients. J Am Coll Surg 2007;204(5):784–92.

[36] Miller PR, Meredith JW, Johnson JC, et al. Prospective evaluation of vacuum-assisted fascial closure after open abdomen: planned ventral hernia rate is substantially reduced. Ann Surg 2004;239(5):608–14.

[37] Smith JW, Matheson PJ, Franklin GA, et al. Randomized Controlled Trial Evaluating the Efficacy of Peritoneal Resuscitation in the Management of Trauma Patients Undergoing Damage Control Surgery. J Am Coll Surg 2017;224(4):396–404.

[38] Dubose JJ, Scalea TM, Holcomb JB, et al. Open abdominal management after damage-control laparotomy for trauma: a prospective observational American Association for the Surgery of Trauma multi-center study. J Trauma Acute Care Surg 2013;74(1):113–20.

[39] Fox N, Crutchfield M, LaChant M, et al. Early abdominal closure improves long-term outcomes after damage-control laparotomy. J Trauma Acute Care Surg 2013;75(5):854–8.

[40] Sharrock AE, Barker T, Yuen HM, et al. Management and closure of the open abdomen after damage control laparotomy for trauma. A systematic review and meta-analysis. Injury 2016;47(2):296–306.

[41] Volpin G, Cohen M, Assaf M, et al. Cytokine levels (IL-4, IL-6, IL-8 and TGFbeta) as potential biomarkers of systemic inflammatory response in trauma patients. Int Orthop 2014;38(6):1303–9.

[42] Ayala A, Wang P, Ba ZF, et al. Differential alterations in plasma IL-6 and TNF levels after trauma and hemorrhage. Am J Physiol 1991;260(1 Pt 2):R167–71.

[43] Hunter CA, Jones SA. IL-6 as a keystone cytokine in health and disease. Nat Immunol 2015;16(5):448–57.

[44] Marshall JC, Cook DJ, Christou NV, et al. Multiple organ dysfunction score: a reliable descriptor of a complex clinical outcome. Crit Care Med 1995;23(10):1638–52.

[45] Smith JW, Neal Garrison R, Matheson PJ, et al. Adjunctive treatment of abdominal catastrophes and sepsis with direct peritoneal resuscitation: indications for use in acute care surgery. J Trauma Acute Care Surg 2014;77(3):393–8.
[46] Weber DG, Bendinelli C, Balogh ZJ. Damage control surgery for abdominal emergencies. Br J Surg 2014;101(1):e109–18.
[47] Ferrara A, MacArthur JD, Wright HK, et al. Hypothermia and acidosis worsen coagulopathy in the patient requiring massive transfusion. Am J Surg 1990;160(5):515–8.
[48] Bergstralh E, Kosanke J. GMATCH Software. Developed by Mayo Clinic Division of Biomedical Statistics and Informatics. 2003.
[49] Austin PC. A critical appraisal of propensity-score matching in the medical literature between 1996 and 2003. Stat Med 2008;27(12):2037–49.
[50] Knaus WA, Draper EA, Wagner DP, et al. APACHE II: a severity of disease classification system. Crit Care Med 1985;13(10):818–29.
[51] Knaus WA, Wagner DP, Draper EA, et al. The APACHE III prognostic system. Risk prediction of hospital mortality for critically ill hospitalized adults. Chest 1991;100(6):1619–36.
[52] Vincent JL, de Mendonca A, Cantraine F, et al. Use of the SOFA score to assess the incidence of organ dysfunction/failure in intensive care units: results of a multi-center, prospective study. Working group on "sepsis-related problems" of the European Society of Intensive Care Medicine. Crit Care Med 1998;26(11):1793–800.
[53] Moreno R, Morais P. Outcome prediction in intensive care: results of a prospective, multicentre, Portuguese study. Intensive Care Med 1997;23(2):177–86.
[54] Livingston BM, MacKirdy FN, Howie JC, et al. Assessment of the performance of five intensive care scoring models within a large Scottish database. Crit Care Med 2000;28(6):1820–7.
[55] Le Gall JR, Lemeshow S, Saulnier F. A new Simplified Acute Physiology Score (SAPS II) based on a European/North American multi-center study. JAMA 1993;270(24):2957–63.
[56] Holcomb JB, del Junco DJ, Fox EE, et al. The prospective, observational, multi-center, major trauma transfusion (PROMMTT) study: comparative effectiveness of a time-varying treatment with competing risks. JAMA Surg 2013;148(2):127–36.
[57] Holcomb JB, Tilley BC, Baraniuk S, et al. Transfusion of plasma, platelets, and red blood cells in a 1:1:1 vs a 1:1:2 ratio and mortality in patients with severe trauma: the PROPPR randomized clinical trial. JAMA 2015;313(5):471–82.
[58] Smith JW, Matheson PJ, Morgan G, et al. Addition of direct peritoneal lavage to human cadaver organ donor resuscitation improves organ procurement. J Am Coll Surg 2015;220(4):539–47.
[59] Santivasi WL, Strand JJ, Mueller PS, et al. The Organ Transplant Imperative. Mayo Clin Proc 2017;92(6):940–6.
[60] Malinoski DJ, Daly MC, Patel MS, et al. Achieving donor management goals before deceased donor procurement is associated with more organs transplanted per donor. J Trauma 2011;71(4):990–5, ; discussion 996.
[61] Patel MS, Zatarain J, De La Cruz S, et al. The impact of meeting donor management goals on the number of organs transplanted per expanded criteria donor: a prospective study from the UNOS Region 5 Donor Management Goals Workgroup. JAMA Surg 2014;149(9):969–75.
[62] Hagan ME, McClean D, Falcone CA, et al. Attaining specific donor management goals increases number of organs transplanted per donor: a quality improvement project. Prog Transpl 2009;19(3):227–31.
[63] Franklin GA, Santos AP, Smith JW, et al. Optimization of donor management goals yields increased organ use. Am Surg 2010;76(6):587–94.
[64] Scientific Registry of Transplant Recipients. Available at: www.SRTR.org. Accessed January 1, 2022.

Advances in Surgery 56 (2022) 247–258

ADVANCES IN SURGERY

What is the Best Inguinal Hernia Repair?

Jennwood Chen, MD[a,b,*],
Robert E. Glasgow, MD, MBA, FACS[a,c]

[a]Univeristy of Utah, Department of Surgery, 50 Medical Dr N, Salt Lake City, UT 84132, USA; [b]Veterans Affairs, Department of Surgery, 550 Foothill Dr, Salt Lake City, UT 84113, USA; [c]Huntsman Cancer Institute, 1950 Circle of Hope, Salt Lake City, UT 84112, USA

Keywords

• Inguinal hernia • Hernia repair • Quality • Value • Mesh • Laparoscopy • Lichtenstein repair • Review

Key points

- Use of mesh, when possible, in inguinal hernia repair decreases recurrence.
- A minimally invasive approach to inguinal hernia repair decreases incisional and chronic pain.
- The best inguinal hernia repair is one that optimizes durability, decreases chronic pain, and optimizes quality of life, all at a minimum overall cost to the health care system.
- Currently, laparoscopic inguinal hernia repair is the best repair.

INTRODUCTION

Somewhat debated, the etymologic origins of "hernia" have been traced back to the Latin word *hirnia*, meaning "a rupture," and to the Greek word *hernios*, meaning "offshoot or bud" [1,2]. Nonetheless, inguinal hernias are an ancient disease with the first written accounts of occurrence dating back to antiquity [1–4].

Inguinal hernias include indirect, direct, femoral, and obturator hernias. Two-thirds of these hernias are indirect, making an indirect hernia the most common groin hernia in both sexes [5]. The cause of inguinal herniation is considered to be multifactorial. In the adult population, weakening or widening

*Corresponding author. 30 North 1900 East, SOM 3B115, Salt Lake City, UT 84132. *E-mail addresses:* Jennwood.Chen@hsc.utah.edu (J.C.); Robert.Glasgow@hsc.utah.edu (R.E.G.)

https://doi.org/10.1016/j.yasu.2022.02.007
0065-3411/22/Published by Elsevier Inc.

of the internal ring may make an asymptomatic patent *processus vaginalis* symptomatic [6,7]. A direct hernia occurs through a defect or weakness in the posterior wall of the inguinal canal (Hesselbach triangle), usually through the transversalis fascia, and thus, increased intraabdominal pressures are thought to be a predisposing factor [8].

Inguinal herniorrhaphy (hernia + *-rrhaphy:* meaning "suture") is one of the most common surgeries performed with nearly 20 million world-wide procedures conducted annually, 800,000 of which occur in the United States [9,10]. It is estimated that 27% to 43% of men and 3% to 6% of women will develop an inguinal hernia during their lifetime [9,11,12].

The history of inguinal hernia surgery is lengthy. However, our evolution of surgical techniques has been contingent on our elucidation and understanding of inguinal anatomy, and thus, the contributions of many great surgeon-anatomists such as Hunter, Cooper, Hesselbach, Camper, Scarpa, Richter, and Gimbernat should not be forgotten. That said, the modern era of inguinal hernia surgery can be attributed to Edoardo Bassini when, in 1887, he described his landmark, tissue-based procedure that allowed for reconstruction of the posterior wall of the inguinal canal and removal of the hernia sac [1]. His revolutionary surgical technique required no additional reinforcement or prosthesis and laid the foundation of modern-day inguinal herniorrhaphy [13].

Since Bassini's epoch-making contribution, more than 100 various techniques for repair of inguinal hernias have been described [14]. Driven in large part by surgical technology, these repairs are broadly characterized by tissue, open mesh, and minimally invasive techniques.

Furthermore, as our health care delivery model continues to evolve from a "quantity" to a "quality" model, so too has our understanding of what constitutes a "successful procedure." Thus, to answer the question "What is the best repair for inguinal hernias?", one must identify and evaluate the interests of the main stakeholders of health care delivery, namely (1) the patient, (2) the provider, and (3) the payor. As patients are the main beneficiary of health care delivery, prioritizing metrics that optimize quality in this framework, we must consider durability, postoperative pain, quality of life (QoL), generalizability, and cost [15,16].

It is important to understand that there is a plethora of considerations that will influence a surgeon's approach to inguinal hernia repair such as surgeon experience, primary versus recurrent, unilateral versus bilateral, previous violation of dissection planes, body habitus, surgical history, and concomitant medical comorbidities, such that the most concise answer to "What is the best repair for inguinal hernias?" is "It depends…". This "cheeky" response, however, is entirely unhelpful. Therefore, in an effort to increase the probability of arriving at a definitive answer, the following discussion will assume a clinical scenario of primary, unilateral inguinal hernias. Furthermore, we will also assume "laparoscopic inguinal hernia repair" to mean both transabdominal preperitoneal (TAPP) and totally extraperitoneal (TEP) approaches, whereas "robotic inguinal hernia repair" will consider only the TAPP approach.

RECURRENCE

Perhaps the most critical and obvious measure of success when one considers the myriad of approaches to inguinal herniorrhaphy is the durability of the repair.

Mesh versus nonmesh

Following the adoption and wide spread practice of the Bassini repair, surgeons soon discovered that forcefully suturing anatomic structures that are not normally in apposition increases tension and hence, hernia recurrence. The quest for a "tension-free" repair thus began in the early twentieth century [4,17]. Surgeons such as Wölfer, Halsted, Tanner, and McVay contributed their modifications by introducing various relaxing incisions; over time, many more iterations of tissue-based repairs were created [18]. Of these, the Shouldice repair deserves special mention, as it is often considered the best "nonmesh based method" when considering recurrence rates and durability [19].

The Canadian Shouldice repair, more commonly referred to as "the Shouldice repair," is a modern resurrection and direct descendant of the Bassini procedure [20]. Developed during the 1950s by Shouldice, Obney, and Ryan, the Shouldice technique is unique among tissue-based repairs, as it is a multilayer reconstruction of the posterior inguinal wall, by imbricating rather than abutting the layers; moreover, the procedure describes excision of the weakened transversalis fascia [4,17,19,20]. In specialist centers, the reported recurrence rates of the Shouldice repair have been reported as low as 0.6% to 1.4% [21–23]. That said, in nonspecialist centers, the recurrence rate approaches 10%, which likely speaks to the technical complexity of the procedure and thus steeper learning curve [24–29].

Another strategy to circumvent the adverse effects of suture line tension is to use a foreign material to create a tensionless repair [1,2,30]. In 1890, Theodor Billroth suggested that the ideal way to repair a hernia defect is with a prosthetic material [31,32]. Today, our understanding of the role of impaired collagen metabolism in the pathogenesis of groin hernias and its role in surgical failure vindicates the near century quest for an adequate xenoprosthetic to be used in inguinal hernia repair, as the use of an already weakened tissue plane to repair a defect, particularly under tension, is a violation of basic surgical principles [33,34].

The evolution of prosthetics in inguinal hernia repair culminated in the 1980s into what is now eponymously called the Lichtenstein repair, which is synonymous with "tension-free" hernioplasty [30,35]. It should be noted that what makes a *hernioplasty* different from *herniorrhaphy* is the use of prosthetic mesh.

Between 1984 and 1988, Irving Lichtenstein refined his hernioplasty technique with the main goal of achieving a completely tension-free repair, not only intraoperatively in a supine position but also postoperatively despite factors such as intraabdominal pressure gradient and contraction of the mesh. The basic tenet of a Lichtenstein repair is to reinforce the entire inguinal floor by insertion of a prosthetic mesh, as opposed to forcefully combining, by way of suture, anatomic structures not normally in juxtaposition [30]. Because a repair under tension predisposes to recurrence, Lichtenstein's tension-free approach theoretically improves recurrence rates. Indeed, since its inception, the Lichtenstein hernioplasty has undergone thorough evaluation, and there is strong evidence that the use of mesh in open inguinal hernia repair is associated with a reduction in the risk of recurrence of between 50% and 75% [36]. Currently, the recommendation from societal guidelines is to incorporate mesh, when possible, in inguinal hernia repairs [37,38].

Open mesh versus minimally invasive

Much of what drives surgical innovation and technique is the interplay between improving patient outcomes and technological advances. Perhaps the most striking example of this is the use of video laparoscopy. Incredibly, the roots of laparoscopic surgery can be traced back to the late nineteenth century [39]. However, the practical use of laparoscopy did not become realized until the 1980s when Kurt Semm performed the first laparoscopic appendectomy [40]. In 1983, John Wicker established a department of *Minimally Invasive Surgery* at the Institute for Urological Surgery, thus coining the term [41]. What transpired in the following decades can only be described as a revolution in general surgery. By the 1990s, virtually every abdominal surgery was attempted via a "minimally invasive approach."

Since the addition of the laparoscopic approach into the armamentarium of hernia repairs, minimally invasive techniques have undergone considerable evolution and have been the source of much controversy. The benefits of a "minimally invasive" approach to inguinal hernia with respect to incisional pain are self-evident. However, the data concerning recurrence after laparoscopic inguinal hernioplasty are conflicting.

In a 1996 prospective study, comparing 100 patients with hernias treated laparoscopically with 108 patients with hernias treated with an open mesh repair, the investigators found an 8% versus 0% rate of recurrence, respectively [42]. Similarly, a 1999 study randomized 79 patients to laparoscopic versus open inguinal repair with mesh. Mean follow-up was 34 months. The rate of recurrence following laparoscopic repair was 12.5% compared with 1.9% with an open approach ($P = .04$). The investigators rightfully concluded "With regard to recurrence rates, the open preperitoneal prosthetic mesh repair remains the best repair" [43]. The case against laparoscopic inguinal hernia in favor of an open mesh approach was further mounted with the publication of a multicenter, randomized controlled study in the Veteran's Affairs system in 2004. More than 2000 Veterans were randomized to either open mesh or laparoscopic mesh repair. The primary endpoint was recurrence at 2 years. Investigators found that recurrence was significantly more common after laparoscopic repair than after open repair of primary hernias (10.1% vs 4.0%) and concluded that the open technique is superior [44]. Ostensibly, the coup de grâce against laparoscopic inguinal hernia repair was delivered in 2012 with the publication of a meta-analysis of 27 randomized controlled trials (RCTs). The analysis included studies published between 1993 and 2010 and involved a total of 7161 patients. Compared with an open mesh approach, laparoscopic inguinal hernia repair was associated with a significant risk of recurrence with an odds ratio (OR) of 2.06 (95% confidence interval [CI] = 1.26 to 3.37, $P = .004$) [45].

As stated, the data regarding recurrence following laparoscopic inguinal hernia repair is mixed, and indeed, evidence to support the counterargument that recurrence rates are no different when compared with an open approach is equally robust.

An analysis of 12 RCTs with 3966 patients spanning the year of 2003 to 2016 showed no significant differences in recurrence rates between the laparoscopic and open groups (OR 1.14, 95% CI 0.51 to 2.55, $P = .76$) [46]. A Cochrane review of 41 RCTs involving 4165 patients concluded that the use of a mesh for repair reduced the risk of hernia recurrence rather than the method of placement (open or laparoscopic surgery) [47]. A review and Bayesian network meta-analysis of 16 studies involving 51,037 patients compared laparoscopic approaches with open mesh repairs. In the subgroup analysis of 12 RCTs, the investigators found no significant difference with respect to hernia recurrence [48].

One study in particular that may help to clarify the variability in hernia recurrence outcomes following laparoscopic and open approaches is a prospective, multicentered RCT randomizing 666 patients to laparoscopic versus an open mesh repair. Patients were followed-up to 5 years. In this study, surgeon experience was stratified into 3 levels: level 1 (<10 procedures), level 2 (10–25 procedures), and level 3 (>25 procedures). There were no significant differences in cumulative hernia recurrence at 5 years (4.9% after laparoscopic and 8.1% after open repair [$P = .10$]). However, when considering only procedures performed by level 3 surgeons, significantly lower hernia recurrence rates were seen after laparoscopic compared with open repairs (0.5% vs 4.2%, $P = .04$) [49]. This observed phenomenon highlights the importance between the correlation of a learner's performance on a task and the number of attempts or time required to complete the task, more commonly known as "the learning curve."

The adoption of a laparoscopic approach to inguinal hernia repair calls on the surgeon to assimilate an entirely new set of technical and cognitive skills, different than those used in the traditional open approach. Not only are the anatomic relationships of the inguinal region near diametric in the laparoscopic view but they are also 2-dimensional (2D). Furthermore, conventional rigid laparoscopic instruments offer 5° of freedom (DOF) [50]. In contrast, the human hand offers 27 DOF [51]. In other words, laparoscopic inguinal hernioplasty is more technically challenging, and indeed, there is evidence that the learning curve to achieve comparable recurrence rates to open is upward of 250 cases [44]. The technical demand of a laparoscopic approach is further illustrated by the trend that recurrence rates have consistently improved over time, presumably from increased global repetition, from a near prohibitive frequency of 25% in the early 1990s, to as good as or better than the open approach [52,53].

In short, laparoscopic inguinal hernia repair is more technically challenging, with a steeper learning curve than its open counter-part; however, in experienced hands, recurrence rates are likely equivalent.

Minimally invasive inguinal hernia repair is not confined to laparoscopy only, and over the last decade, there has been exponential growth in the practice of robotic inguinal hernia repair [54]. Still, the data looking at long-term recurrence rates are hardly robust. In a mixed treatment comparison analysis of 16 studies contrasting open, laparoscopic, and robotic inguinal hernia repairs, the investigators found that short-term recurrence following robotic repairs were comparable to an open approach (risk ratio [RR] 0.98%; 95% CI 0.45–2.10) [48]. A meta-analysis of 12 single-center studies found the short-term, approximately 1-year, pooled recurrence rate following robotic inguinal hernia repair was 0.18% (95% CI 0.00–0.84) [55]. Finally, a 2019 review and meta-analysis of 19, nearly all single-centered, retrospective studies found a recurrence rate of 1.2%. Comparative meta-analysis outcomes found no statistical difference compared with an open or laparoscopic approach [56].

From a purely anatomic consideration, there is no reason to believe that the recurrence rate following robotic inguinal hernia repair should differ significantly from a laparoscopic approach. That said, there is a paucity of level 1 evidence regarding this matter, and further studies are needed to confirm this presumption.

CHRONIC GROIN PAIN

Chronic postoperative inguinal pain (CPIP), also known as inguinodynia, is groin pain or discomfort lasting greater than 3 months after surgery [57]. With a reported frequency of up to 75% in some studies, CPIP is one of the most significant complications following inguinal hernia repair [58–61]. In fact, as recurrence rates have steadily decreased, CPIP has become the more prevalent and critical concern and is particularly worrisome, as many patients presenting for elective hernia repair either have minimal or no pain at baseline or are seeking repair to relieve pain and discomfort [62].

Although there are likely several overlapping mechanisms responsible for CPIP, some investigators have postulated that inflammatory tissue reactions after mesh repair may lead to a prolonged healing process that may last longer than 3 months [63]. However, inguinodynia has been described long before modern mesh-based techniques, and indeed, there is evidence that an open mesh repair is associated with less postoperative pain compared with tissue-based repairs [58,59,64]. This finding likely speaks to the fact that tension not only increases the risk of recurrence but also causes pain.

As previously mentioned, the benefit of a minimally invasive approach to inguinal hernia repair with regard to incisional pain is self-evident. That said, whether minimal access trauma translates into less *chronic* groin pain is perhaps a less intuitive conclusion. It is hypothesized that minimally invasive placement of mesh preserves the natural embedding of the inguinal nerves, whereas open mesh implantation often interferes with the ilioinguinal nerve (IIN) [62]. Interestingly, an analysis of 9 RCTs investigating elective division of the IIN during open mesh repair found no significant reduction of CPIP beyond 6 months, which argues against the emphasis on IIN interference [65]. Still, irrespective of the exact mechanism, the data firmly support the notion that minimally invasive approaches to hernia repairs are associated with less CPIP. A longitudinal RCT of 660 patients randomized to either laparoscopic or open inguinal repair reported a significant increase in CPIP in the open mesh group at 5 years, (28% vs 14.9%; $P = .004$) [49]. In a subgroup analysis of a multidata base study of 29 prospective trials, the investigators reported a significant decrease (OR 0.61 [0.49–0.77]) in chronic pain when the repair was performed laparoscopically rather than open with mesh [61]. Recently, an analysis of 58 unique RCTs involving 17,510 randomly assigned patients found that laparoscopic hernia repair was associated with significantly less postoperative pain in 3-time intervals: from 2 weeks to 6 months after surgery (RR 0.74, 95% CI = 0.62–0.88), 6 months to 1 year (RR 0.74, 95% CI = 0.59–0.93), and 1 year onwards (RR 0.62, 95% CI = 0.47–0.82) [66].

With regard to the benefits of robotic inguinal hernioplasty on CPIP, it is tempting to extrapolate data from studies of laparoscopic hernia repair. However, similar to the question of recurrence, there is a paucity of strong evidence to conclude that robotic inguinal hernioplasty offers the same advantages on chronic pain as does laparoscopy.

In addition to reductions in chronic pain, minimally invasive inguinal hernia repairs have been shown to be superior to open inguinal hernia repairs with respect to QoL, quicker return to work, faster normalization of functional status and activities of daily living, and patient satisfaction [49,66–73].

In summary, laparoscopic inguinal hernia repair is associated with less chronic groin pain, earlier return to work, faster recovery, and improved QoL when compared with an open approach.

COST AND VALUE

As one moves from an open to laparoscopic to robotic repair of unilateral inguinal hernia, one sees incremental additions to the cost of performing the surgery. In a recent analysis of 100 consecutive contemporary procedures for each type of inguinal hernia repair, both variable and fixed costs were evaluated [74]. Variable costs include direct material costs, direct labor costs, and variable overhead costs on a per case basis. Fixed costs included capital equipment and associated service contracts.

When accounting for all sources of variable cost on per case basis, the overall variable costs for laparoscopic inguinal hernia repair were 1.02X higher than an open repair (95% CI [0.9,1.15], $P = .78$). Overall variable costs of a robotic inguinal hernia repair, however, were 2.11X compared with open repair (95% CI [1.87,2.39], $P < .001$) and 2.06X compared with laparoscopic repair.

When fixed costs of the capital equipment and associated service contracts for the surgical equipment are allocated on a per case usage basis using full absorption costing, the differences in costs become more dramatic. A laparoscopic repair was 1.03X more costly, whereas robotic inguinal hernia repair was 3.18X more costly than an open repair.

Value is defined as quality divided by cost [75]. Assuming equivalent recurrence rates for each repair, the differences in value are driven by differences in cost. In this analysis, when considering just variable costs, a laparoscopic hernia repair reduces value by 2% and robotic repair by 53% compared with an open repair. When considering both variable and fixed costs, a laparoscopic hernia repair reduces value by 3% compared with an open repair. A robotic repair reduces the value of inguinal hernia repair by 69%. The optimization of value in surgical care requires improving quality while decreasing cost of delivering care. Using recurrence as the primary outcome of interest to the patient, the factor driving the reduction in value is the added cost of using incrementally more technology as one moves from open to laparoscopic to robotic surgery to achieve the same patient outcome [76].

Variable and fixed costs of a laparoscopic approach were not significantly different than an open approach in this study. As such, when one adds the improvement in patient-reported outcomes noted earlier for a laparoscopic approach to the equivalent recurrence rates, one must conclude that a laparoscopic approach provides more value to the patient than an open approach and certainly more value than a robotic approach [74].

DISCUSSION

Inguinal hernias are an age-old malady and have likely plagued humanity since the beginning of recorded history or even before. With a lifetime risk of inguinal hernia development of 43% for men and 6% for women, yielding more than 20 million world-wide patients yearly, and representing more than 2 billion dollars in US health care expenditures per annum, there is enormous incentive to identify the "best" repair. However, as inguinal hernia repair has evolved over the centuries, so too has our metrics of success. From simply "fixing the hernia" to considerations of durability, pain, QoL, and resource utilization, the answer to "What is the best repair for inguinal hernias?" is unsurprisingly nuanced, delivered with caveats, and is a moving target. Moreover, if one were to also consider factors such as recurrence, laterality, surgeon experience, previous tissue plane violation, patient comorbidities, and so forth, the complexity of the discussion would assuredly outweigh the utility of the answer. Therefore, similar to the rationale of neglecting air resistance when discussing the physics of projectiles, the authors aimed to simplify the discussion and consequently the answer, by assuming only primary, unilateral inguinal hernias. They further simplified the discussion by disregarding anatomic approach (ie, TEP vs TAPP) when considering laparoscopic and robotic repairs.

With these assumptions and based on current and available evidence, the inguinal hernia repair that optimizes durability, decreases chronic pain, optimizes QoL, and expediates postoperative functionality, all at a minimum overall cost to the health care system, is a laparoscopic one.

CLINICS CARE POINTS

- The use of mesh in inguinal hernia repair objectively reduces recurrence.
- In experience hands, laparoscopic inguinal hernia repair has equivalent recurrence rates as compared with open.
- Minimally invasive inguinal hernia repair is associated with decreased rates of CPIP.
- A robotic approach reduces the value of inguinal hernia repair by nearly 70%.

DISCLOSURE

The authors have nothing to disclose.

References

[1] Hori T, Yasukawa D. Fascinating history of groin hernias: comprehensive recognition of anatomy, classic considerations for herniorrhaphy, and current controversies in hernioplasty. World J Methodol 2021;11(4):160–86.
[2] Lau WY. History of treatment of groin hernia. World J Surg 2002;26(6):748–59.
[3] Major RH. The papyrus ebers. Ann Med Hist 1930;2(5):547–55.
[4] Legutko J, Pach R, Solecki R, et al. [The history of treatment of groin hernia]. Folia Med Cracov 2008;49(1–2):57–74.
[5] Wei K, Lu C, Ge L, et al. A study of incidence of different types of groin hernias in adults. Medicine 2018;97(16):e0423.
[6] Bendavid R, Sanjay P, Woodward A. (2007) Single strenuous event: does it predispose to inguinal herniation? Hernia 11:493–496. Hernia 2008;12(4):443.
[7] Ramanan B, Maloley BJ, Fitzgibbons RJ. Inguinal hernia follow or repair? Serono Sym 2014;48(1):1–11.
[8] Ng AY, Lin J, Ching SS, et al. Does primary closure of direct inguinal hernia defect during laparoscopic mesh repair reduce the risk of early recurrence? Hernia 2020;24(5):1093–8.
[9] Kingsnorth A, LeBlanc K. Hernias: inguinal and incisional. Lancet 2003;362(9395):1561–71.
[10] Murphy BL, Ubl DS, Zhang J, et al. Trends of inguinal hernia repairs performed for recurrence in the United States. Surgery 2018;163(2):343–50.
[11] Burcharth J, Pedersen M, Bisgaard T, et al. Nationwide prevalence of groin hernia repair. PLoS One 2013;8(1):e54367.
[12] Köckerling F, Simons MP. Current concepts of inguinal hernia repair. Visc Med 2018;34(2):145–50.
[13] Tan WP, Lavu H, Rosato EL, et al. Edoardo bassini (1844–1924): father of modern-day hernia surgery. Am Surg 2013;79(11):1131–3.
[14] Bendavid R. New techniques in hernia repair. World J Surg 1989;13(5):522–31.

[15] Marzorati C, Pravettoni G. Value as the key concept in the health care system: how it has influenced medical practice and clinical decision-making processes. J Multidiscip Healthc 2017;10:101–6.
[16] Porter ME, Teisberg EO. How physicians can change the future of health care. JAMA 2007;297(10):1103–11.
[17] Read RC. The centenary of Bassini's contribution to inguinal herniorrhaphy. Am J Surg 1987;153(3):324–6.
[18] Halsted WS. The radical cure of hernia. J Am Med Assoc 1889;XIII(5):179–80.
[19] Amato B, Moja L, Panico S, et al. Shouldice technique versus other open techniques for inguinal hernia repair. Cochrane Database Syst Rev 2012;4(4):CD001543.
[20] Bendavid R. The shouldice repair. Published online 1995:122-134. doi:10.1159/000423919
[21] Schumpelick V, Treutner KH, Arlt G. Inguinal hernia repair in adults. Lancet 1994;344(8919):375–9.
[22] Glassow F. The shouldice hospital technique. Int Surg 1986;71(3):148–53.
[23] Wantz GE. The Canadian repair: personal observations. World J Surg 1989;13(5):516–21.
[24] Arlt G, Schumpelick V. The shouldice repair for inguinal hernia technique and results. Zentralbl Chir 2007;127(7):565–9.
[25] Töns C, Klinge U, Kupczyk-Joeris D, et al. [Controlled study of cremaster resection in Shouldice repair of primary inguinal hernia]. Zentralbl Chir 1991;116(12):737–43.
[26] Kux M, Fuchsjäger N, Feichter A. [Lichtenstein patch versus Shouldice technique in primary inguinal hernia with a high risk of recurrence]. Chirurg 1994;65(1):59–62 [discussion: 63].
[27] Hoffmann R, Frick T, Attinger B, et al. [Bassini or Shouldice operation?]. Helv Chir Acta 1991;58(1–2):207–12.
[28] Tran VK, Pütz T, Rohde H. A randomized controlled trial for inguinal hernia repair to compare the Shouldice and the Bassini-Kirschner operation. Int Surg 1992;77(4):235–7.
[29] Aust JB, Kingsnorth AN, Murray GD. Prospective randomized trial comparing the Shouldice technique and plication darn for inguinal hernia. Br J Surg 1993;80(6):807.
[30] Amid PK. Lichtenstein tension-free hernioplasty: Its inception, evolution, and principles. Hernia 2004;8(1):1–7.
[31] T B. The medical sciences in the German Universities. A study in the history of civilization. In: Welch, editor13. Macmillan; 1924; https://doi.org/10.1001/archneurpsyc.1925.02200120131012.
[32] Baylón K, Rodríguez-Camarillo P, Elías-Zúñiga A, et al. Past, Present and Future of Surgical Meshes: A Review. Membranes 2017;7(3):47; https://doi.org/10.3390/membranes7030047.
[33] Desarda MP. Surgical physiology of inguinal hernia repair - a study of 200 cases. BMC Surg 2003;3(1):2.
[34] Rosch R, Klinge U, Si Z, et al. A role for the collagen I/III and MMP-1/-13 genes in primary inguinal hernia? BMC Med Genet 2002;3(1):2.
[35] Wantz GE. Experience with the tension-free hernioplasty for primary inguinal hernias in men. J Am Coll Surg 1996;183(4):351–6.
[36] Scott N, Go PMNYH, Graham P, et al. Open Mesh versus non-Mesh for groin hernia repair. Cochrane Db Syst Rev 2001;3:CD002197.
[37] Group TH. International guidelines for groin hernia management. Hernia 2018;22(1):1–165.
[38] AlMarzooqi R, Tish S, Huang LC, et al. Review of inguinal hernia repair techniques within the Americas Hernia Society Quality Collaborative. Hernia 2019;23(3):429–38.
[39] Kelley WE. The evolution of laparoscopy and the revolution in surgery in the decade of the 1990s. JSLS 2008;12(4):351–7.
[40] Semm K. Endoscopic appendectomy. Endoscopy 1983;15(02):59–64.

[41] Litynski GS. Endoscopic surgery: the history, the pioneers. World J Surg 1999;23(8): 745–53.
[42] Horeyseck G, Roland F, Rolfes N. Die "spannungsfreie" Reparation der Leistenhernie: laparoskopisch (TAPP) versus offen (Lichtenstein). Der Chir 1996;67(10):1036–40.
[43] Beets GL, Dirksen CD, Go PMNYH, et al. Open or laparoscopic preperitoneal mesh repair for recurrent inguinal hernia? Surg Endosc 1999;13(4):323–7.
[44] Neumayer L, Giobbie-Hurder A, Jonasson O, et al. Investigators VACSP 456. Open mesh versus laparoscopic mesh repair of inguinal hernia. N Engl J Med 2004;350(18): 1819–27.
[45] O'Reilly EA, Burke JP, O'Connell PR. A meta-analysis of surgical morbidity and recurrence after laparoscopic and open repair of primary unilateral inguinal hernia. Ann Surg 2012;255(5):846–53.
[46] Bullen NL, Massey LH, Antoniou SA, et al. Open versus laparoscopic mesh repair of primary unilateral uncomplicated inguinal hernia: a systematic review with meta-analysis and trial sequential analysis. Hernia 2019;23(3):461–72.
[47] McCormack K, Scott N, Go PMNYH, et al. Laparoscopic techniques versus open techniques for inguinal hernia repair. Cochrane Db Syst Rev 2003;2010(1):CD001785.
[48] Aiolfi A, Cavalli M, Micheletto G, et al. Primary inguinal hernia: systematic review and Bayesian network meta-analysis comparing open, laparoscopic transabdominal preperitoneal, totally extraperitoneal, and robotic preperitoneal repair. Hernia 2019;23(3): 473–84.
[49] Eker HH, Langeveld HR, Klitsie PJ, et al. Randomized clinical trial of total extraperitoneal inguinal hernioplasty vs lichtenstein repair: a long-term follow-up study. Arch Surg 2012;147(3):256–60.
[50] Dewaele F, Pauw TD, Kalmar A, et al. Is the human brain capable of controlling seven degrees of freedom? J Surg Res 2019;238:1–9.
[51] Lin J, Wu Y, Huang TS. Modeling the constraints of human hand motion. Proc Work Hum Motion 2000;121–6.
[52] Corbitt JD. Transabdominal preperitoneal herniorrhaphy. Surg Laparosc Endosc 1993;3(4):328–32.
[53] Ortenzi M, Williams S, Solanki N, et al. Laparoscopic repair of inguinal hernia: retrospective comparison of TEP and TAPP procedures in a tertiary referral center. Minerva Chir 2020;75(5):279–85.
[54] George EI, Brand TC, LaPorta A, et al. Origins of robotic surgery: from skepticism to standard of care. JSLS 2018;22(4):e2018.00039.
[55] Aiolfi A, Cavalli M, Micheletto G, et al. Robotic inguinal hernia repair: is technology taking over? Systematic review and meta-analysis. Hernia 2019;23(3):509–19.
[56] Qabbani A, Aboumarzouk OM, ElBakry T, et al. Robotic inguinal hernia repair: systematic review and meta-analysis. Anz J Surg 2021;91(11):2277–87.
[57] Classification of chronic pain. Descriptions of chronic pain syndromes and definitions of pain terms. Prepared by the International Association for the Study of Pain, Subcommittee on Taxonomy. Pain Suppl 1986;3:S1–226.
[58] Poobalan AS, Bruce J, Smith WCS, et al. A review of chronic pain after inguinal herniorrhaphy. Clin J Pain 2003;19(1):48–54.
[59] Aasvang E, Kehlet H. Chronic postoperative pain: the case of inguinal herniorrhaphy. Br J Anaesth 2005;95(1):69–76.
[60] Manangi M, Shivashankar S, Vijayakumar A. Chronic pain after inguinal hernia repair. Int Sch Res Notices 2014;2014:839681.
[61] Nienhuijs S, Staal E, Strobbe L, et al. Chronic pain after mesh repair of inguinal hernia: a systematic review. Am J Surg 2007;194(3):394–400.
[62] Reinpold W. Risk factors of chronic pain after inguinal hernia repair: a systematic review. Innovative Surg Sci 2017;2(2):61–8.

[63] Cunningham J, Temple WJ, Mitchell P, et al. Cooperative hernia study: pain in the postrepair patient. Ann Surg 1996;224(5):598–602.

[64] Grant A. Erratum to: open mesh versus non-mesh repair of groin hernia: meta-analysis of randomised trials based on individual patient data. Hernia 2002;6(4):204.

[65] Charalambous MP, Charalambous CP. Incidence of chronic groin pain following open mesh inguinal hernia repair, and effect of elective division of the ilioinguinal nerve: meta-analysis of randomized controlled trials. Hernia 2018;22(3):401–9.

[66] Patterson TJ, Beck J, Currie PJ, et al. Meta-analysis of patient-reported outcomes after laparoscopic versus open inguinal hernia repair. Br J Surg 2019;106(7):824–36.

[67] Corthals S, Cleven S van, Uyttebroek O, et al. Quality of life after open versus laparoscopic preperitoneal mesh repair for unilateral inguinal hernias. Asian J Surg 2021;44(10): 1266–73.

[68] Myers E, Browne KM, Kavanagh DO, et al. Laparoscopic (TEP) versus lichtenstein inguinal hernia repair: a comparison of quality-of-life outcomes. World J Surg 2010;34(12): 3059–64.

[69] Langeveld HR, van't Riet M, Weidema WF, et al. Total extraperitoneal inguinal hernia repair compared with lichtenstein (the LEVEL-Trial). Ann Surg 2010;251(5):819–24.

[70] IV JGB, Cesnik LW, Kirwan T, et al. Patient perceptions of acute pain and activity disruption following inguinal hernia repair: a propensity-matched comparison of robotic-assisted, laparoscopic, and open approaches. J Robotic Surg 2018;12(4):625–32.

[71] LeBlanc K, Dickens E, Gonzalez A, et al. Prospective, multicenter, pairwise analysis of robotic-assisted inguinal hernia repair with open and laparoscopic inguinal hernia repair: early results from the Prospective Hernia Study. Hernia 2020;24(5):1069–81.

[72] Iraniha A, Peloquin J. Long-term quality of life and outcomes following robotic assisted TAPP inguinal hernia repair. J Robotic Surg 2018;12(2):261–9.

[73] Froylich D, Haskins IN, Aminian A, et al. Laparoscopic versus open inguinal hernia repair in patients with obesity: an American College of Surgeons NSQIP clinical outcomes analysis. Surg Endosc 2017;31(3):1305–10.

[74] Glasgow RE, Mulvihill SJ, Pettit JC, et al. Value analysis of methods of inguinal hernia repair. Ann Surg 2021;274(4):572–80.

[75] Porter ME. What is value in health care? N Engl J Med 2010;363(26):2477–81.

[76] Sorenson C, Drummond M, Khan BB. Medical technology as a key driver of rising health expenditure: disentangling the relationship. Clinicoecon Outcomes Res 2013;5:223–34.

Advances in Surgery 56 (2022) 259–273

ADVANCES IN SURGERY

Do all Patients Get the Same Care Across Hospitals?

Adrian Diaz, MD, MPH[a,b,1],
Timothy M. Pawlik, MD, MPH, MTS, PhD[a,*]

[a]Department of Surgery, The Ohio State University Wexner Medical Center and James Comprehensive Cancer Center, 395 West 12th Avenue, Suite 670, Columbus, OH 43210, USA; [b]Center for Healthcare Outcomes and Policy, University of Michigan, Ann Arbor, MI, USA

Keywords

• Surgical care • Variation • Outcomes • Utilization • Disparities • Quality of care

Key points

- There is significant variation in utilization rates of surgery across the United States.
- Surgical outcomes vary by hospital characteristics, including procedure-specific volume, for many operations.
- Not all surgical procedures demonstrate significant variation across hospitals.
- There is significant evidence there is variation in access and outcomes from surgery that is attributable to race and social determinants of health.

Concern with variation in surgical outcomes across hospitals and providers is arguably as old as the practice of surgery itself. Perhaps one of the first rigorous studies of variation in patient care across hospitals may be attributed to the Hungarian physician Ignaz Semmelweis. While working in Vienna General Hospital's First Obstetrical Clinic in 1847, Semmelweis [1] demonstrated that the doctors' ward had 3 times higher mortality than that of the midwives' ward. This observation would ultimately lead Semmelweis to propose the novel idea of handwashing. Semmelweis would go on to demonstrate that wherever handwashing was implemented mortality was reduced to less than 1%, albeit to the chagrin of the medical opinion of the times. This work was the foundation for the surgeon Joseph Lister, who would pioneer

[1]Present address: 293 Reinhard Avenue. Columbus. OH 43206.

*Corresponding author. *E-mail address:* tim.pawlik@osumc.edu

https://doi.org/10.1016/j.yasu.2022.03.005

antiseptic surgery. Similar to Semmelweis, Lister [2,3] documented remarkable reductions in postoperative infections wherever antiseptic techniques were implemented across Europe. At the time, neither individual received the recognition they deserved, but today both are distinguished as two of the founders of modern surgery. Perhaps equally as important, Semmelweis and Lister pioneered the concept to investigate variation in care across different settings and to study positive deviants as a mechanism for improving care.

If Semmelweis and Lister pioneered the study of health outcomes, Ernest Codman cemented it as a rigorous science. Credited with the "End Result Idea," Ernest Codman established the practice in which hospital staff would follow every patient treated long enough to determine whether the treatment was successful and then learn from any failures to avoid those situations in the future [4]. Codman [5] is credited with establishing one of the first surgical registries and has come to be known as the father of surgical outcomes research. Surprisingly controversial at the time, the "Idea" was the basis for the Hospital Standardization movement founded by the American College of Surgeons, and the precursor to the Joint Commission on Accreditation of Hospitals formed in 1951. Today, known as The Joint Commission, the topic of quality assurance and control remains vital to American and all health care systems worldwide [6].

More recently, the modern era of surgical outcomes research has greatly benefited from 2 advances: big data and advanced statistical modeling. Because of the advent of the medicoindustrial complex and the electronic health record, surgeons today have more data to understand variation than Semmelweis, Lister, and Codman could have ever dreamed. Broadly speaking, these large databases can be categorized into either clinical registries or administrative case registries. Furthermore, advances in statistical modeling and computing power have provided surgeons and researchers readily availability to tools to analyze large amounts of data quickly and reliably while accounting for confounders and differential risk across patient populations.

CLINICAL REGISTRIES

Similar to the databases of the past, modern clinical registries serve to evaluate and improve outcomes for a given population defined by a particular condition, disease, or exposure. Most clinical registries were established either for clinical research or for quality improvement. Strengths of clinical registries include clinical granularity and large sample size. Weaknesses include the fact that the data often lag in availability, reliance on abstractors or other data capture methods that may create variability, and resource intensiveness to create and maintain these databases. Examples of commonly used databases are the American College of Surgeons National Surgical Quality Improvement program [7], the National Cancer Data Base [8], and the National Trauma Data Bank [9].

ADMINISTRATIVE DATA

Administrative databases are large, often population-based sources of data generated for purposes other than clinical research. Oftentimes, these databases are generated from billing claims, but may also be generated for regulatory or certification purposes. Strengths of administrative databases are derived from the data being often population based with very large sample sizes. Furthermore, these databases are often relatively inexpensive and readily available. Weaknesses of administrative data include the lack of clinical detail, as the data are often collected for billing or other purposes. As such, these databases can be subject to inaccurate or variable coding. Examples of commonly used administrative databases include the Medicare Provider Analysis and Review [10], The Veterans Affairs National Patient Care Database [11], IBM Research Databases [12], and several national and state level databases from the health care cost and utilization project [13].

ADVANCED STATISTICAL MODELING

In addition to large clinical registries and administrative data sets, advanced statistical techniques have given surgeons and researchers the tools to enhance causal inference from these large data sets. Multivariable regression is the conventional method of data analysis in observational studies. These regression models may take many forms depending on the structure of the data set and the distribution of the variables. For example, the most commonly used models include linear regression for continuous outcomes, logistic regression for dichotomous outcomes, proportional hazard models for time-to-event studies, and Poisson regression for count data. These models can be used to disentangle the relationship between covariates and outcomes. Regression models can control for differences between groups by providing estimates of effect when other covariates are held fixed. In large data set analysis, outcomes are generally risk-adjusted to account for patient factors, such as age, sex, race, and known comorbidities.

In investigating variation across hospitals and specifically whether patients receive the same care, risk-adjustment with conventional multivariable regression models remains subject to accuracy and validity. In particular, when the outcome is rare (ie, death) or when sample size is small (ie, uncommon operation), it is hard to know whether high or low probabilities are due to chance or true differences. As such, reliability adjustment, an application of hierarchical modeling, allows for quantification and removal of this statistical noise using empirical Bayes techniques [14,15]. More specifically, this technique filters out statistical "noise" by shrinking the observed rate toward the average rate. The degree of shrinkage is proportional to the reliability of the measure, which is largely a function of sample size (ie, hospital caseload) [16]. This approach has been increasingly applied to health care, including in the public reporting of hospital outcomes for medical conditions and is becoming exceedingly important to consider when investigating whether all patients get the same care at all hospitals [17,18].

VARIATION IN UTILIZATION

The study of surgical utilization variation began in the 1970s when Bunker [19] examined the differences in the number of surgeons relative to surgical operations within the United States and England. In this seminal work, the investigator characterized the relationship between the supply of surgeons and the number of operations. Specifically, there was a greater number of operations performed in a fee-for-service environment in the United States versus in a nationalized health care setting such as England. Building on this work, Wennberg [20] studied variation in surgical utilization specially related to small area variation. In particular, Wennberg created a new unit of analysis, hospital service area, by examining where patients sought surgical care. Of interest, there was marked variation, up to 12 times, in the utilization of operations, including tonsillectomy, appendectomy, prostatectomy, and hysterectomy, among hospital service areas in the same state. Furthermore, more physicians and hospitals in a given service area were associated with more services provided. In addition, these relationships existed despite no major differences in patients across a given service area [20]. Building on this work, Birkmeyer and colleagues [21] studied the utilization of common procedures across the entire United States. Similar to the initial study on variation within a single state, Birkmeyer and colleagues reported dramatic variation in the utilization of common surgical procedures across hospital referral regions. For example, rates of carotid endarterectomy varied nearly three-fold across different regions. Importantly, there were certain operations in which there was little variation, whereas other operations demonstrated dramatic variation. The investigators suggested that procedures with the highest degree of variation reflected areas of surgical practice in which there was substantial disagreement on both diagnosis and treatment. This study became the foundation for what would later become the Dartmouth Atlas Project, which has documented dramatic variations in how medical resources are distributed and used in the United States [22].

After these publications in the 1990s, researchers spent the next 3 decades refining analytical methods to investigate variation in the provision of surgical care. For example, Gawande and colleagues [23] investigated surgical care in the last year of life and demonstrated that nearly one-third of patients underwent a surgical procedure in the last year of life and that the intensity of procedures at the end of life was highly correlated with the number of hospital beds in a region rather than with patient characteristics. Beyond utilization of certain surgical operations, there has been recent focus on variation in spending as a marker of utilization. Specifically, patients may undergo the same operation yet have wide variation in episode spending, suggesting variation in the utilization of health care (eg, more tests, longer length of stay) around a given surgical episode [24]. For example, among patients undergoing bariatric surgery, episode cost can vary by almost $2000 among the highest and lowest quintile hospitals despite similar outcomes and patient characteristics [25]. Similar findings have been reported for complex cancer operations, in which the surgical episode can vary by as much as $5000 despite similar outcomes [26].

Most recently, hospital networks have expanded with the promise of higher-value care [27]. Emerging evidence suggests, however, that even within hospital networks significant variation in utilization persists [17,28,29]. For example, Chhabra and colleagues [29] reported that even within the same hospital network, discharge destination and utilization of postacute care varied dramatically across hospitals.

VARIATION IN OUTCOMES

In a seminal article published in 2002 in the *New England Journal of Medicine*, Birkmeyer and colleagues [30] demonstrated that hospital volume was inversely correlated with procedure mortality: as hospital volume increased, mortality decreased. Interestingly, the relative importance of volume has been noted to vary according to the type of procedure. Specifically, generally high-risk operations, such as pancreatectomy and esophagectomy, had a stronger volume-outcome relationship than low- and moderate-risk operations [31]. A similar volume-outcome relationship has been observed among surgeons in that for some high-risk operations not only the hospital but also individual surgeon volume drive outcomes [32]. In fact, similar variations in outcomes across hospitals based on procedure volume have been noted for nearly every surgical subspecialty, including cardiac, vascular, and oncology [33–36]. Based on research that has demonstrated volume-based variation in mortality across hospitals and surgeons, patient and advocacy groups have advocated for specific guidelines to establish minimum volume standards for certain high-risk procedures [37]. Eventually, many top hospitals and health systems joined the "Volume Pledge" vowing not to perform any operation that did not meet certain minimum hospital volume standards [38].

Variation in mortalities across hospitals has subsequently been examined relative to other patient outcomes. For example, Ghaferi and colleagues [39] reported on mortality after several common general and vascular surgery procedures and noted significant variation in mortality. Perhaps of more interest, the investigators noted that, although the incidence of complications was similar among many centers, the difference in patient mortality was largely due to differences in the ability of the hospital and staff to rescue the patient from the complication [39]. Coined "failure to rescue," this metric has been established as an important means to assess quality of postoperative outcomes, as well as define variation of outcomes among patients following surgery [39]. In fact, variation in failure to rescue has been documented following a wide range of operations, including many general surgery and oncologic operations [40–43].

Although the analysis of individual outcome measures, such as mortality, morbidity, length of stay, and readmission, has advantages, composite benchmarks of surgical quality may be more relevant and helpful [44–46]. In particular, data on any given single indicator do not necessarily reflect the whole surgical process and may not reliably measure overall hospital quality [47,48]. Composite measures combine information from multiple domains into a single summary measure and therefore may be superior to individual measures for the analysis of hospital performance [49,50]. One such composite measure is textbook outcome (TO), which provides a comprehensive summary of hospital performance [51]. Specifically, TO includes multiple desirable postoperative outcomes that, when achieved, represent the ideal hospitalization. In this manner, TO reflects overall quality across all domains of performance. In addition, TO may be easier for both patients and clinicians to interpret when analyzing quality trends, rather than trying to interpret different individual performance indicators. As a result, TO may be a more patient-centered benchmark to determine the ideal hospitalization from the patient perspective. To that effect, variation in TO among hospitals has been examined for a host of operations. Similar to individual metrics, investigators have demonstrated marked variation in rates of TO among hospitals for aneurysm repair, hepatopancreatobiliary, and colon cancer operations [52–55]. Because TO is a patient-centric composite outcome, it may be a better means for patients and payers alike to examine variation that exists in the value provided by hospitals [56].

DISPARITIES IN SURGICAL CARE

Variation in utilization of surgical services, as well as perioperative outcomes, has also been strongly associated with a range of social determinants of health (Fig. 1A–D). For example, in the United States, black patients fare worse than their white counterparts after undergoing surgery. Specifically, black patients who undergo surgical procedures have an estimated 20% to 50% higher risk of mortality compared with white patients [57–61]. (Fig. 2) Although the reasons for racial disparities related to surgical care are complicated and multifactorial, the data suggest that black patients are more likely to present later in the course of their care, be more likely to need emergent surgery, as well as be treated at lower-volume centers that have worse quality of care [62–65]. Although the gap in surgical mortality among white and black patients has narrowed over the last decade, significant disparities still exist [66].

In addition to racial disparities, other social determinants of health have been demonstrated to impact utilization and outcomes following surgery. Social determinants of health have been defined as various facets of an individual's life that can influence their health and well-being, including economic stability, neighborhood and physical environment, education, and food [67–69]. In particular, the neighborhood in which you live can impact patient access to quality surgical care, as well as drive disparities in postoperative outcomes as much as hospital factors in which the procedure was performed [70–72]. The relationship among race/ethnicity, socioeconomic status, insurance status, and other factors associated with disparities across health conditions, including surgical outcomes, is intertwined and nuanced. For example, patients residing in communities characterized by a high social vulnerability index were less likely to undergo high-risk cancer surgery at a high-volume hospital [73,74]. Although postoperative complications and mortality increased as social vulnerability index increased, some of the risk appeared to be mitigated by having surgery at a high-volume hospital [74,75]. Among patients undergoing a colon resection for either diverticulitis or cancer, patients from high social vulnerability areas were more likely to undergo a nonelective operation compared

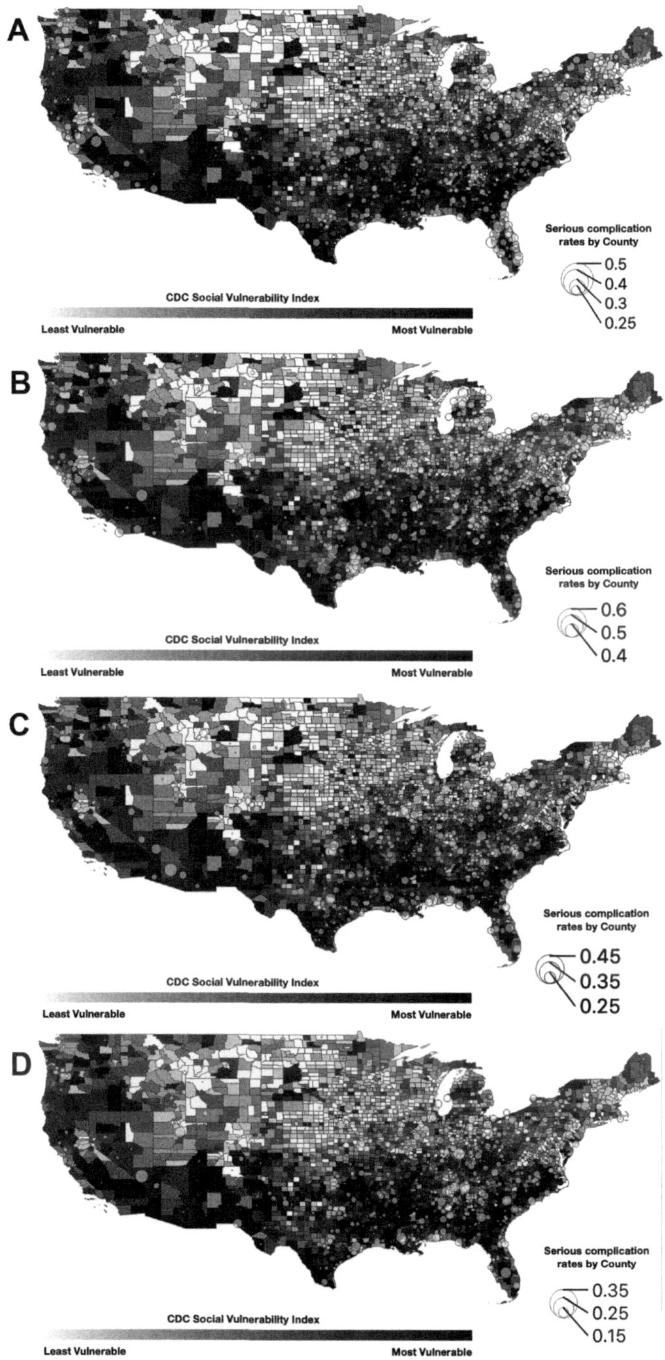

Fig. 1. Serious complication rates by county for each operation examined. CDC, Centers for Disease Control and Prevention.

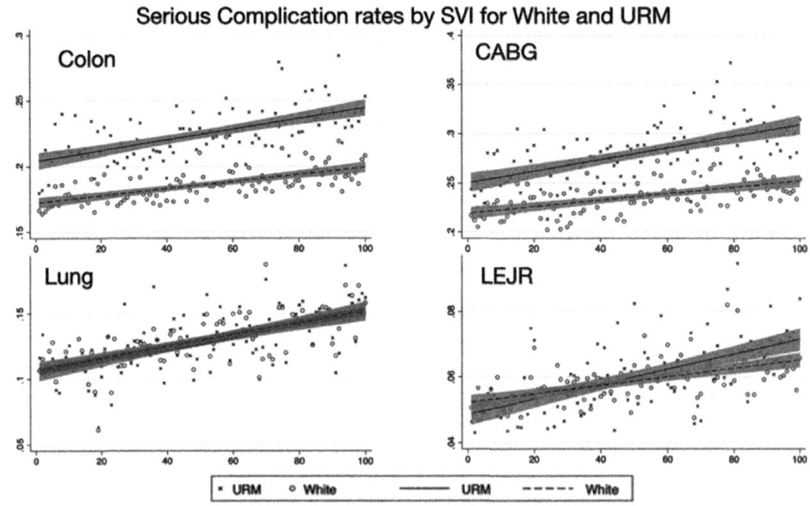

Fig. 2. Serious complication rates relative to SVI level for each operation examined stratified according to race/ethnicity. CABG, coronary artery bypass grafting; LEJR, lower extremity joint replacment; URM, underrepresented minority.

with their counterparts residing in low social vulnerability areas [76]. Similarly, Carmichael and colleagues [77] demonstrated that patients from high social vulnerability were more likely to undergo emergent cholecystectomy compared with their counterparts from low social vulnerability areas. Azap and colleagues [78] also reported that social vulnerability index (SVI) was associated with patient risk of having lower odds to undergo resection/transplant for early-stage hepatocellular carcinoma (HCC). The data suggested that patients who live in highly vulnerable counties and communities were less likely to have access to surgical care and receive surgical intervention for early-stage HCC. Collectively, these studies demonstrated that patients from areas with high vulnerability and low socioeconomic status have disparate access to timely, high-quality surgical care, thereby exacerbating disparities in surgical outcomes and overall health.

Overall, patient social vulnerability has also been strongly associated with the risk of adverse postoperative outcomes following colon or lung resection, coronary artery bypass, and hip and knee replacement [77]. Specifically, patients residing in vulnerable communities characterized by a high social vulnerability generally had worse postoperative outcomes. Of note, the impact of social vulnerability was most pronounced among black/minority patients, rather than white individuals. Social determinants of health, including social vulnerability, have also been associated with a decreased probability of achieving a TO following many different surgical procedures for colon, rectal, esophageal, or lung cancer [71]. Social vulnerability was associated with lower attainment of TO and an increased risk of adverse postoperative surgical outcomes after hepatopancreatic surgery [79].

Importantly, Paro and colleagues [80] demonstrated that not all social determinants of health are equal. For example, despite similar overall aggregate social vulnerability index scores, cluster analysis was able to discriminate various social determinants of health subthemes among patients who resided in "average" vulnerability communities that stratified patients relative to risk of adverse postoperative events. Most recently, residential segregation, the spatial separation of population groups along racial or ethnic lines, has also been associated with surgical outcomes [81–83]. Patients who resided in counties with a lower integration index were less likely to have an optimal TO following resection of cancer compared with patients who resided in more integrated counties [81]. The data highlight the importance of increasing residential racial diversity and integration as a means to improve patient outcomes. The relationship between neighborhoods, social determinants of health, and variation in surgical outcomes still needs to be better elucidated to understand if and why patients from varying social demographics and geography may have variation in access to and differences in outcomes following surgery.

REDUCING VARIATION AND OPPORTUNITIES FOR IMPROVING SURGICAL CARE

Despite demonstrated differences in surgical outcomes across hospitals, the likelihood of variation in outcomes seems to be also related to the procedure being performed. For example, for less complex operations, there appears to be less of a volume-outcome relationship versus high-risk operations [30]. To this point, Ibrahim and colleagues [84] reported no differences in outcomes among patients following common general surgery procedures treated at critical access hospitals versus noncritical access centers. Similar findings were also observed among patients undergoing emergency colectomy procedures. These findings suggest that there may be less variation in outcomes for select, common, low-risk general surgery operations. To this point, although treatment at high-volume, National Cancer Institute cancer centers has been associated with superior surgical outcomes for complex procedures and rare cancers, Lansing and colleagues reported no difference in surgical outcomes for select patients with cancer and operations. Specifically, among patients undergoing a colectomy for cancer without metastatic disease, surgical mortality, complications, and readmissions were comparable among smaller rural hospitals and large urban centers. In light of these data from Ibrahim and colleagues and Lansing and colleagues, surgical variation may not be as pronounced for certain common operations as previously thought. Rather, most variation in surgical care and outcomes likely relates to low-volume, high-risk surgery, and these procedures should be the main focus of centralization.

Of note, health care trends have led to an acceleration of hospital consolidation with more than 70% of hospitals now belonging to larger health systems [85,86]. Proponents of hospital mergers tout the potential to improve outcomes and reduce health spending by standardizing care, eliminating redundancy, and achieving economies of scale [27]. However, there is conflicting evidence as to whether expanding hospital systems actually reduce health spending [87–90]. Furthermore, wide variation in surgical outcomes within health systems has been observed [29,91]. For example, Sheetz and colleagues [92] demonstrated that surgical outcomes for colectomy, coronary artery bypass graft, and hip replacement varied widely across hospitals affiliated with the *US News & World Report* Honor Roll hospitals. Similarly, Diaz and colleagues [17] demonstrated wide variation in utilization and spending for high-risk cancer surgery across and within hospital networks. Despite an opportunity for health systems and hospital networks to standardize care and reduce variation, early evidence suggests that expanding health networks are not delivering on this promise.

Addressing disparities and achieving equity in health care care delivery and outcomes is perhaps this generation's biggest challenge. As such, when searching for interventions aimed at improving outcomes in at-risk populations, one must take a nuanced approach and consider each point in a patient's care continuum. There is sufficient evidence to demonstrate that there are at-risk, socially vulnerable populations that live in close proximity to high-quality hospitals but fail to receive care at these hospitals [73,93]. For this cohort of high-risk patients, further investigation is warranted to help elucidate which barriers, including but not limited to health literacy, insurance networks, and/or patient preference, contribute to patients bypassing high-quality hospitals. As such, triaging high-risk patients to local, high-quality hospitals within small geographic areas may serve as a template for improving the value of surgical care [94]. For patients who live further away from a high-quality hospital, the travel burden to the nearest high-quality hospital may prove a greater challenge. Nevertheless, as health systems become larger with a wider geographic footprint, these systems must consider innovative ways (eg, coordinating travel and boarding, disseminating knowledge, partnering with corporations) to ensure high-risk patients undergoing complex operations are referred to centers of excellence [95]. Measuring and reporting outcomes by race and socioeconomic status has been helpful, yet we must go beyond just reporting disparate care. Many payers and providers have begun to issue "equity reports" in which outcomes by race, ethnicity, sex, and socioeconomic status are routinely reported [96–99]. Providers and hospitals should expect to be measured not only by their overall outcomes but also by how equitable the health care they provide is.

SUMMARY

Overall, there is an extensive body of research demonstrating significant variation in the utilization of surgery and outcomes from surgery, including differences in mortality, complications, readmission, and failure to rescue. The literature suggests that these variations exist across as well as within small area geographies in the United States. Furthermore, there is variation in access and outcomes from surgery that is attributable to race and social determinants of health. Among the many challenges of studying and understanding variation in surgical care is the fact that by definition there will be high and low performers. Moving forward, patients, clinicians, payers, and policymakers will need to work together to determine which surgical utilization rate is "optimal" and how much variation in outcomes is acceptable.

CLINICS CARE POINTS

- In caring for patients, social determinants of health and a patient's lived environment are just as likely to impact outcomes as are patient demographics and clinical factors.
- There is significant evidence that racial minorities and patients from neighborhoods with poor social determinants of health are more likely to have adverse outcomes.
- For some high-risk procedures, centralization to high-volume centers improves outcomes and reduces adverse outcomes; however, for many moderate- and low-risk procedures, there is little to no difference in outcomes between high- and low-volume centers as well as rural and urban centers.

Disclosure

The authors have nothing to disclose.

References

[1] Semmelweis I, Semmelweis IF. The etiology, concept, and prophylaxis of childbed fever. Univ of Wisconsin Press; 1983.
[2] Lister J. On the effects of the antiseptic system of treatment upon the salubrity of a surgical hospital. Lancet 1870;95(2418):4–6.
[3] Lister J. On the antiseptic principle in the practice of surgery. Br Med J 1867;2(351):246–8.
[4] Kaska SC, Weinstein JN. Ernest Amory Codman, 1869-1940: a pioneer of evidence-based medicine: the end result idea. Spine 1998;23(5):629–33.
[5] Codman EA. The classic: the Registry of Bone Sarcomas as an example of the end-result idea in hospital organization. Clin Orthop Relat Res 2009;467(11):2766.
[6] Ernest A, Codman MD. FACS (1869-1940). American College of Surgeons. Available at: http://www.facs.org/about-acs/archives/pasthighlights/codmanhighlight. Accessed October 31, 2021.
[7] ACS National Surgical Quality Improvement Program. American College of Surgeons. Available at: https://www.facs.org/quality-programs/acs-nsqip. Accessed May 28, 2020.
[8] National Cancer Database. American College of Surgeons. Available at: http://www.facs.org/quality-programs/cancer/ncdb. Accessed October 31, 2021.
[9] About NTDB. American College of Surgeons. Available at: http://www.facs.org/quality-programs/trauma/tqp/center-programs/ntdb/about. Accessed October 31, 2021.
[10] MEDPAR I CMS. Available at: https://www.cms.gov/Research-Statistics-Data-and-Systems/Statistics-Trends-and-Reports/MedicareFeeforSvcPartsAB/MEDPAR. Accessed October 31, 2021.
[11] Wang XQ, Vincent BM, Wiitala WL, et al. Veterans Affairs patient database (VAPD 2014–2017): building nationwide granular data for clinical discovery. BMC Med Res Methodol 2019;19(1):94.
[12] IBM MarketScan Research Databases for Life Sciences Researchers. :15.
[13] HCUP-US Databases. Available at: https://www.hcup-us.ahrq.gov/databases.jsp. Accessed October 31, 2021.

[14] Dimick JB, Ghaferi AA, Osborne NH, et al. Reliability adjustment for reporting hospital outcomes with surgery. Ann Surg 2012;255(4):703–7.
[15] Dimick JB, Staiger DO, Birkmeyer JD. Ranking hospitals on surgical mortality: the importance of reliability adjustment. Health Serv Res 2010;45(6 Pt 1):1614–29.
[16] Normand SLT, Glickman ME, Gatsonis CA. Statistical methods for profiling providers of medical care: issues and applications. J Am Stat Assoc 1997;92(439):803–14.
[17] Diaz A, Chhabra KR, Dimick JB, et al. Variations in surgical spending within hospital systems for complex cancer surgery. Cancer 2021;127(4):586–97; https://doi.org/10.1002/cncr.33299.
[18] Grenda TR, Krell RW, Dimick JB. Reliability of hospital cost profiles in inpatient surgery. Surgery 2016;159(2):375–80.
[19] Bunker JP. Surgical manpower. A comparison of operations and surgeons in the United States and in England and Wales. N Engl J Med 1970;282(3):135–44.
[20] Wennberg J. Gittelsohn null. Small area variations in health care delivery. Science 1973;182(4117):1102–8.
[21] Birkmeyer JD, Sharp SM, Finlayson SR, et al. Variation profiles of common surgical procedures. Surgery 1998;124(5):917–23.
[22] Home. Dartmouth Atlas of Health Care. Available at: https://www.dartmouthatlas.org/. Accessed November 3, 2021.
[23] Kwok AC, Semel ME, Lipsitz SR, et al. The intensity and variation of surgical care at the end of life: a retrospective cohort study. Lancet 2011;378(9800):1408–13.
[24] Newhouse JP, Garber AM. Geographic variation in health care spending in the United States: insights from an Institute of Medicine report. JAMA 2013;310(12):1227–8.
[25] Grenda TR, Pradarelli JC, Thumma JR, et al. Variation in hospital episode costs with bariatric surgery. JAMA Surg 2015;150(12):1109–15.
[26] Diaz A, Nuliyalu U, Dimick JB, et al. Variation in surgical spending among the highest quality hospitals for cancer surgery. Ann Surg 2021; https://doi.org/10.1097/SLA.0000000000004641.
[27] Dafny LS, Lee TH. The good merger. N Engl J Med 2015;372(22):2077–9.
[28] Sheetz KH, Ryan AM, Ibrahim AM, et al. Association of hospital network participation with surgical outcomes and Medicare expenditures. Ann Surg 2019;270(2):288–94.
[29] Chhabra KR, Sheetz KH, Regenbogen SE, et al. Wide variation in surgical spending within hospital systems: a missed opportunity for bundled payment success. Ann Surg 2019;1; https://doi.org/10.1097/SLA.0000000000003741.
[30] Birkmeyer JD, Siewers AE, Finlayson EVA, et al. Hospital volume and surgical mortality in the United States. N Engl J Med 2002;346(15):1128–37.
[31] Finks JF, Osborne NH, Birkmeyer JD. Trends in hospital volume and operative mortality for high-risk surgery. N Engl J Med 2011;364(22):2128–37.
[32] Birkmeyer JD, Stukel TA, Siewers AE, et al. Surgeon volume and operative mortality in the United States. N Engl J Med 2003;349(22):2117–27.
[33] Nathan H, Cameron JL, Choti MA, et al. The volume-outcomes effect in hepato-pancreato-biliary surgery: hospital versus surgeon contributions and specificity of the relationship. J Am Coll Surg 2009;208(4):528–38.
[34] Alsfasser G, Leicht H, Günster C, et al. Volume-outcome relationship in pancreatic surgery. Br J Surg 2016;103(1):136–43.
[35] O'Donnell TF, Boitano LT, Deery SE, et al. Hospital volume matters: the volume-outcome relationship in open juxtarenal AAA repair. J Vasc Surg 2019;69(4):1323–4.
[36] Kalfa D, Chai P, Bacha E. Surgical volume-to-outcome relationship and monitoring of technical performance in pediatric cardiac surgery. Pediatr Cardiol 2014;35(6):899–905.
[37] The Leapfrong Group. Surgeon volume and surgical appropriateness. leapfrog. 2017. Available at: http://www.leapfroggroup.org/surgeon-volume. Accessed March 10, 2019.

[38] Urbach DR. Pledging to eliminate low-volume surgery. N Engl J Med 2015;373(15): 1388–90.
[39] Ghaferi AA, Birkmeyer JD, Dimick JB. Variation in hospital mortality associated with inpatient surgery. N Engl J Med 2009;361(14):1368–75.
[40] Ghaferi AA, Birkmeyer JD, Dimick JB. Complications, failure to rescue, and mortality with major inpatient surgery in Medicare patients. Ann Surg 2009;250(6):1029–34.
[41] Amini N, Spolverato G, Kim Y, et al. Trends in hospital volume and failure to rescue for pancreatic surgery. J Gastrointest Surg 2015;19(9):1581–92.
[42] Buettner S, Gani F, Amini N, et al. The relative effect of hospital and surgeon volume on failure to rescue among patients undergoing liver resection for cancer. Surgery 2016;159(4): 1004–12.
[43] Spolverato G, Ejaz A, Hyder O, et al. Failure to rescue as a source of variation in hospital mortality after hepatic surgery. Br J Surg 2014;101(7):836–46.
[44] Rössler F, Sapisochin G, Song G, et al. Defining benchmarks for major liver surgery: a multicenter analysis of 5202 living liver donors. Ann Surg 2016;264(3):492–500.
[45] Donabedian A. Twenty years of research on the quality of medical care: 1964-1984. Eval Health Prof 1985;8(3):243–65.
[46] Dimick JB, Staiger DO, Baser O, et al. Composite measures for predicting surgical mortality in the hospital. Health Aff 2009;28(4):1189–98.
[47] Dimick JB, Welch HG. The zero mortality paradox in surgery. J Am Coll Surg 2008;206(1): 13–6.
[48] Dimick JB, Welch HG, Birkmeyer JD. Surgical mortality as an indicator of hospital quality: the problem with small sample size. JAMA 2004;292(7):847–51.
[49] Dimick JB, Birkmeyer NJ, Finks JF, et al. Composite measures for profiling hospitals on bariatric surgery performance. JAMA Surg 2014;149(1):10–6.
[50] Dimick JB, Staiger DO, Osborne NH, et al. Composite measures for rating hospital quality with major surgery. Health Serv Res 2012;47(5):1861–79.
[51] Kolfschoten NE, Kievit J, Gooiker GA, et al. Focusing on desired outcomes of care after colon cancer resections; hospital variations in 'textbook outcome. Eur J Surg Oncol 2013;39(2):156–63.
[52] Karthaus E, Lijftogt N, Busweiler LA, et al. Textbook outcome: a composite measure for quality of elective aneurysm surgery. Ann Surg 2017;266(5):898–904.
[53] Sweigert PJ, Eguia E, Baker MS, et al. Assessment of cancer center variation in textbook oncologic outcomes following colectomy for adenocarcinoma. J Gastrointest Surg 2021;25(3):775–85.
[54] Merath K, Chen Q, Bagante F, et al. Textbook outcomes among Medicare patients undergoing hepatopancreatic surgery. Ann Surg 2020;271(6):1116–23.
[55] Merath K, Chen Q, Bagante F, et al. A multi-institutional international analysis of textbook outcomes among patients undergoing curative-intent resection of intrahepatic cholangiocarcinoma. JAMA Surg 2019;154(6):e190571.
[56] Shah R, Diaz A, Tripepi M, et al. Quality Versus Costs Related to Gastrointestinal Surgery: Disentangling the Value Proposition. J Gastrointest Surg 2020;24(12):2874–83.
[57] Rangrass G, Ghaferi AA, Dimick JB. Explaining racial disparities in outcomes after cardiac surgery: the role of hospital quality. JAMA Surg 2014;149(3):223–7.
[58] Osborne NH, Upchurch GR, Mathur AK, et al. Explaining racial disparities in mortality after abdominal aortic aneurysm repair. J Vasc Surg 2009;50(4):709–13.
[59] Morris AM, Rhoads KF, Stain SC, et al. Understanding racial disparities in cancer treatment and outcomes. J Am Coll Surg 2010;211(1):105–13.
[60] Haider AH, Scott VK, Rehman KA, et al. Racial disparities in surgical care and outcomes in the United States: a comprehensive review of patient, provider, and systemic factors. J Am Coll Surg 2013;216(3):482–92.e12.
[61] Lucas FL, Stukel TA, Morris AM, et al. Race and surgical mortality in the United States. Ann Surg 2006;243(2):281–6.

[62] Tsai TC, Joynt KE, Orav EJ, et al. Variation in surgical-readmission rates and quality of hospital care. N Engl J Med 2013;369(12):1134–42.
[63] Birkmeyer JD, Dimick JB. Understanding and reducing variation in surgical mortality. Annu Rev Med 2009;60:405–15.
[64] Dimick J, Ruhter J, Sarrazin MV, et al. Black patients more likely than whites to undergo surgery at low-quality hospitals in segregated regions. Health Aff (Millwood) 2013;32(6): 1046–53.
[65] Scarborough JE, Bennett KM, Pietrobon R, et al. Trends in the utilization of high-volume hospitals by minority and underinsured surgical patients. Am Surg 2010;76(5):529–38.
[66] Mehtsun WT, Figueroa JF, Zheng J, et al. Racial disparities in surgical mortality: the gap appears to have narrowed. Health Aff (Millwood) 2017;36(6):1057–64.
[67] Alderwick H, Gottlieb LM. Meanings and misunderstandings: a social determinants of health lexicon for health care systems. Milbank Q 2019;97(2):407–19.
[68] Adler NE, Glymour MM, Fielding J. Addressing social determinants of health and health inequalities. JAMA 2016;316(16):1641–2.
[69] Social determinants of health I Healthy People. 2020. Available at: https://www.healthypeople.gov/2020/topics-objectives/topic/social-determinants-of-health. Accessed September 7, 2020.
[70] Diaz A, Hyer JM, Barmash E, et al. County-level social vulnerability is associated with worse surgical outcomes especially among minority patients. Ann Surg 2021; https://doi.org/10.1097/SLA.0000000000004691.
[71] Hyer JM, Tsilimigras DI, Diaz A, et al. High social vulnerability and "textbook outcomes" after cancer surgery. J Am Coll Surgeons 2020 In press.
[72] Diaz A, O'Reggio R, Norman M, et al. Association of historic housing policy, modern day neighborhood deprivation and outcomes after inpatient hospitalization. Ann Surg 2021; https://doi.org/10.1097/SLA.0000000000005195.
[73] Diaz A, Chavarin D, Paredes AZ, et al. Association of neighborhood characteristics with utilization of high-volume hospitals among patients undergoing high-risk cancer surgery. Ann Surg Oncol 2021;28(2):617–31.
[74] Diaz A, Hyer JM, Azap R, et al. Association of social vulnerability with the use of high-volume and magnet recognition hospitals for hepatopancreatic cancer surgery. Surgery 2021;170(2):571–8.
[75] Diaz A, Beane JD, Hyer JM, et al. Impact of hospital quality on surgical outcomes in patients with high social vulnerability: association of textbook outcomes and social vulnerability by hospital quality. Surgery 2021;0(0); https://doi.org/10.1016/j.surg.2021.10.021.
[76] Diaz A, Barmash E, Azap R, et al. Association of County-Level Social Vulnerability with Elective Versus Non-elective Colorectal Surgery. J Gastrointest Surg 2021;25(3):786–94.
[77] Carmichael H, Moore A, Steward L, et al. Using the social vulnerability index to examine local disparities in emergent and elective cholecystectomy. J Surg Res 2019;243:160–4.
[78] Azap RA, Hyer JM, Diaz A, et al. Association of county-level vulnerability, patient-level race/ethnicity, and receipt of surgery for early-stage hepatocellular carcinoma. JAMA Surg 2021;156(2):197–9.
[79] Azap RA, Paredes AZ, Diaz A, et al. The association of neighborhood social vulnerability with surgical textbook outcomes among patients undergoing hepatopancreatic surgery. Surgery 2020;168(5):868–75.
[80] Paro A, Hyer JM, Diaz A, et al. Profiles in social vulnerability: the association of social determinants of health with postoperative surgical outcomes. Surgery 2021;26; https://doi.org/10.1016/j.surg.2021.06.001.
[81] Paro A, Dalmacy D, Madison Hyer J, et al. Impact of residential racial integration on postoperative outcomes among Medicare beneficiaries undergoing resection for cancer. Ann Surg Oncol 2021;28(12):7566–74.

[82] Diaz A, Dalmacy D, Herbert C, et al. Association of county-level racial diversity and likelihood of a textbook outcome following pancreas surgery. Ann Surg Oncol 2021;28(13): 8076–84.
[83] Diaz A, Dalmacy D, Hyer JM, et al. Intersection of social vulnerability and residential diversity: postoperative outcomes following resection of lung and colon cancer. J Surg Oncol 2021;124(5):886–93.
[84] Ibrahim AM, Hughes TG, Thumma JR, et al. Association of hospital critical access status with surgical outcomes and expenditures among Medicare beneficiaries. JAMA 2016;315(19): 2095–103.
[85] TrendWatch Chartbook 2019 I AHA. American Hospital Association. Available at: https://www.aha.org/guidesreports/2019-10-25-trendwatch-chartbook-2019. Accessed February 11, 2020.
[86] Snapshot of U.S Health Systems, 2016. Available at: https://www.ahrq.gov/sites/default/files/wysiwyg/snapshot-of-us-health-systems-2016v2.pdf. Accessed February 11, 2020.
[87] Schmitt M. Do hospital mergers reduce costs? J Health Econ 2017;52:74–94.
[88] Dafny L, Ho K, Lee RS. The price effects of cross-market mergers: theory and evidence from the hospital industry. RAND J Econ 2019;50(2):286–325.
[89] Cooper Z, Craig SV, Gaynor M, et al. The price ain't right? Hospital prices and health spending on the privately insured. Q J Econ 2019;134(1):51–107.
[90] White C, Whaley C. Prices paid to hospitals by private health plans are high relative to Medicare and vary widely: findings from an employer-led transparency initiative. 2019. Available at: https://www.rand.org/pubs/research_reports/RR3033.html. Accessed April 16, 2020.
[91] Sheetz KH, Chhabra K, Nathan H, et al. The quality of surgical care at hospitals associated with America's highest-rated medical centers. Ann Surg 2020;271(5):862–7.
[92] Sheetz KH, Ibrahim AM, Nathan H, et al. Variation in surgical outcomes across networks of the highest-rated US hospitals. JAMA Surg 2019;154(6):510.
[93] Diaz A, Burns S, Paredes AZ, et al. Accessing surgical care for pancreaticoduodenectomy: patient variation in travel distance and choice to bypass hospitals to reach higher volume centers. J Surg Oncol 2019;120(8):1318–26.
[94] Smith ME, Shubeck SP, Nuliyalu U, et al. Local referral of high-risk patients to high-quality hospitals: surgical outcomes, cost savings, and travel burdens. Ann Surg 2020;271(6): 1065–71.
[95] Ibrahim A, Dimick JB. Redesigning the delivery of specialty care within newly formed hospital networks. Catalyst Carryover 2017;3(2); https://doi.org/10.1056/CAT.17.0503.
[96] Humana Highlights Commitment to Addressing Health Equity in 2020 Corporate Responsibility Report. Available at: https://press.humana.com/news/news-details/2021/Humana-Highlights-Commitment-to-Addressing-Health-Equity-in-2020-Corporate-Responsibility-Report/default.aspx. Accessed November 15, 2021.
[97] Equity in health care quality I Disparities Solutions Center. DSC. Available at: https://www.mghdisparitiessolutions.org/equity-in-health-care-quality. Accessed November 15, 2021.
[98] WHO Commission on Social Determinants of Health, World Health Organization. In: Closing the gap in a generation: health equity through action on the social determinants of health: commission on social determinants of health final report. World Health Organization, Commission on Social Determinants of Health; 2008.
[99] Health equity report I Blue Cross Blue Shield of Massachusetts. Available at: https://www.bluecrossma.org/myblue/equity-in-health-care/health-equity-report. Accessed November 15, 2021.

Advances in Surgery 56 (2022) 275–286
ADVANCES IN SURGERY

What Is the Role of Neoadjuvant Endocrine Therapy for Breast Cancer?

Anna Weiss, MD[a], Tari A. King, MD[b,*]

[a]Division of Breast Surgery, Brigham and Women's Hospital, Dana-Farber/Brigham Cancer Center, Harvard Medical School, 450 Brookline Avenue, YC 1220, Boston, MA, USA; [b]Division of Breast Surgery, Brigham and Women's Hospital, Dana-Farber/Brigham Cancer Center, Harvard Medical School, 450 Brookline Avenue, YC 1220, Boston, MA, USA

Keywords

• Hormone receptor-positive breast cancer • Neoadjuvant endocrine therapy
• Neoadjuvant hormonal therapy

Key points

- Neoadjuvant chemotherapy (NAC) is falling out of favor for hormone receptor-positive breast cancer, and neoadjuvant endocrine therapy (NET) is gaining popularity.
- NET effectively downsizes breast tumors, allowing for breast conservation in postmenopausal patients.
- There is an opportunity to develop axillary management strategies specific to NET.

INTRODUCTION

Reasons to use preoperative (neoadjuvant) systemic therapy for the treatment of breast cancer include downsizing breast tumors [1–3], downstaging nodal disease [4–7], and assessing response as a means of prognostication and guide for adjuvant therapies [8,9]. The ideal neoadjuvant therapy is one from which the patient would derive long-term benefit. Recent large randomized controlled trials using genomic recurrence scores (RS) have demonstrated that many patients with hormone receptor-positive, human epidermal growth factor receptor 2-negative (HR + HER2-) breast cancer do not benefit from adjuvant chemotherapy and as such, neoadjuvant chemotherapy (NAC) is falling out of favor

*Corresponding author. *E-mail address:* tking7@bwh.harvard.edu

https://doi.org/10.1016/j.yasu.2022.02.008
0065-3411/22/

[10,11]. The TAILORx trial [10] randomized 6711 pre and postmenopausal patients with HR + HER2-node-negative tumors and Oncotype DX RS between 11 and 25 to endocrine therapy versus chemo-endocrine therapy; invasive disease-free survival for those treated with endocrine therapy was noninferior to those treated with chemo-endocrine therapy, with a hazard ratio of 1.08 (95% confidence interval [CI] 0.94 to 1.24; $P = .26$). Of note, 70% of the tumors tested had an Oncotype DX RS$\leq$ 25, indicating that many node-negative patients could be spared adjuvant chemotherapy. Similarly, the RxPONDER trial [11] randomized 5083 women with HR + HER2-breast cancer, 1 to 3 positive lymph nodes, and Oncotype DX RS$\leq$25 to endocrine therapy versus chemo-endocrine therapy. Among the 3350 postmenopausal patients, the hazards ratio for invasive disease-free survival was not significant for chemo-endocrine versus endocrine therapy alone (0.97, 95% CI 0.78–1.22; $P = .82$), indicating that most postmenopausal patients with HR + HER2-node-positive disease do not benefit from adjuvant chemotherapy. In contrast, the data for most premenopausal women continue to support adjuvant chemotherapy.

If a patient is not going to gain a survival benefit from adjuvant chemotherapy, using NAC solely to downsize a breast tumor and achieve breast-conserving therapy (BCT) is not indicated; as such, several clinical trials have compared neoadjuvant endocrine therapy (NET) to NAC directly. A phase II trial randomized 239 postmenopausal women with stage IIA–IIIB HR + HER2-breast cancer to NET (aromatase inhibitors [AI] anastrozole or exemestane) or NAC (doxorubicin and paclitaxel). Objective response rates were 64% in each group, and BCT rates were 33% and 24%, respectively ($P = .058$) [12]. The GEICAM/2006-03 trial [13] was another phase II trial that randomized 95 pre and postmenopausal women with HR + HER2-breast cancer to NET (exemestane) or NAC (epirubicin and cyclophosphamide followed by docetaxel). Clinical response rates were 48% and 66%, respectively ($P = .075$) and BCT rates were 56% and 47%, respectively ($P = .2369$). According to a meta-analysis by Spring and colleagues [14], NET has a lower toxicity profile than NAC but equal if not greater efficacy converting patients to BCT, which is one of the major goals of neoadjuvant systemic therapy, making it an attractive option for the neoadjuvant treatment of patients with HR + HER2-postmenopausal breast cancer.

Background–primary endocrine therapy

The Cancer Research Campaign trial [15] randomized 381 women over 70 with operable breast cancer to tamoxifen alone or surgery plus tamoxifen. At an initial follow-up of 34 months, there were no differences in survival or quality of life measures; however, patients on the tamoxifen arm more frequently required surgical intervention for local progression (35/183 [19%] compared with 15/171 [9%] in the surgery group, $P = .001$). Though the survival curves were no different at 3 years, patients in the tamoxifen arm had increased overall (hazard ratio 1.29, 95% CI 1.04–1.59) and breast cancer-specific (hazard ratio 1.68, 95% CI 1.15–2.47) mortality at 12.7 years and tamoxifen provided significantly less local control (hazard ratio 17.24, 95% CI 6.41–47.62 and 5.99, 95% CI 4.12–8.70 for mastectomy and BCT compared with tamoxifen, respectively) [16].

The Group for Research on Endocrine Therapy in the Elderly (GRETA) trial [17] randomized 473 women over 70 with operable breast cancer to tamoxifen alone or surgery plus tamoxifen. At a median follow-up of 36 months, patients treated with tamoxifen alone had increased rates of local progression (60/236 [25%] vs 15/237 [6%], $P < .0001$) but survival and rates of distant metastases were similar ($P = .67$ and .058, respectively). In contrast to the Cancer Research Campaign trial, survival findings were durable at a median follow-up of 80 months (no difference between tamoxifen and surgery, $P = .89$) and 95 (41.6%) patients had a complete or partial response to tamoxifen alone (defined as a decrease of >50% of the largest 2 tumor dimensions by mammogram) [18]. These findings indicate that primary endocrine therapy is a reasonable option but should be reserved for patients with severe comorbidities and/or limited life expectancy.

DISCUSSION

The ability of neoadjuvant endocrine therapy to downsize breast tumors

Building on studies of primary endocrine therapy, several clinical trials were then designed to assess the ability of NET to downsize breast tumors to achieve BCT (Table 1) [19–22]. The P024 trial [19] randomized 337 postmenopausal patients with HR + HER2-breast cancer who were not eligible for BCT to letrozole or tamoxifen. Objective response rates were 55% and 36%, respectively ($P < .001$), and BCT rates were 45% and 35%, respectively ($P = .022$). The Immediate Preoperative Anastrozole, Tamoxifen, or Combined with Tamoxifen (IMPACT) trial [20] randomized 330 postmenopausal women with HR + HER2-breast cancer to anastrozole, tamoxifen, or a combination of the 2. Objective tumor response rates by caliper measurement were 37%, 36% and 39%, respectively ($P = .61$) but in a subgroup analysis of 124 patients who were mastectomy-only candidates at presentation, 46% converted to BCT-eligible after treatment with anastrozole compared with

Table 1
Rates of breast tumor downsizing in landmark clinical trials of NET

Trial	Pretreatment	Posttreatment
P024 [19]	Inoperable & mastectomy-only patients	35–45%[a] BCT performed
IMPACT [20]	Mastectomy-only patients	31–44%[a] BCT performed
PROACT [21]	Inoperable patients	36–41%[a] operable
ACOSOG Z1031 [22]	Mastectomy-only patients	51% BCT candidates
	Marginal for BCT	83% BCT candidates

Abbreviations: BCS, breast-conserving surgery; BCT, breast-conserving therapy.
[a]Ranges are listed for the various neoadjuvant agents tested in that trial.

22% with tamoxifen (odds ratio of BCT 2.94 [95% CI 1.11, 7.81]; $P = .03$). Lastly, the Pre-Operative "Arimidex" Compared to Tamoxifen (PROACT) trial [21] randomized 451 postmenopausal women with HR + HER2-breast cancer to anastrozole or tamoxifen. Objective response rates were 39.5% and 35.4%, respectively ($P = .29$); however, conversion from inoperable or BCT-ineligible to operable or BCT-eligible favored anastrozole (43.0% vs 30.8%, $P = .04$). These trials established the superiority of AI over tamoxifen for use as NET. Subsequently, the ACOSOG Z1031 trial [22] aimed to determine the best AI and randomized 377 postmenopausal women to letrozole, anastrozole, or exemestane. Clinical response rates were similar at 74.8%, 69.1%, and 62.9%, respectively. Across all treatment groups, 51% of those who were considered mastectomy-only candidates and 83% of those who were considered marginal for BCT were considered BCT candidates after NET.

When downsizing a breast tumor, multi-modal breast imaging can be helpful to monitor response to neoadjuvant therapy and determine BCT candidacy, though data are limited following NET. In a meta-analysis of 5272 individual patients treated with NAC, magnetic resonance imaging (MRI) more accurately correlated with pathologic tumor size than ultrasonography and mammography [23]. A prospective study of 57 women demonstrated that MRI tumor measurement was similarly accurate for patients treated with NET and those treated with NAC ($P = .46$) [24]. As such, it is the authors' view that MRI should be considered pre- and post-NET to assess response and plan for BCT.

Axillary lymph node response to neoadjuvant endocrine therapy

Pathologic complete response (pCR; ypT0/is ypN0) to NAC is associated with improved survival. However, it is well known that overall [4] and nodal [25,26] pCR rates following NAC are lower among patients with HR + HER2-breast cancer as compared with other breast cancer subtypes. Additionally, this association of pCR and outcome is robust for the more aggressive subtypes (HER2+ and TNBC) but less so for HR + HER2-disease [27]. In the CTNeoBC pooled analysis, the hazard ratio of event-free survival was 0.25 (95% CI 0.18–0.34) for patients with HR-HER2+ who experienced a pCR and 0.24 (95% CI 0.18–0.33) for patients with TNBC who experienced a pCR compared with those who did not [27]. In contrast, the hazard ratio for patients with HR + HER2- with grade 1/2 disease was 0.63 (95% CI 0.38–1.04). Thus, the likelihood of experiencing a pCR is much lower in patients with HR + HER2-, and the lack of pCR does not correlate with inferior disease outcomes.

There is modest but mounting evidence that nodal pCR rates after NET are similar, or even lower than after NAC. In a National Cancer Database (NCDB) study, 76/571 (13%) of clinically node-positive (cN1) patients treated with NET experienced a nodal pCR compared with 1420/6233 (23%) of patients with cN1 treated with NAC ($P < .001$) [28]. In a single-institution series of 30 patients with cN1 who converted to clinically node-negative (cN0) after NET, 1 (3%)

experienced a nodal pCR [29]. In a single-institution study out of Memorial Sloan Kettering, of 38 patients with biopsy-proven cN1 who converted to cN0 after NET, 4 (11%) experienced a nodal pCR compared with 60/338 (18%) treated with NAC ($P = .37$) [30]. In a series out of the Mayo Clinic, 84 patients with biopsy-proven cN1 were treated with NET and 4 (5%) experienced a nodal pCR [31]. Lastly, the "Neo-adjuvant Study of Chemotherapy versus Endocrine Therapy" (Korean Breast Cancer Study Group 012) or "NEST" trial [32] randomized 187 patients with HR + HER2-node-positive premenopausal breast cancer to 24 weeks of NET or NAC and found nodal pCR rates of 4/83 (5%) following NET and 12/87 (14%) following NAC ($P < .005$). These trials are summarized in Table 2.

In contrast to breast imaging, the use of axillary imaging to assess response to systemic therapy is of limited value. This has been demonstrated in both the ACOSOG Z1071 [33] and SN FNAC [34] clinical trials, 2 large multi-institution prospective clinical trials that performed sentinel lymph node biopsy (SLNB) with planned completion axillary lymph node dissection (ALND) after NAC in patients who converted from cN1 to cN0. In both trials, relying on the normalization of axillary ultrasound findings would have led to numerous unnecessary ALNDs. Similar data regarding the accuracy of axillary imaging after NET are lacking.

Axillary surgery after neoadjuvant endocrine therapy

In the National Comprehensive Cancer Network (NCCN) guidelines for axillary management after neoadjuvant therapy [35], patients with NET are grouped with patients with NAC. However, patients selected for NET tend to be

Table 2
Nodal pCR and ALND rates following NET

Study	Setting	Total N treated with NET	Nodal pCR rate among cN1 treated with NET	ALND rates among those treated with NET who are ypN + by SLNB
Weiss et al, [28] 2019	NCDB	2138	76/571 (13%)	cN0: 152/403 (38%) cN1: 68/135 (50%)
Hammond et al, [29] 2020	Single institution	39	1/30 (3%)[a]	cN1: 26/29 (90%)
Montagna et al, [30] 2020	Single institution	127	4/38 (11%)[b]	NR
Murphy et al, [31] 2021	Single institution	194	4/84 (5%)	cN0: 17/28 (61%) cN1: 68/80 (85%)
Kim et al, [32] 2020	RCT	87	4/83 (5%)	NR

Abbreviations: ALND, axillary lymph node dissection; pCR, pathologic complete response; NCDB, national cancer database; NET, neoadjuvant endocrine therapy; NR, not reported; RCT, randomized controlled trial; SLNB, sentinel lymph node biopsy.
[a]Among those who converted to cN0.
[b]Among those with biopsy-proven cN1 disease.

older, with different disease biology and subsequently different expected response rates [28,30]. This selection bias is further demonstrated by the frequent omission of ALND despite ypN + disease after NET (see Table 2). For example, in an NCDB analysis of patients with stage II–III HR + HER2-breast cancer, only 68/135 (50%) patients with ypN + disease discovered on SLNB after NET were treated with completion ALND [28].

As indications for NET broaden, data are needed to determine if this practice of omitting ALND is safe. Given that patients treated with NET have received only a small fraction of their overall treatment, we hypothesized that minimal residual nodal disease burden after NET would not have a detrimental impact on long-term outcomes. To determine the prognostic significance of residual nodal disease after NET we interrogated an NCDB cohort of patients with HR + HER2-cT1-3, N0-1 breast cancer selected for NET and axillary surgery between 2010 and 2016. In a propensity score-matched analysis, patients with cN0 and cN1 with residual nodal disease after NET had similar 5-year adjusted overall survival as patients who proceeded to upfront surgery and were found to have nodal disease (*P* values were >0.05 for all nodal categories compared: ypN0(i+), ypN1mi, 1 to 2 positive nodes, ≥3 positive nodes) [36].

To examine the nodal disease burden in patients selected for NET, we interrogated both the NCDB (2012–2016) and our prospectively maintained, single-institution database (2015–2018) for patients with HR + HER2-stage I–III breast cancer treated with NET (N = 3640 and 95, respectively). Most patients with cN0 who underwent axillary surgery had a low volume of nodal disease (0, 1, or 2 positive nodes): 2945/3227 (91%) and 44/46 (96%), respectively. In contrast, only 342/675 (51%) and 7/23 (30%) respective patients with cN1 had a low volume of nodal disease. In a subsequent analysis of patients with cN0 and cN1 in the NCDB cohort, there was no difference in 5-year overall survival by type of axillary surgery (SLNB vs ALND), regardless of the volume of nodal disease [37]. A recent single-institution study of regional recurrence rates in patients with residual nodal disease after NET treated with SLNB alone lends further support to the safety of omitting ALND [31]. A total of 194 HR + HER2-breast cancers were evaluated, 84 of which had biopsy-proven nodal metastases. Among 110 patients with cN0, 99 had axillary surgery, 28/99 (28%) had ypN + disease and 11/28 (39%) underwent SLNB alone. Among the 84 patients with cN1, 80 had residual nodal disease and 12/80 (15%) underwent SLNB alone. There were no regional recurrences at a median follow-up of 35 months. Although follow-up is limited in both the NCDB cohort and the single-institution study, taken together, these data suggest that most patients selected for NET have a low nodal disease burden, and choice of axillary surgery may not impact survival outcomes.

Careful consideration of these data has led our group to draw several conclusions regarding nodal response rates and management of the axilla after NET (Fig. 1). We do not expect a nodal pCR to NET; the prognostic significance of residual nodal disease after NET seems similar to nodal disease detected in upfront surgery patients; and type of axillary surgery may not impact long-term outcomes. These conclusions are supported by the fact that

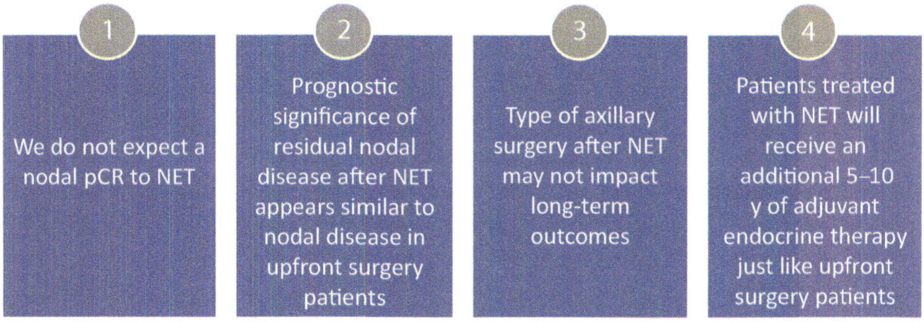

Fig. 1. Assumptions regarding axillary lymph node surgery that can be made for patients being treated with NET. HR, hormone receptor; NET, neoadjuvant endocrine therapy; y, years.

patients selected for NET have not received their full complement of systemic therapy at the time of surgery, that is, they will receive an additional 5 to 10 years of adjuvant endocrine therapy, just like upfront surgery patients. As such, axillary management strategies used in upfront surgery patients may be appropriate for patients selected for NET, thereby avoiding overtreatment, and minimizing the morbidity of axillary surgery. It should be noted, however, that these data are drawn from highly selected patient populations, and any decision to omit ALND in patients with nodal disease after NET should be considered in the context of the multi-disciplinary team.

Remaining questions

There are several remaining questions regarding NET use, but those most relevant to surgeons include how to select patients for NET, and how to best measure response to NET.

Patient selection

Traditional factors used to select patients for NET treatment, both on- and off-trial, include menopausal status, strength of estrogen or progesterone receptor staining, and histologic grade. Some clinical trials made more rigorous attempts to select patients with favorable tumor biology. For example, GEICAM [13] enrolled only luminal A patients, defined as estrogen and progesterone receptor-positive, HER2-, and cytokeratin 8 and 18 positive. Many believe that genomic assays can further improve patient selection for NET or NAC and there is growing evidence that genomic assays can be reliably performed on core biopsy specimens [38,39]. Bear and colleagues [40] performed a feasibility trial testing a patient's willingness to accept treatment allocation based on Oncotype DX RS. Postmenopausal patients with RS$\leq$ 11 were assigned to NET, those with RS between 11 and 25 were randomized to NET or NAC, and those with RS$\geq$25 were assigned to NAC. Only 15% refused their treatment allocation, lower than their predesignated 33% unacceptable rate. BCT rates were 75% for patients with RS$\leq$ 11 treated with NET, 72% and 64% for patients with RS 11 to 25 treated with NET and NAC, respectively, and 57% for RS greater than 25 treated with NAC. The TransNEOS study [41] examined 295 postmenopausal patients with HR + HER2-node-negative breast cancer who were treated with 6 months of letrozole to determine whether RS could predict response to NET. Clinical response rates among patients with RS less than 18, 18 to 30 and $\geq$ 31 were 54%, 42%, and 22%, respectively ($P < .001$). In summary, pretreatment genomic assays performed on core needle biopsy specimens can and should be considered to triage patients to the appropriate neoadjuvant regimen, and patients are accepting this approach.

Few groups have examined NET for premenopausal women. In 2012, the phase III STAGE trial [42] randomized 197 premenopausal women to 24 weeks of NET (tamoxifen or anastrozole) with ovarian suppression (OS). Clinical response rates were 50.5% and 70.4%, respectively (estimated difference 19.9%, 95% CI 6.5–33.3; $P = .004$), confirming the superiority of AI + OS over tamoxifen + OS as NET for premenopausal women. However, when compared directly to NAC, NET has not performed well in the premenopausal cohort. In an unplanned analysis of 51 premenopausal women (of 95 total) enrolled in the GEICAM/2006-03 trial [13], objective response rates measured by MRI were 75% after NAC and 44% after NET ($P = .027$). The NEST trial [32], a phase III clinical trial, randomized 187 premenopausal women to 24 weeks of NET (tamoxifen and OS with goserelin) or standard NAC. Higher response rates were observed following NAC than NET in both MRI (83.7% vs 52.9%, respectively; estimated difference 30.8%, 95% CI 17.6–44.0, $P < .001$) and caliper measurements (83.9% vs 71.3%, respectively; estimated difference 12.6%, 95% CI 0.4–24.9, $P = .046$). These findings make NET less attractive for premenopausal women until additional data are available.

Measures of response to neoadjuvant endocrine therapy

Given the limited prognostic significance of pCR in HR + HER2-breast cancer as described above, groups have examined other measures of disease response to NET such as changes in Ki67 staining levels and the preoperative endocrine prognostic index (PEPI). Among 158 patients with paired samples from the IMPACT trial, higher Ki67 staining levels after 2 weeks of NET were associated with inferior recurrence-free survival (log-rank $P = .008$) [43]. PEPI [44] was developed in the P024 trial cohort [19] and independently validated in the IMPACT trial [20] and includes 4 factors significantly associated with improved recurrence-free survival: high estrogen receptor Allred score (3–8), low Ki67 staining levels ($\leq$2.7%), small pathologic tumor size (ypT1-2) and pathologic nodal status (ypN0). In the independent validation, there was a separation of the relapse-free survival curves of the 3 PEPI groups (0, 1–3, $\geq$4; $P = .002$) and no patients with a PEPI score of 0 recurred at a median follow-up of 60.3 months. Despite the prognostic significance of these measures of response, none as yet have implications for local therapy.

SUMMARY

The role of NET in HR + HER2-breast cancer is to effectively downsize breast tumors in women who desire BCT. Outside of a clinical trial, current data only support the use of NET in postmenopausal patients, and pretreatment genomic RS performed on core needle biopsy specimens should be considered to select patients for this approach; if there is no role for adjuvant chemotherapy, there is no role for NAC. Upfront surgery axillary management algorithms may be considered for patients with NET with residual nodal disease in properly selected patients.

CLINICS CARE POINTS

- Neoadjuvant endocrine therapy (NET) downsizes breast tumors, thereby allowing for breast conservation with equal efficacy as neoadjuvant chemotherapy (NAC) in postmenopausal patients.
- Genomic assays can be used to guide both adjuvant and neoadjuvant treatment strategies.
- More research is needed to determine if NET can be used in premenopausal patients.
- Axillary surgical management following NET is not well-described, but early data suggest that patients selected for NET may be treated per upfront surgery algorithms.

DISCLOSURE

There is no funding for this work. AW reports unrelated institutional research funding from Myriad Laboratories, Inc.

References

[1] Fisher B, Brown A, Mamounas E, et al. Effect of preoperative chemotherapy on local-regional disease in women with operable breast cancer: findings from National surgical adjuvant breast and bowel project B-18. J Clin Oncol 1997;15(7):2483–93.

[2] van der Hage JA, van de Velde CJ, Julien JP, et al. Preoperative chemotherapy in primary operable breast cancer: results from the European Organization for Research and Treatment of Cancer trial 10902. J Clin Oncol 2001;19(22):4224–37.

[3] Gianni L, Baselga J, Eiermann W, et al. Phase III trial evaluating the addition of paclitaxel to doxorubicin followed by cyclophosphamide, methotrexate, and fluorouracil, as adjuvant or primary systemic therapy: European cooperative trial in operable Breast Cancer. J Clin Oncol 2009;27(15):2474–81.

[4] Boughey JC, Suman VJ, Mittendorf EA, et al. Sentinel lymph node surgery after neoadjuvant chemotherapy in patients with node-positive breast cancer: the ACOSOG Z1071 (Alliance) clinical trial. JAMA 2013;310(14):1455–61.

[5] Kuehn T, Bauerfeind I, Fehm T, et al. Sentinel-lymph-node biopsy in patients with breast cancer before and after neoadjuvant chemotherapy (SENTINA): a prospective, multicentre cohort study. Lancet Oncol 2013;14(7):609–18.

[6] Boileau JF, Poirier B, Basik M, et al. Sentinel node biopsy after neoadjuvant chemotherapy in biopsy-proven node-positive breast cancer: the SN FNAC study. J Clin Oncol 2015;33(3):258–64.

[7] Classe JM, Loaec C, Gimbergues P, et al. Sentinel lymph node biopsy without axillary lymphadenectomy after neoadjuvant chemotherapy is accurate and safe for selected patients: the GANEA 2 study. Breast Cancer Res Treat 2019;173(2):343–52.

[8] von Minckwitz G, Huang CS, Mano MS, et al. Trastuzumab emtansine for residual invasive HER2-positive breast cancer. N Engl J Med 2019;380(7):617–28.
[9] Masuda N, Lee SJ, Ohtani S, et al. Adjuvant capecitabine for breast cancer after preoperative chemotherapy. N Engl J Med 2017;376(22):2147–59.
[10] Sparano JA, Gray RJ, Makower DF, et al. Adjuvant chemotherapy guided by a 21-gene expression assay in breast cancer. N Engl J Med 2018;379(2):111–21.
[11] Kalinsky K, Barlow WE, Meric-Bernstam F, et al. Abstract GS3-00: First results from a phase III randomized clinical trial of standard adjuvant endocrine therapy (ET) +/- chemotherapy (CT) in patients (pts) with 1-3 positive nodes, hormone receptor-positive (HR+) and HER2-negative (HER2-) breast cancer (BC) with recurrence score (RS) < 25: SWOG S1007 (RxPonder). Cancer Res 2021;81(4 Supplement):GS3-00-GS3-00.
[12] Semiglazov VF, Semiglazov VV, Dashyan GA, et al. Phase 2 randomized trial of primary endocrine therapy versus chemotherapy in postmenopausal patients with estrogen receptor-positive breast cancer. Cancer 2007;110(2):244–54.
[13] Alba E, Calvo L, Albanell J, et al. Chemotherapy (CT) and hormonotherapy (HT) as neoadjuvant treatment in luminal breast cancer patients: results from the GEICAM/2006-03, a multicenter, randomized, phase-II study. Ann Oncol 2012;23(12):3069–74.
[14] Spring LM, Gupta A, Reynolds KL, et al. Neoadjuvant endocrine therapy for estrogen receptor-positive breast cancer: a systematic review and meta-analysis. JAMA Oncol 2016;2(11):1477–86.
[15] Bates T, Riley DL, Houghton J, et al. Breast cancer in elderly women: a cancer research Campaign trial comparing treatment with tamoxifen and optimal surgery with tamoxifen alone. The elderly breast cancer working party. Br J Surg 1991;78(5):591–4.
[16] Fennessy M, Bates T, MacRae K, et al. Late follow-up of a randomized trial of surgery plus tamoxifen versus tamoxifen alone in women aged over 70 years with operable breast cancer. Br J Surg 2004;91(6):699–704.
[17] Mustacchi G, Milani S, Pluchinotta A, et al. Tamoxifen or surgery plus tamoxifen as primary treatment for elderly patients with operable breast cancer: The G.R.E.T.A. Trial. Group for Research on Endocrine Therapy in the Elderly. Anticancer Res 1994;14(5B):2197–200.
[18] Mustacchi G, Ceccherini R, Milani S, et al. Tamoxifen alone versus adjuvant tamoxifen for operable breast cancer of the elderly: long-term results of the phase III randomized controlled multicenter GRETA trial. Ann Oncol 2003;14(3):414–20.
[19] Eiermann W, Paepke S, Appfelstaedt J, et al. Preoperative treatment of postmenopausal breast cancer patients with letrozole: A randomized double-blind multicenter study. Ann Oncol 2001;12(11):1527–32.
[20] Smith IE, Dowsett M, Ebbs SR, et al. Neoadjuvant treatment of postmenopausal breast cancer with anastrozole, tamoxifen, or both in combination: the Immediate Preoperative Anastrozole, Tamoxifen, or Combined with Tamoxifen (IMPACT) multicenter double-blind randomized trial. J Clin Oncol 2005;23(22):5108–16.
[21] Cataliotti L, Buzdar AU, Noguchi S, et al. Comparison of anastrozole versus tamoxifen as preoperative therapy in postmenopausal women with hormone receptor-positive breast cancer: the Pre-Operative "Arimidex" Compared to Tamoxifen (PROACT) trial. Cancer 2006;106(10):2095–103.
[22] Ellis MJ, Suman VJ, Hoog J, et al. Randomized phase II neoadjuvant comparison between letrozole, anastrozole, and exemestane for postmenopausal women with estrogen receptor-rich stage 2 to 3 breast cancer: clinical and biomarker outcomes and predictive value of the baseline PAM50-based intrinsic subtype–ACOSOG Z1031. J Clin Oncol 2011;29(17):2342–9.
[23] Gu YL, Pan SM, Ren J, et al. Role of magnetic resonance imaging in detection of pathologic complete remission in breast cancer patients treated with neoadjuvant chemotherapy: a meta-analysis. Clin Breast Cancer 2017;17(4):245–55.
[24] Takeda K, Kanao S, Okada T, et al. MRI evaluation of residual tumor size after neoadjuvant endocrine therapy vs. neoadjuvant chemotherapy. Eur J Radiol 2012;81(9):2148–53.

[25] Laws A, Hughes ME, Hu J, et al. Impact of residual nodal disease burden on technical outcomes of sentinel lymph node biopsy for node-positive (cN1) breast cancer patients treated with neoadjuvant chemotherapy. Ann Surg Oncol 2019;26(12):3846–55.
[26] Mamtani A, Barrio AV, King TA, et al. How often does neoadjuvant chemotherapy avoid axillary dissection in patients with histologically confirmed nodal metastases? results of a prospective study. Ann Surg Oncol 2016;23(11):3467–74.
[27] Cortazar P, Zhang L, Untch M, et al. Pathological complete response and long-term clinical benefit in breast cancer: the CTNeoBC pooled analysis. Lancet 2014;384(9938):164–72.
[28] Weiss A, Wong S, Golshan M, et al. Patterns of Axillary management in stages 2 and 3 hormone receptor-positive breast cancer by initial treatment approach. Ann Surg Oncol 2019;26(13):4326–36.
[29] Hammond JB, Parnall TH, Scott DW, et al. Gauging the efficacy of neoadjuvant endocrine therapy in breast cancer patients with known axillary disease. J Surg Oncol 2020;122(4):619–22; https://doi.org/10.1002/jso.26047.
[30] Montagna G, Sevilimedu V, Fornier M, et al. How effective is neoadjuvant endocrine therapy (NET) in downstaging the axilla and achieving breast-conserving surgery? Ann Surg Oncol 2020;27(12):4702–10.
[31] Murphy BM, Hoskin TL, Degnim AC, et al. Surgical management of axilla following neoadjuvant endocrine therapy. Ann Surg Oncol 2021;28(13):8729–39.
[32] Kim HJ, Noh WC, Lee ES, et al. Efficacy of neoadjuvant endocrine therapy compared with neoadjuvant chemotherapy in pre-menopausal patients with oestrogen receptor-positive and HER2-negative, lymph node-positive breast cancer. Breast Cancer Res 2020;22(1):54.
[33] Boughey JC, Ballman KV, Hunt KK, et al. Axillary ultrasound after neoadjuvant chemotherapy and its impact on sentinel lymph node surgery: results from the american college of surgeons oncology group Z1071 Trial (Alliance). J Clin Oncol 2015;33(30):3386–93.
[34] Morency D, Dumitra S, Parvez E, et al. Axillary lymph node ultrasound following neoadjuvant chemotherapy in biopsy-proven node-positive breast cancer: results from the SN FNAC Study. Ann Surg Oncol 2019;26(13):4337–45.
[35] National Comprehensive Cancer Network (NCCN). Clinical practice guidelines in oncology. breast cancer (Version 8.2021). Available at: https://www.nccn.org/professionals/physician_gls/pdf/breast.pdf. Accessed March 15, 2022.
[36] Kantor O, Wong S, Weiss A, et al. Prognostic significance of residual nodal disease after neoadjuvant endocrine therapy for hormone receptor-positive breast cancer. NPJ Breast Cancer 2020;6:35.
[37] Kantor O, Wakeman M, Weiss A, et al. Axillary management after neoadjuvant endocrine therapy for hormone receptor-positive breast cancer. Ann Surg Oncol 2021;28(3):1358–67; https://doi.org/10.1245/s10434-020-09073-6.
[38] Qi P, Yang Y, Bai QM, et al. Concordance of the 21-gene assay between core needle biopsy and resection specimens in early breast cancer patients. Breast Cancer Res Treat 2021;186(2):327–42.
[39] Orozco JIJ, Chang SC, Matsuba C, et al. Is the 21-gene recurrence score on core needle biopsy equivalent to surgical specimen in early-stage breast cancer? A comparison of gene expression between paired core needle biopsy and surgical specimens. Ann Surg Oncol 2021;28(10):5588–96.
[40] Bear HD, Wan W, Robidoux A, et al. Using the 21-gene assay from core needle biopsies to choose neoadjuvant therapy for breast cancer: A multicenter trial. J Surg Oncol 2017;115(8):917–23.
[41] Iwata H, Masuda N, Yamamoto Y, et al. Validation of the 21-gene test as a predictor of clinical response to neoadjuvant hormonal therapy for ER+, HER2-negative breast cancer: the TransNEOS study. Breast Cancer Res Treat 2019;173(1):123–33.
[42] Masuda N, Sagara Y, Kinoshita T, et al. Neoadjuvant anastrozole versus tamoxifen in patients receiving goserelin for premenopausal breast cancer (STAGE): a double-blind, randomised phase 3 trial. Lancet Oncol 2012;13(4):345–52.

[43] Dowsett M, Smith IE, Ebbs SR, et al. Short-term changes in Ki-67 during neoadjuvant treatment of primary breast cancer with anastrozole or tamoxifen alone or combined correlate with recurrence-free survival. Clin Cancer Res 2005;11(2 Pt 2):951s-8s.
[44] Ellis MJ, Tao Y, Luo J, et al. Outcome prediction for estrogen receptor-positive breast cancer based on postneoadjuvant endocrine therapy tumor characteristics. J Natl Cancer Inst 2008;100(19):1380–8.

Advances in Surgery 56 (2022) 287–304

ADVANCES IN SURGERY

What Is the Best Treatment for Acute Limb Ischemia?

Elizabeth G. King, MD, Alik Farber, MD*

Division of Vascular & Endovascular Surgery, Boston University School of Medicine 85 East Concord Street, Suite 3000, Boston, MA 02118, USA

Keywords

• Acute limb ischemia (ALI) • Embolectomy • Pharmacomechanical thrombectomy • Catheter-directed thrombolysis

Key points

- Acute limb ischemia (ALI) is a vascular emergency associated with high rates of limb loss and mortality.
- In situ thrombosis is the most common cause of lower-extremity ischemia, whereas upper-extremity ischemia more frequently occurs owing to embolic events.
- ALI is graded using the Rutherford classification based on the neurologic and vascular examination of the affected limb and is used to stratify urgency of intervention.
- Management of ALI includes immediate anticoagulation, expeditious revascularization using open or endovascular techniques, followed by identification and appropriate treatment of the underlying cause.
- Approach to revascularization depends on the severity of ischemia at presentation, time to reperfusion, chance of recovery, underlying cause, location of occlusion, procedural risks, and comorbid conditions.

BACKGROUND/OVERVIEW

Acute limb ischemia (ALI) is a common vascular emergency that results from the interruption of blood flow to the limb and hypoperfusion of downstream tissue of less than 2 weeks duration. ALI affects between 15 and 26 patients per 100,000 each year in the United States and is associated with high rates

*Corresponding author. Department of Surgery, 85 East Concord St, Suite 3000, Boston, MA 02118. *E-mail address:* Alik.Farber@bmc.org

https://doi.org/10.1016/j.yasu.2022.03.004
0065-3411/22/

of morbidity and mortality [1]. Previous studies cite perioperative mortality and limb loss rates of 20% to 40% and 12% to 50%, respectively, in cases of lower-extremity ALI [2,3]. Upper-extremity ALI occurs less commonly, accounting for approximately 17% of cases of ALI, with amputation and mortality rates ranging from 0% to 18% and 0% to 19%, respectively [4].

ALI presents a challenge for the surgeon because of both the consequences of potential tissue injury and the associated medical comorbidities inherent to this patent population. The prospective population-based Oxford Vascular Study observed that 42% of patients presenting with ALI had preexisting peripheral arterial disease (PAD), and 40% had known atherosclerotic risk factors [5].

The diagnosis of ALI can be made by a comprehensive history and physical examination and confirmed with selective use of diagnostic imaging. Management of ALI includes immediate anticoagulation, expeditious restoration of arterial circulation using open or endovascular techniques, followed by identification and appropriate treatment of the underlying cause.

CLASSIFICATION AND CAUSE

ALI presents with similar symptoms regardless of etiology; however, determination of its cause is important to guide management. In the lower extremity, ALI is most commonly a result of in situ thrombosis, owing to high prevalence of arterial occlusive disease; in the upper extremity, embolism is the most common cause of ALI. Other causes of ALI include trauma, iatrogenic injury, hypercoagulable states, arterial dissection, phlegmasia, hemodynamic perturbations, including low-flow states, such as cardiogenic and septic shock, as well as arterial vasospasm (Table 1).

Table 1
Causes of acute limb ischemia

Classification	Approximate frequency, %
In situ thrombosis	41
Embolism	38
• Cardiac 80%	
• Noncardiac 15%	
• Unknown 5%	
Occlusion of bypass/intervention	15
Thrombosis of popliteal aneurysm	3
Trauma	2
Iatrogenic	2

Adapted from Knowles M and Timaran CH. Epidemiology of Acute Critical Limb Ischemia. In: Dieter RS, Dieter Jr. RA, Dieter III RA, Nanjundappa A. (eds) Critical Limb Ischemia. Springer, Cham. 2017; Tan T, Farber A. The management of peripheral arterial emboli. In: Cameron JL, Cameron AM, eds. Current Surgical Therapy. 11th ed. Philadelphia: Elsevier;2014:903-909.

Thrombosis

Most cases of ALI are the result of in situ arterial thrombosis, often developing as a complication of atherosclerotic plaque or aneurysm. It can be caused by hypercoagulability or stenosis within a native artery, bypass graft, or stent. In cases of preexisting atherosclerotic disease, vessels become progressively narrowed, allowing for the development of collaterals, which may result in a less severe degree of acute ischemia, but a more complicated revascularization. Hypercoagulable states can also induce thrombus formation in arteries without atherosclerotic disease.

Emboli

When an embolus that originated in the proximal arterial tree travels to and lodges in a distal artery or arteriole, it causes interruption of blood flow to downstream tissue, resulting in ischemic injury to muscles, nerves, and skin. Anatomically, emboli lodge at bifurcations with the lower extremities more commonly affected than the upper extremities (Fig. 1). Cardiac causes account for approximately 80% of all cases of peripheral arterial embolism. These include emboli originating in the left atrium of patients with atrial arrhythmias, left ventricular thrombus in the setting of a recent myocardial infarction (MI), prosthetic heart valves, valvular heart disease owing to rheumatic fever or endocarditis, and atrial myxomas (Fig. 2). Noncardiac causes account for 15% to 20% of peripheral arterial emboli. Sources of emboli include arterial aneurysms, most commonly involving the aorta or popliteal artery, atherosclerotic plaques, trauma, and paradoxic emboli from deep venous thrombosis in patients with a patent foramen ovale (Fig. 3). Prompt anticoagulation and intervention are required to prevent formation of thrombus proximal and distal to the embolus.

CLINICAL PRESENTATION

The "Six Ps": pain, pulselessness, poikilothermia , paresthesia, pallor, and paralysis characterize ALI. Depending on the location and duration of the occlusion, extent of collateral circulation owing to existing arterial occlusive disease, and underlying cause, the clinical presentation may vary.

History and physical examination help to elucidate cause of the ischemic event. Pertinent history includes prior embolic episodes, history of PAD, recent MI, arrhythmias, valvular heart disease, aneurysmal disease, dissection, prior vascular interventions, and hypercoagulable states. A critical detail to note is the duration of symptoms, as irreversible muscle and nerve injury starts after 6 to 8 hours of severe acute ischemia.

Acute onset of ischemic pain in a patient without preexisting symptoms of PAD and normal distal pulses of the nonischemic limb suggests an embolic event. Such patients are often able to pinpoint the exact onset of symptoms, and the degree of limb ischemia is usually severe. A history of atrial arrhythmias, prior MI, or valvular disease is commonly present. In contrast, patients with a history of claudication, rest pain, or nonhealing ulcers are likely to

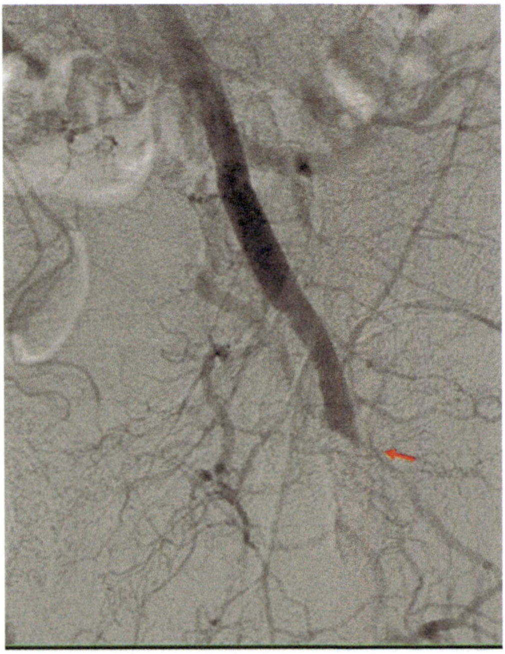

Fig. 1. An abrupt cutoff of the left common femoral artery consistent with the appearance of an embolus (*arrow*).

have preexisting PAD, and symptoms usually reflect in situ thrombosis of a diseased vessel, ipsilateral bypass graft, or stent. Pulses in the nonischemic limb are often absent. In patients with an acute-on-chronic process, the established collateral circulation may limit the severity of ischemia. Despite these findings, it can be difficult to reliably distinguish between embolic and thrombotic causes, especially in older patients with coexistent PAD.

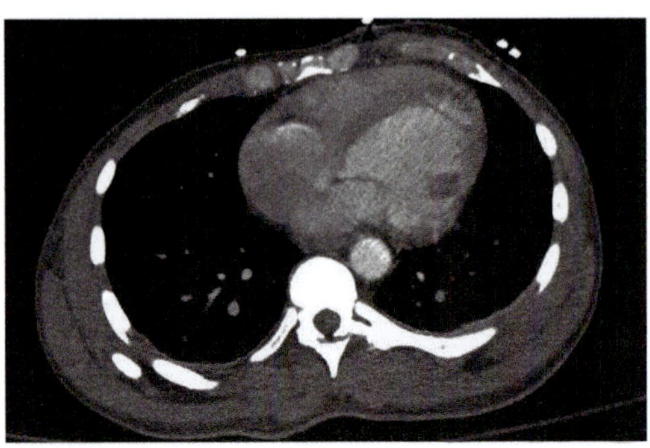

Fig. 2. Left ventricular thrombus in patient presenting with bilateral femoral artery occlusions.

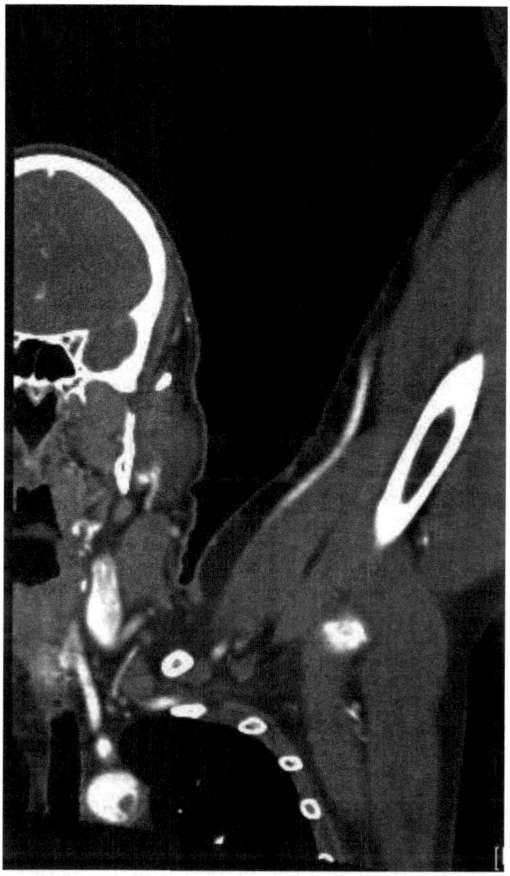

Fig. 3. Aortic thrombus in patient presenting with acute left upper-extremity ischemia.

Physical examination is used to determine the severity of ALI and level of occlusion, which aids in determining the most appropriate management. On physical examination, the affected limb is cool and pale and with varying degree of sensory and motor loss. Distal pulses are not palpable. The temperature level (border of coolness and warmth) and presence of proximal pulses suggest the location of the occluded vessel. Continuous-wave Doppler evaluation of peripheral signals is imperative to assess the degree of ischemia. ALI is graded using the Rutherford classification based on the neurologic and vascular examination of the affected limb and is used to stratify urgency of intervention (Table 2).

DIAGNOSTIC EXAMINATION

Imaging may help to elucidate the cause by identifying the responsible ulcerative plaque, dissection, thrombosed aneurysm, or acute thrombosis of an

Table 2
Clinical categories of acute limb ischemia

		Findings		Doppler signals	
Category	Description/ prognosis	Sensory loss	Muscle weakness	Arterial	Venous
I. Viable	Not immediately threatened	None	None	Audible	Audible
II. Threatened					
a. Marginally	Salvageable if promptly treated	Minimal (toes)/ none	None	Absent	Audible
b. Immediately	Salvageable with immediate revascularization	More than toes, associated rest pain	Mild, moderate	Absent	Audible
III. Irreversible	Major tissue loss or permanent neurologic damage	Profound, anesthetic	Profound, paralysis (rigors)	Absent	Absent

Modified from Rutherford RB, et al. Recommended standards for reports dealing with lower extremity ischemia: Revised version, Journal of Vascular Surgery, 26 (3), 1997, 517-538.

atherosclerotic vessel, bypass graft, or stent, as well as to aid in operative planning. Current imaging modalities include duplex ultrasonography, magnetic resonance angiography, computed tomographic angiography (CTA), and digital subtraction angiography. CTA of the chest, abdomen, or pelvis with lower-extremity runoff is preferred, as it can be performed expeditiously at most centers. However, imaging should not delay the need for emergent revascularization in patients with profound ischemia given the risk of irreversible muscle and peripheral nerve damage.

MANAGEMENT

When ALI is suspected, initial management includes intravenous fluid resuscitation and anticoagulation. In the absence of contraindications to therapeutic anticoagulation, a loading bolus of intravenous heparin, followed by initiation of a continuous infusion, should be administered to prevent propagation of the thrombus and maintain patency of collateral vessels. Direct thrombin inhibitors, lepirudin or argatroban, may be used in patients with intolerance to heparin. The use of anticoagulation alone may be considered in unstable patients or nonambulatory patients without limb-threatening ALI (Rutherford I) [6].

Selection of operative approach

The 2 primary approaches for revascularization in ALI are open surgical techniques and percutaneous endovascular therapy, including catheter-directed thrombolysis (CDT), pharmacomechanical, and aspiration thrombectomy. Hybrid approaches using both open and endovascular techniques may also be considered. When selecting the approach to revascularization, severity of ischemia at presentation, time to reperfusion, chance of recovery, underlying cause, location of occlusion, procedural risks, and comorbid conditions should be considered.

In purely embolic events, successful extraction of the embolus by endovascular or open techniques may reveal a widely patent arterial system with no need for further intervention. More commonly, thrombosis of an already stenotic atherosclerotic lesion is observed. Once the thrombus is removed, the underlying stenosis or occlusion must be treated to minimize the risk of rethrombosis. Discrete atherosclerotic lesions may be treated with balloon angioplasty or open surgical endarterectomy with patch angioplasty, whereas more extensive lesions may require stenting or bypass.

Endovascular revascularization

An endovascular approach, which can be performed under local anesthesia, should be considered in patients with a viable or marginally threatened limb (Rutherford I and IIa), those at medically high risk for open surgery, and in the setting of a thrombotic occlusion [7]. Patients with distal emboli, as observed in patients with normal femoral but absent distal pulses, may benefit from an initial angiogram and CDT or mechanical thrombectomy. This strategy may be more effective in establishing reperfusion of smaller distal vessels, as well as elucidating concomitant atherosclerotic lesions which may be treated using endovascular techniques, such as angioplasty and stenting.

Catheter-directed thrombolysis

With the advent of angiography and endovascular techniques, CDT emerged as a less-invasive alternative to open surgery in the management of ALI. In CDT, a multiside hole catheter is percutaneously placed across the thrombus to deliver a localized infusion of a thrombolytic agent, which enzymatically dissolves the thrombus through fibrin degradation. Thrombolysis is typically administered over a period of 24 to 48 hours as the patient is admitted to a monitored setting, such as an intensive care unit (ICU).

As the CDT approach gained in popularity, several landmark trials in the 1990s sought to compare outcomes of CDT with open surgery. A 2013 Cochrane meta-analysis of 5 prospective randomized controlled trials, including the Rochester, Surgery versus Thrombolysis for Ischemia of the Lower Extremities (STILE), and TOPAS (Thrombolysis or Peripheral Artery Surgery) trials, compared CDT using recombinant tissue plasminogen activator or urokinase with open surgical revascularization in patients with ALI. One-year death and limb-salvage rates were similar between the groups; however, significantly higher rates of stroke (1.3% vs 0%), major bleeding (8.8% vs 3.3%), and distal embolization (12.3% vs 0%) were observed in patients who underwent thrombolysis [8].

Disadvantages of CDT are the relatively longer time periods required to achieve tissue reperfusion and risk of potential bleeding complications. A systematic review by Ebben and colleagues [9] of 106 studies using CDT for lower-extremity arterial occlusions demonstrated a 75% angiographic patency rate and 91% freedom from amputation, but an 18% incidence of bleeding complications. Other studies have demonstrated that lower doses of fibrinolytics resulted in similar rates of success with fewer bleeding complications, but at a cost of longer treatment duration [10]. Older age, female sex, and cardiac comorbidities have been identified as factors that increase the risk of bleeding [11].

Given bleeding risk, CDT is contraindicated in certain patients. Absolute contraindications to pharmacologic thrombolysis include active bleeding, stroke or neurosurgical procedure within 3 months, malignant intracranial neoplasm, or history of hemorrhagic stroke. Relative contraindications include uncontrolled hypertension, central nervous system tumors or known intracranial pathologic condition, recent gastrointestinal bleed, trauma, pregnancy, major surgery within 3 weeks, and recent eye surgery.

Percutaneous mechanical thrombectomy

Percutaneous mechanical thrombectomy (PMT) techniques of thrombus extraction were developed to address the shortcomings of CDT, namely prolonged infusion times and bleeding complications. Although CDT may take 24 to 72 hours to restore vessel patency, the aim of PMT is to resolve the occlusion and restore patency during the index procedure, thereby reducing the need for multiple procedures required for successful thrombolysis, decreasing the amount of tPA required, and reducing the need for ICU admissions. The ability to rapidly restore perfusion also allows for its potential utilization in more severe cases of ischemia.

Under ideal circumstances, PMT expeditiously reduces overall clot burden and can increase the surface area of exposed clot to enable more effective pharmacologic lysis. Numerous devices have been designed to use suction, rotational infusion, ultrasound, or a high-velocity rheolytic jet to achieve mechanical thrombectomy. Pharmacomechanical thrombolysis combines thrombolytic therapy with mechanical thrombectomy. The percutaneous device is used to first lace the thrombus with a bolus of thrombolytic agent, after which mechanical thrombectomy is performed. The AngioJet Thrombectomy System (Boston Scientific, Marlborough, MA, USA) is one such device, which works on the premise of Bernoulli's principle. Circumferentially oriented pressurized saline jets fragment the thrombus with creation of a low-pressure zone, facilitating the removal of the resultant thrombotic debris through catheter side holes.

Outcomes of PMT for ALI have demonstrated acceptable limb salvage and survival rates. In the PEARL (Peripheral Use of AngioJet Rheolytic Thrombectomy) multicenter registry, successful outcome, as defined as completion of the procedure without need for revascularization, bypass, or amputation and absence of substantial or complete occlusion in any vessel, was achieved in

83% of ALI patients with use of the AngioJet device. More than half of the patients (52%) did not require adjunctive CDT, and 1-year amputation-free survival and overall survival were 81% and 91%, respectively. Location of the occlusion was found to be significant, as patients with infrapopliteal artery involvement demonstrated worse outcomes with a 1-year amputation-free survival of 69%, as compared with 87% in patients without infrapopliteal involvement [12].

AngioJet pharmacomechanical thrombolysis, combined with thrombus maceration with balloon angioplasty, followed by stenting for refractory stenosis ($\geq$30%) is described by Ascher and colleagues [13] as a "fast-track thrombolysis protocol." This technique resulted in satisfactory thrombolysis with widely patent arterial inflow and outflow at discharge in 81% of patients with a median postoperative length of stay (LOS) of 1 day (mean LOS, 3.1 $\pm$ 4.5 days).

In comparing PMT with CDT, a single-center retrospective review by de Athayde Soares and colleagues [14] reported similar limb salvage (87.8% vs 89.7%), overall survival (84.7% vs 69.2%), and secondary patency (81.9% vs 78.8%) rates at 1.9 years, but higher 30-day mortality in the CDT group. In addition, it was observed that within the pharmacomechanical thrombectomy group, patients with longer duration of mechanical thrombolysis with AngioJet (>150 cycles per second) had higher rates of hematuria, myoglobinuria, acute renal failure, and death. Previous studies have also shown that use of Angiojet is an independent risk factor for acute kidney injury, related to the resulting red blood cell hemolysis [15].

With the widespread adoption of various PMT devices, several studies have compared more contemporary endovascular techniques with surgical revascularization in ALI. Higher rates of mortality, postoperative complications, and amputation were reported by Taha and colleagues [16] in patients undergoing open surgery for ALI, but in the subgroup of patients with Rutherford II ALI, amputation rates were comparable between the endovascular and open repair groups at 30 days (7% vs 10%) and 1 year (13% vs 16%). When stratified by cause of ischemia, a trend toward improved limb salvage with an endovascular approach was observed in patients with a failed stent or native artery thrombosis. A meta-analysis published in 2020 by Veenstra and colleagues [17] included 4689 patients across 25 studies and concluded that catheter-driven thrombolysis techniques had comparable limb salvage rates to open surgery albeit with higher risk of hemorrhagic complications. However, conclusions regarding the use of a hybrid approach or comparisons between various endovascular techniques could not be made.

Aspiration mechanical thrombectomy is another endovascular technique for thrombus removal and can be used in patients with a contraindication to thrombolytic medication. This technology, available in the United States since 2008 for cerebral revascularization in acute ischemic stroke, uses a catheter delivered to the site of occlusion, through which continuous vacuum suction is applied to extract the thrombus. Two single-center retrospective studies using the Indigo aspiration catheter (Penumbra Inc, Alameda, CA, USA) in

ALI demonstrated 51% to 53.3% technical success rates, without the need to initiate CDT or proceed with open surgery [18,19].

Open surgical revascularization

Open surgical techniques have long been the mainstay of management of ALI, especially in patients with an immediately threatened limb (Rutherford IIb) owing to the critical importance of the time to revascularization. Open surgery has also been preferred in patients with a contraindication to fibrinolytic therapy. Newer advances in endovascular techniques, however, allow for rapid reperfusion of the ischemic extremity and can be achieved without the use of lytic medications.

The anatomic location and the cause of the ALI are important in determining the most appropriate revascularization strategy. In cases of ALI owing to an embolic cause, especially if lodged within the proximal limb or above the inguinal ligament, an open approach has been advocated [20,21]. The balloon embolectomy catheter, introduced by Thomas J. Fogarty and colleagues in 1963, remains the primary open surgical technique in the treatment of acute peripheral arterial embolism. The Fogarty embolectomy catheter allows for thromboembolic material to be extracted distal and proximal to the arteriotomy site and is most effective when used in larger, nondiseased vessels. Embolectomy has decreased success in the smaller tibial vessels, as well as in the presence of atherosclerotic disease and risks iatrogenic vessel injury; thus, in these cases an endovascular approach should be considered [22]. Upper-extremity ALI, which is most often embolic in cause, is commonly managed with an open approach owing to relatively nondiseased vessels, ease, and speed to reperfusion with few complications (Fig. 4).

Ideally, open surgical cases are performed in a hybrid operating room, which allows for use of angiography and adjunctive endovascular techniques. Completion angiography after thromboembolectomy has been recommended to evaluate for incomplete restoration of perfusion, residual thrombus, distal embolization, iatrogenic vessel injury, and underlying steno-occlusive lesions [23,24]. de Donato and colleagues [25] advocate for a hybrid approach in which endovascular techniques of angioplasty, stenting, thrombolysis, and mechanical thrombectomy are used to treat any residual lesions identified on selective completion angiogram after open thromboembolectomy. With this hybrid technique, primary patency was reported to be 87.1% at 5 years, as compared with 66.3% with thromboembolectomy alone, and freedom from reintervention was 89% at 5 years, as compared with 74%.

In the setting of acute-on-chronic limb-threatening ischemia, bypass may be preferable in patients with more extensive atherosclerotic disease burden, particularly patients with a life expectancy beyond 2 years. Native artery occlusions treated with surgical revascularization in the STILE trial were found to have more durable long-term outcomes than CDT, notably in patients with femoral-popliteal occlusions, diabetes, or critical ischemia, with lower rates of recurrent ischemia (35% vs 64%) and amputation (0% vs 10%) at 1 year

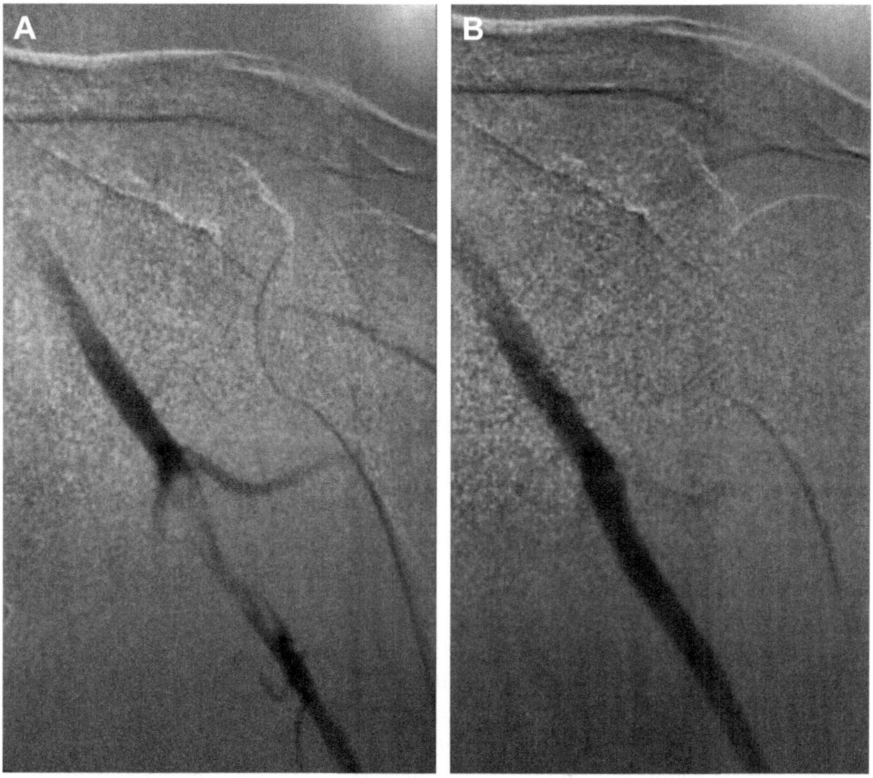

Fig. 4. Axillary artery embolus resulting in upper-extremity ALI (*A*) and postembolectomy completion angiogram (*B*). (Image courtesy of KC Zamor.)

[26]. In addition, the post hoc analysis of the BASIL (Bypass vs Angioplasty in Severe Ischaemia of the Leg) trial demonstrated reduced risk of future amputation and death in patients alive with their leg intact at 2 years who were randomized to the surgery-first group to treat critical limb ischemia [27]. However, the applicability of these trials is limited given more contemporary endovascular practices. The BEST-CLI trial will provide more information on durability of revascularization strategy in patients with critical limb ischemia from PAD [28].

Outcomes after infrainguinal bypass performed in the setting of ALI as compared with other indications for lower-extremity bypass were examined by Baril and colleagues [29] using Vascular Study Group of New England data. Of the 5712 lower-extremity bypass procedures included, 5.7% was performed for ALI. Patients undergoing bypass for ALI more commonly had a history of prior ipsilateral endovascular or open revascularization procedures, longer operative times with higher blood loss, greater use of prosthetic conduit, and increased in-hospital major adverse events. Graft patency rates were equivalent between groups, but higher rates of major amputation (22.4% vs 9.7%) and mortality (20.9% vs 13.1%) at 1 year occurred in ALI patients. On multivariable analysis, ALI was demonstrated to be an independent predictor of major amputation and mortality.

Predictors of amputation

Prior studies have examined factors predictive of amputation in patients presenting with ALI with varied results, but most commonly amputation has been associated with severe ischemia. A retrospective review of ALI patients treated at Harborview Medical Center identified multiple attempts at limb salvage, higher Rutherford class, multilevel occlusion, more proximal levels of occlusion, and necrotic muscle at the time of fasciotomy as predictive of limb loss [30]. Genovese and colleagues [31] found advanced ischemia (Rutherford IIb), thrombosed bypass, and failure of initial revascularization procedure to be associated with an increased risk of amputation. In the US Medicare population, predictors of amputation included advanced age, male gender, black race, diabetes, and history of PAD [2].

SPECIAL CONSIDERATIONS

Occluded lower-extremity bypass grafts

Comerota and colleagues [32] examined the subset of patients with ALI from the STILE trial with bypass graft occlusions. Patients with occluded grafts for greater than 14 days had better outcomes with surgical management, with a new bypass reported to be the most successful strategy. Among patients with occlusion less than 14 days in duration, successful CDT decreased limb loss at 1 year compared with surgical patients (20% vs 48%) and reduced the magnitude of the planned surgical procedure. Following successful lysis, an underlying critical lesion was revealed in 81% of grafts, highlighting a role for thrombolysis in determining a culprit lesion in cases of thrombotic occlusion. In comparing autogenous and prosthetic grafts, patients with occluded prosthetic grafts experienced more major morbidity, but once patency was restored with thrombolysis or surgery, both groups had similar 1-year patency rates. In addition, it was noted that 50% of grafts initially opened with thrombolysis were occluded at 1 year. Similar rates of amputation among patients undergoing thrombolysis for bypass graft occlusion less than 30 days were reported by Koraen and colleagues [33] with 75% 1-year amputation-free survival. Independent risk factors for major amputation were technical failure, increased age, and use of synthetic conduit.

These studies support the use of thrombolysis in acute bypass graft occlusion, particularly vein bypasses, which were observed to have more benefit. However, CDT was the primary method of endovascular treatment, with PMT only used as an adjunct in a limited number of patients. The study by Taha and colleagues [16], which included both CDT and PMT, reported higher technical success with open surgical repair for thrombosed bypass grafts, but similar rates of amputation at 1 year (23% vs 23%). In this study, 75% of the bypasses was prosthetic, possibly suggesting that open surgical revascularization may be the preferred option for failed prosthetic grafts. Further studies evaluating the efficacy of newer pharmacomechanical thrombectomy techniques in the management of occluded lower-extremity autogenous and prosthetic bypass grafts are needed.

Popliteal artery aneurysms

Popliteal artery aneurysms are the most common peripheral arterial aneurysm (>70%), yet are rare in the general population, occurring with a reported incidence of 7.4 per 100,000 men and 1.0 per 100,000 women [34]. Acute ischemia can result from emboli to the tibial vessels with or without thrombosis of the aneurysm (Fig. 5). ALI in this situation commonly results from occlusion of all major outflow vessels below the knee and is associated with a 14% early amputation rate [35].

In 2021, the Society for Vascular Surgery issued clinical practice guidelines on the management of popliteal artery aneurysms. In the absence of immediate limb threat, thrombolysis or pharmacomechanical interventions are recommended in patients with Rutherford I and IIa ALI to restore patency of the tibial outflow vessels in advance of endovascular or open repair. In cases of isolated aneurysm thrombosis and patent inflow and outflow vessels, there is no

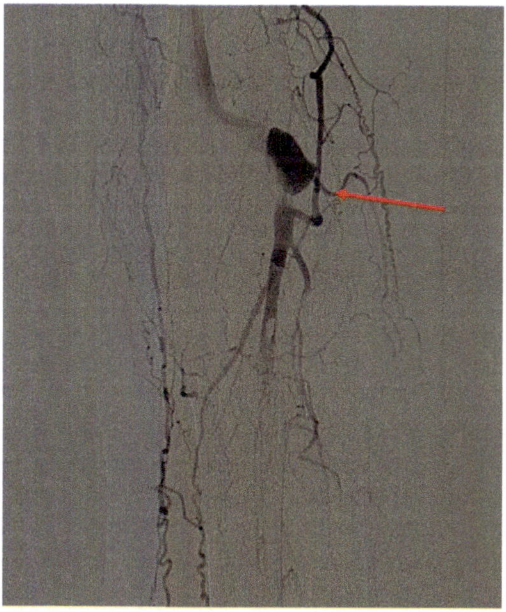

Fig. 5. Embolic obliteration of all tibial outflow vessels secondary to a popliteal artery aneurysm (*arrow*).

indication for lysis before definitive repair [36]. Immediate revascularization with open surgical bypass or endovascular aneurysm exclusion is recommended in patients with severe limb ischemia (Rutherford IIb), as the additional time required to allow for CDT cannot be tolerated. However, mechanical or aspiration thrombectomy may be used as adjuncts to clear distal runoff vessels [37].

Irreversible ischemia

Patients who present with complete loss of motor and sensory function, inaudible arterial and venous Doppler signals, and presence of livedo reticularis have irreversible ischemia (Rutherford III). Revascularization may cause life-threatening physiologic changes owing to reperfusion with little chance of functional limb salvage. A primary amputation in this setting is preferable to avoid multiple organ failure and death [38]. Depending on the level of occlusion, revascularization to allow for a more distal amputation or to improve wound healing potential postamputation may be considered.

POSTOPERATIVE MANAGEMENT

Despite successful revascularization, limb loss may occur from development of acute compartment syndrome, as previously ischemic tissue swells within the confined fascial space of the calf or forearm. The more severe the ischemia, the more likely a reperfusion compartment syndrome is to develop. In patients with a history of prolonged ischemia (>6 hours) and those with limb edema observed after reperfusion, prophylactic fasciotomies are recommended [39]. Patients who have not undergone fasciotomy are followed closely with serial examinations, and compartment syndrome is suspected in those who develop a tense swollen extremity with pain on passive motion, weakness, or decreased sensation. In sedated, neurologically impaired, or uncooperative patients who cannot be followed with serial examinations, direct compartment pressures can be measured. Fasciotomy should be performed if compartment pressures are elevated (>30 mm Hg), if the difference between the diastolic pressure and compartment pressure is less than 10 mm Hg, or if there is high clinical suspicion despite normal compartment pressures. Delay in diagnosis and management of compartment syndrome has devastating consequences and can lead to both limb loss and mortality.

Hemodynamic monitoring, routine laboratory analysis with correction of acidosis and electrolyte imbalance resulting from intracellular potassium leak and hydrogen ion release, and serial neurovascular examinations are necessary. Rhabdomyolysis, a systemic effect of muscle ischemia, can cause acute tubular necrosis and renal failure. Aggressive resuscitation with intravenous fluids is the main treatment modality. Urine alkalinization with bicarbonate may also be required in patients with significant tissue damage and increasing creatine phosphokinase.

The need for continued postoperative antithrombotic therapy is dependent on the cause of the acute ischemic event. Patients with an embolic source are anticoagulated with heparin and converted to warfarin or a direct oral anticoagulant, as the risk of recurrent peripheral arterial embolism approaches 30%. Patients are maintained on lifelong anticoagulation in the setting of cardiogenic embolism and in cases when the source of embolism is not surgically correctable or cannot be identified. Anticoagulation is also recommended in acute thrombosis of a native artery associated with a hypercoagulable state.

In cases of thrombosis resulting from an atherosclerotic plaque or occluded bypass, and for embolic events resulting from a thrombosed aneurysm, long-term antiplatelet therapy is recommended to preserve patency after repair [7]. The addition of low-dose rivaroxaban may also be considered. The Vascular Outcomes Study of ASA (acetylsalicylic acid) Along with Rivaroxaban in Endovascular or Surgical Limb Revascularization for PAD (VOYAGER PAD) trial found that low-dose rivaroxaban (2.5 mg twice a day) reduced the risk of ALI by 33% (absolute risk reduction 2.6% at 3 years) in patients undergoing lower-extremity revascularization for symptomatic PAD when compared with placebo [40]. In addition, a meta-analysis of pooled data from both the COMPASS (Cardiovascular Outcomes for People Using Anticoagulation Strategies) and VOYAGER trials found low-dose rivaroxaban plus aspirin to be superior to aspirin alone in reducing adverse cardiovascular outcomes, acute limb ischemia, and major amputation in patients with PAD. The 32% reduction (hazard ratio: 0.68) in major adverse limb events comes with an absolute risk increase of 0.6% per year of major bleeding events, but not significantly higher rates of fatal or critical organ bleeding [41].

SUMMARY

ALI is a vascular emergency associated with high rates of limb loss and mortality. Expeditious diagnosis, anticoagulation, and revascularization are of utmost importance in reducing morbidity. Management of these patients is challenging given the severe systemic illness resulting from tissue ischemia and the high incidence of preexisting comorbid conditions and underlying PAD. Approach to revascularization depends on the severity of ischemia, location of occlusion, underlying cause, chance of recovery, procedural risks, comorbidities, and access to operating rooms or angiography suites.

Open surgical approaches have historically been used to address immediately threatened limbs (Rutherford IIb) or in patients with contraindications to thrombolysis. The development of rheolytic, mechanical, and aspiration thrombectomy techniques, however, allows for rapid endovascular revascularization, allowing for application in more severe cases of ischemia, and can be performed with or without the use of lytic medications. Open embolectomy is best used to address embolic causes of ALI occurring in larger, nondiseased vessels, and ALI of the upper extremity. In the setting of severe multilevel atherosclerotic disease, open surgical bypass may be indicated in the presence of a distal target.

Endovascular techniques are selected in thrombotic occlusions of atherosclerotic native vessels, bypass grafts, or stents in patients with a marginally threatened limb (Rutherford IIa). CDT frequently results in exposure of an underlying culprit lesion that can be managed with angioplasty or stenting. CDT may also be more effective in establishing reperfusion of smaller distal vessels, or in the case of occluded tibial runoff in the setting of a popliteal artery aneurysm. More contemporary endovascular techniques, including pharmacomechanical thrombectomy, wwhicl h hich which allow for revascularization during the index procedure, have an increasing role in the management of ALI and have demonstrated acceptable limb salvage and survival rates when compared with open surgery.

In patients with irreversible ischemia (Rutherford III), primary amputation is commonly performed to mitigate the life-threatening physiologic changes that can occur with revascularization of severely ischemic tissue in an extremity with little chance of functional limb salvage.

Once the acute ischemic episode and its sequelae have been managed, the underlying cause should be further investigated and treated. Depending on the cause and revascularization strategy, long-term anticoagulation or antithrombotic therapy may be indicated.

CLINICS CARE POINTS

- In the absence of contraindications, therapeutic anticoagulation should be initiated as the initial step in the management of acute limb ischemia.
- History and physical examination findings are critical to determine duration, severity, level of occlusion, and possible cause.
- Open embolectomy is best used to address embolic causes of acute limb ischemia occurring in larger, nondiseased vessels and acute limb ischemia of the upper extremity.
- Consider the use of endovascular interventions, including catheter-directed thrombolysis and pharmacomechanical thrombectomy, in patients with thrombotic occlusions of atherosclerotic vessels, bypass grafts, or stents in patients with a marginally threatened limb (Rutherford IIa).
- Four-compartment fasciotomies should be performed in patients with prolonged ischemia (>6 hours), limb edema after reperfusion, or elevated compartment pressures (>30 mm Hg).

Disclosure

The authors have nothing to disclose.

References

[1] Gilliland C, Shah J, Martin JG, et al. Acute limb ischemia. Tech Vasc Interv Radiol 2017;20(4):274–80.
[2] Baril DT, Ghosh K, Rosen AB. Trends in the incidence, treatment, and outcomes of acute lower extremity ischemia in the United States Medicare population. J Vasc Surg 2014;60(3):669–77.e2.

[3] Wang JC, Kim AH, Kashyap VS. Open surgical or endovascular revascularization for acute limb ischemia. J Vasc Surg 2016;63(1):270–8.
[4] Eyers P, Earnshaw JJ. Acute non-traumatic arm ischaemia. Br J Surg 1998;85(10):1340–6.
[5] Howard DP, Banerjee A, Fairhead JF, et al. Population-based study of incidence, risk factors, outcome, and prognosis of ischemia peripheral arterial events: implications for prevention. Circulation 2015;132:1805–15.
[6] O'Connell JB, Quinones-Baldrich WJ. Proper evaluation and management of acute embolic versus thrombotic limb ischemia. Semin Vasc Surg 2009;22(1):10–6.
[7] Creager MA, Kaufman JA, Conte MS. Acute limb ischemia. N Engl J Med 2012;366(23):2198–206.
[8] Berridge DC, Kessel DO, Robertson I. Surgery versus thrombolysis for initial management of acute limb ischemia. Cochrane Database Syst Rev 2013;(6):CD002784.
[9] Ebben HP, Jongkind V, Wisselink W, et al. Catheter directed thrombolysis protocols for peripheral arterial occlusions: a systematic review. Eur J Endovasc Surg 2019;57(5):667–75.
[10] Ebben HP, Nederhoed JH, Lely RJ. Low-dose thrombolytics for thromboembolic lower extremity arterial occlusions is effective without major hemorrhagic complications. Eur J Vasc Endovasc Surg 2014;48(5):551–8.
[11] de Athayde Soares R, Matielo MF, Brochado Neto FC, et al. Analysis of the results of endovascular and open surgical treatment of acute limb ischemia. J Vasc Surg 2019;69(3):843–9.
[12] Leung DA, Blitz LR, Nelson T, et al. Rheolytic pharmacomechanical thrombectomy for the management of acute limb ischemia: results from the PEARL registry. J Endovasc Ther 2015;22(4):546–57.
[13] Ascher E, Kibrik P, Rizvi SA, et al. Fast-track thrombolysis protocol for acute limb ischemia. J Vasc Surg 2021;73(3):950–9.
[14] de Athayde Soares R, Matielo MF, Brochado Neto FC, et al. Analysis of the safety and efficacy of the endovascular treatment for acute limb ischemia with percutaneous pharmacomechanical thrombectomy compared with catheter-directed thrombolysis. Ann Vasc Surg 2020;66:470–8.
[15] Escobar GA, Burks D, Abarte MR, et al. Risk of acute kidney injury after percutaneous pharmacomechanical thrombectomy using AngioJet in venous and arterial thrombosis. Ann Vasc Surg 2017;42:238–45.
[16] Taha AG, Byrne RM, Avgerinos ED, et al. Comparative effectiveness of endovascular versus surgical revascularization for acute lower extremity ischemia. J Vasc Surg J Vasc Surg 2015;61(1):147–54.
[17] Veenstra EB, van der Laan MJ, Zeebregts CJ, et al. A systematic review and meta-analysis of endovascular and surgical revascularization techniques in acute limb ischemia. J Vasc Surg 2020;71(2):654–68.
[18] Lopez R, Yamashita TS, Neisen M, et al. Single-center experience with Indigo aspiration thrombectomy for acute lower limb ischemia. J Vasc Surg 2020;72(1):226–32.
[19] Kwok CH, Fleming S, Chan KK, et al. Aspiration thrombectomy versus conventional catheter-directed thrombolysis as first-line treatment for noniatrogenic acute lower limb ischemia. J Vasc Interv Radiol 2018;29(5):607–13.
[20] McNally MM, Univers J. Acute limb ischemia. Surg Clin North Am 2018;98(5):1081–96.
[21] Norgren L, Hiatt WR, Dormandy JA, et al. Inter-society consensus for the management of peripheral arterial disease (TASC II). J Vasc Surg 2007;45(Suppl S):S5–67.
[22] de Donato G, Pasqui E, Setacci F, et al. Acute on chronic limb ischemia: from surgical embolectomy and thrombolysis to endovascular options. Semin Vasc Surg 2018;31(2-4):66–75.
[23] Lipsitz EC, Veith FJ, Wain RA. Digital fluoroscopy as a valuable adjunct to open vascular operations. Semin Vasc Surg 2003;16:280–90.
[24] Parsons RE, Marin ML, Veith FJ, et al. Fluoroscopically assisted thromboembolectomy: an improved method for treating acute arterial occlusions. Ann Vasc Surg 1996;10:201–10.

[25] de Donato G, Setacci F, Sirignano P, et al. The combination of surgical embolectomy and endovascular techniques may improve outcomes of patients with acute lower limb ischemia. J Vasc Surg 2014;59(3):729–36.
[26] Weaver FA, Comerota AJ, Youngblood M, et al. Surgical revascularization versus thrombolysis for nonembolic lower extremity native artery occlusions: results of a prospective randomized trial. The STILE Investigators. J Vasc Surg 1996;24(4):513–21.
[27] Adam DJ, Beard JD, Cleveland T, et al. Bypass versus angioplasty in severe ischemia of the leg (BASIL): multicentre, randomized controlled trial. Lancet 2005;366(9501):1925–34.
[28] Menard MT, Farber A, Assmann SF, et al. Design and rationale of the best endovascular versus best surgical therapy for patients with critical limb ischemia (BEST-CLI) trial. J Am Heart Assoc 2016;5(7):e003219.
[29] Baril DT, Patel VI, Judelson DR, et al. Outcomes of lower extremity bypass for acute limb ischemia. J Vasc Surg 2013;58(4):949–56.
[30] Hemingway J, Emanuels D, Aarabi S, et al. Safety of transfer, type of procedure, and factors predictive of limb salvage in modern series of acute limb ischemia. J Vasc Surg 2019;69(4): 1174–9.
[31] Genovese EA, Chaer RA, Taha AG, et al. Risk factors for long-term mortality and amputation after open and endovascular treatment of acute limb ischemia. Ann Vasc Surg 2016;30: 82–92.
[32] Comerota AJ, Weaver FA, Hosking JD, et al. Results of a prospective, randomized trial of surgery versus thrombolysis for occluded lower extremity bypass grafts. Am J Surg 1996;172(2):105–12.
[33] Koraen L, Kuoppala M, Acosta S, et al. Thrombolysis for lower extremity bypass graft occlusion. J Vasc Surg 2001;54(5):1339–44.
[34] Jacobowitz G, Cayne NS. Lower extremity aneurysms. In: Cronenwett JL, Johnston KW, editors. Rutherford's vascular surgery. 8th edition. Philadelphia: Elsevier Saunders; 2014. p. 2190–205.
[35] Kropman RH, Schrijver AM, Keldar JC, et al. Clinical outcome of acute leg ischemia due to thrombosed popliteal artery aneurysm: systematic review of 895 cases. Eur J Vasc Endovasc Surg 2010;39:452–7.
[36] Pulli R, Dorigo W, Castelli, et al. A multicentric experience with open surgical repair and endovascular exclusion of popliteal artery aneurysms. Eur J Vasc Endovasc Surg 2013;45:357–63.
[37] Farber A, Angle N, Avgerinos E, et al. The Society for Vascular Surgery clinical practice guidelines on popliteal artery aneurysms. J Vasc Surg 2021;S0741-5214(21):00680–7.
[38] Jaffery Z, Thornton SN, White CJ. Acute limb ischemia. Am J Med Sci 2001;342(3): 226–34.
[39] Brooks JD, Shames ML. Acute limb ischemia. In: Cronenwett JL, Farber A, Mitchell EL, editors. Vascular decision making: medical, endovascular, surgical. Philadelphia: Wolters Kluwer; 2021. p. 310–4.
[40] Hess CN, Debus ES, Nehler MR, et al. Reduction in acute limb ischemia with rivaroxaban versus placebo in peripheral artery disease after lower extremity revascularization: insights from VOYAGER PAD. Circulation 2021;144(23):1831–41.
[41] Anand SS, Hiatt W, Dyal L, et al. Low-dose rivaroxaban and aspirin among patients with peripheral artery disease: a meta-analysis of the COMPASS and VOYAGER trials. Eur J Prev Cardiol 2021 zwab128.

Advances in Surgery 56 (2022) 305–319

ADVANCES IN SURGERY

Endovascular Repair of Complex Aortic Aneurysms

Guilherme B.B. Lima, MD, Marina Dias-Neto, MD, MSc, PhD, Emanuel R. Tenorio, MD, PhD, Aidin Baghbani-Oskouei, MD, Gustavo S. Oderich, MD*

McGovern Medical School, The University of Texas Health Science Center at Houston, Houston, 6400 Fannin Street, Suite 2850, Houston, TX 77030, USA

Keywords

• Complex aortic aneurysms • Complex abdominal aortic aneurysm (CAAA)
• Thoracoabdominal aortic aneurysms (TAAA) • Endovascular aortic repair
• Fenestrated-branched endovascular repair
• Fenestrated-branched endovascular aortic repair (FB-EVAR)

Key points

- Fenestrated-branched endovascular aortic repair evolved from an alternative to treat elderly and higher risk patients to the first line of treatment in most patients with suitable anatomy, independent of the clinical risk.
- Anatomic feasibility requires adequate landing zones, target vessels, and iliofemoral access.
- Open surgical repair is an alternative in good risk patients who are not well suited for endovascular approach and patients with genetically triggered aortic diseases.

Abbreviations

SMA	Superior mesenteric artery
LIMA	Left internal mammary artery

*Corresponding author. 6400 Fannin Street Suite 2850, Houston, TX 77030. *E-mail addresses:* guilherme.lima@uth.tmc.edu (G.B.B.L.); Marina.D.Neto@uth.tmc.edu (M.D.-N.); Emanuel.J.RamosTenorio@uth.tmc.edu (E.R.T.); Aidin.Baghbanioskouei@uth.tmc.edu (A.B.-O.); gustavo.oderich@uth.tmc.edu (G.S.O.)

https://doi.org/10.1016/j.yasu.2022.04.002
0065-3411/22/

INTRODUCTION

Aortic aneurysms most often affect the abdominal aorta, with an estimated prevalence of 1.4% among people aged between 50 and 84 years [1]. Prospective randomized studies confirmed several short-term advantages for endovascular aortic repair (EVAR) compared with open surgery, including decreased mortality, morbidity, and shorter hospital stay. However, the survival advantage diminishes during follow-up, and after 2 years, it is similar in patients treated by both techniques [2]. The presence of a segment of normal aorta with a minimum length of 10 mm below the renal arteries is a prerequisite for standard EVAR. Among patients who have shorter sealing zones or involvement of the renal and mesenteric vessels, techniques of endovascular incorporation are indicated. In the last 2 decades, these techniques have evolved from initial attempts to perform extra-anatomic reconstructions coupled with endovascular exclusion of the aneurysm (eg, hybrid repair or debranching) to total endovascular incorporation using parallel fenestrated and branched stent-grafts.

Greenberg and colleagues first described parallel stent-grafts in 2003 to extend the proximal landing zone in patients with short neck infrarenal aneurysms [3]. Indications for the technique were expanded to include arch, thoracoabdominal, and aortoiliac aneurysms, and several terms were coined to describe different configurations, including snorkel, chimney, periscope, sandwich, and octopus grafts [4–10]. A limitation of these techniques is the risk of gutter endoleaks, which is higher with greater than 2 parallel grafts and in patients with a total absence of sealing zones. Therefore, the technique is reserved for urgent cases or patients who are not suitable for fenestrated and branched stent grafts [11].

Fenestrated-branched endovascular aortic repair (FB-EVAR) has gained widespread acceptance as an alternative to open surgical repair in patients with complex aortic aneurysms [12–14]. The first report using physician modified endografts (PMEGs) was by Park and colleagues in 1996 [15]. Subsequently, manufactured fenestrated stent-grafts were developed in Western Australia by Hartley and Lawrence-Brown, with the first implant by John Anderson in 1998. The technique evolved with reinforced fenestrations, diameter reducing ties preloaded systems. Devices with directional branches or cuffs were pioneered by Chuter and colleagues in 2001, leading to the development of off-the-shelf multibranched stent-grafts for the repair of thoracoabdominal aortic aneurysms (TAAAs). Currently, these devices are tailored to the patient anatomy with the options of fenestrated, branched and mixed fenestrated, and branched designs. Reports from single and multicenter experiences and systematic reviews have shown lower mortality and morbidity for FB-EVAR compared with historical results of open surgical repair [12–14,16–21]. The main advantages are noted on mortality, respiratory complications, acute kidney injury, and length of stay. The last clinical practice guidelines from the European Society for Vascular Surgery recommended FB-EVAR as the first line of treatment of patients with complex abdominal aortic aneurysms (CAAAs)

[11]. This article focuses on the latest developments in FB-EVAR techniques and outcomes.

INDICATIONS

The term complex aortic aneurysms is defined an aneurysm that involves major aortic side branches, thereby requiring more extensive open surgical reconstruction or endovascular incorporation. CAAAs and TAAAs involve the renal and mesenteric arteries (Fig. 1). Most patients are asymptomatic and diagnosed incidentally using duplex ultrasound or abdominal imaging. The Society of Vascular Surgery clinical practice guidelines recommend screening with a duplex ultrasound men with a history of tobacco use and aged 65 to 75 years (strong level of recommendation and high quality of evidence) [22].

The aneurysm diameter is the most important determinant of the risk of rupture. The estimated annual risk of rupture is 10% for aneurysms greater than 6 cm, 30% for aneurysms greater than 7 cm, and 50% for aneurysms greater than 8 cm [23,24]. Treatment is recommended in patients with aneurysms 5.5 cm or greater and a life expectancy of at least 2 years. Size threshold is often increased to 6 cm or greater for patients with TAAAs because of the risk of disabling complications such as paralysis or dialysis. Rapid aneurysm enlargement, defined 5 mm or greater in 6 months, is also an indication for

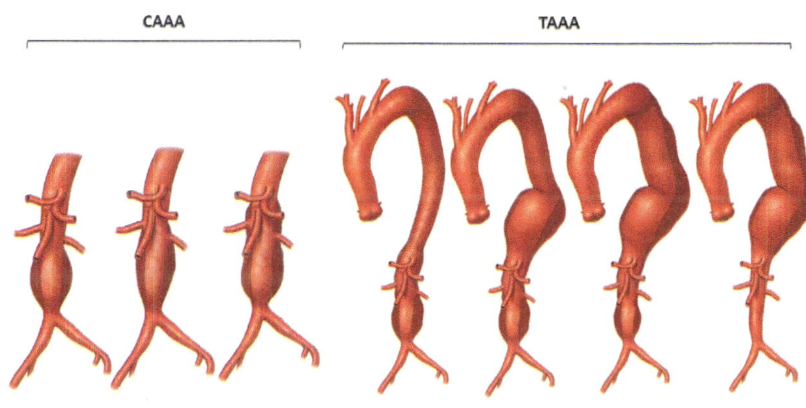

Fig. 1. Classification of CAAAs and TAAAs. Juxta-renal aortic aneurysm: 0 to 4 mm infrarenal neck, pararenal: affect at least one renal artery and extend up to superior mesenteric artery, and paravisceral: affects the renal arteries and the SMA but extend not beyond the celiac axis. *Extent IV* TAAA has extension to the level of the diaphragmatic hiatus with involvement of the celiac axis, SMA, and renal arteries but not into the descending thoracic aorta; *extent III* TAAA starts below T6 and extends to renal arteries; *extent II* TAAA starts above T6 and extends below the level of the renal arteries often to the aortic bifurcation; and *extent I* TAAA involves descending thoracic aorta from above T6 (often up to the left subclavian artery) to the level of the renal arteries. (Reproduced by permission of University of Texas Health Science at Houston for Medical Education and Research. All rights reserved.)

repair. Aneurysms with saccular morphology may have a higher risk of rupture, although this is ill defined [22,25]. Patients with symptoms, including pain, distal embolization (eg, "blue toe syndrome"), and those with ruptured aneurysms should be treated irrespective of the diameter. The use of a fixed diameter is not adequate for all patients. It is recommended to use body surface area to define the optimal threshold for repair, which is lower in women and individuals of shorter stature [26,27]. Finally, the decision to proceed with repair should balance the risk of rupture with the operative risk, which depends on the analysis of results at the institution and clinical risk assessment.

PREOPERATIVE EVALUATION

Preoperative evaluation is individualized based on cardiovascular risk factors. In general, cardiac, pulmonary, renal, and overall clinical status are assessed with physical examination and ancillary tests such as cardiac stress test, laboratory studies, estimation of glomerular filtration rate (eGFR), and pulmonary function test. Patients should be medically optimized before elective repair [11]. Repair may be contraindicated in patients with prohibitively high clinical risk or those with short life expectancy because of advanced stages of pulmonary, cardiac, and renal diseases or malignancies. A medical genetics evaluation is considered in patients with family history, those who are younger than 50 years of age, or have phenotypic features. Genetically triggered aortic diseases (GenTADs) include Marfan syndrome, Turner syndrome, Vascular Ehlers-Danlos syndrome, and Loeys-Dietz syndrome, among others. Patients with GenTADs are treated by open surgical repair, with endovascular repair considered as an alternative in patients who failed prior open repair and developed anastomotic or patch aneurysms or are at high risk for open surgery.

ENDOVASCULAR REPAIR

Patient selection

A computed tomography angiography (CTA) of the chest, abdomen, and pelvis with 1 to2 mm cuts is the single most important study to provide a detailed anatomic assessment. It allows evaluation of cause, the extent of disease, involvement of renal and mesenteric arteries, and arterial access. The risk of contrast-induced nephrotoxicity has been overstated. The most recent consensus recommends prophylactic hydration of patients with an eGFR less than 30 mL/min/1.73 m^2 and for those with an eGFR 30 to 44 mL/min/1.73 m^2 and high-risk circumstances at the discretion of the ordering clinician [28].

The most important anatomic determinants for FB-EVAR are the presence of a proximal and distal landing zone, adequate iliofemoral access, and suitable renal and mesenteric target vessels. The proximal sealing zone should have a maximum diameter of 32 mm for the supraceliac aorta or 42-mm for the thoracic aorta with a minimum length of 25 mm, without thrombus or calcification. The requirements for suitable target vessels are 4 to 11 mm diameter with a minimum length to first branch bifurcation of more than 15 mm. The absence of a proper landing zone or the presence of small or narrow iliac arteries may indicate adjunctive open surgical procedures such as cervical debranching or iliac conduits [29]. Finally, excessive amount of atheromatous debris (shaggy aorta) throughout the aortic arch and thoracoabdominal segments may contraindicate endovascular repair due to high risk of embolization.

Device design

Analysis of the CTA using centerline of flow is performed to determine precise length measurements and the axial location of the target vessels. The minimum recommended effective sealing zone should be 25 mm in length with 360-degree fabric apposition to a normal aortic segment. Most patients have a minimum of 3 or 4 vessels incorporated with a device planned with supraceliac sealing zone, even if the aneurysm extends to the level of the renal arteries [29–32]. Distal sealing is planned in the iliac arteries or less frequently in the infrarenal aorta, when normal [33].

All patent renal and mesenteric arteries are incorporated using the options of scallop, reinforced fenestrations, or a directional branch. Double-wide scallops are typically 20 × 20 mm openings in the uppermost portion of the device and are typically designed to preserve flow into the celiac axis (CA), without the need for stent alignment. Double-wide scallops are usually used for fenestrated devices designed to treat short neck infrarenal or juxtarenal aneurysms but should not be considered part of the effective sealing zone, given that these do not provide 360-degree fabric apposition to the aortic wall. Fenestrations are small circular openings reinforced by a nitinol ring with options of 6 × 6 mm (small) or 8 × 8 mm (large) configurations. These are aligned by a balloon-expandable stent-graft to prevent shuttering with vessel thrombosis and endoleak. Fenestrations are ideally used when the target vessel has origin from a relatively normal aortic segment with a luminal diameter of 30 mm or less. A recent analysis of the distance from the fenestration to the aortic wall indicates that fenestration gaps of 5 mm or greater are associated with an increased risk of target vessel endoleak and instability [34]. Directional branches are presewn cuffs with options of 6 or 8 mm diameter and length of 18 to 22 mm. The branches can be internal or external and oriented caudally (antegrade) or cranially (retrograde). Directional branches are connected to the target vessel using flexible self-expandable or balloon-expandable stent-grafts. Directional branches are ideally suited for caudally oriented vessels with minimum inner aortic luminal diameter of 25 mm. Use of downgoing oriented directional branches for upgoing oriented target vessels may pose significant technical difficulty and result in lower patency rates. In some cases, the design may be compromised by using retrograde branches or a fenestration if the vessel is upgoing and has origin from a wider aortic segment. Fenestrations are planned to be positioned precisely in the middle of the origin of the target vessel, whereas directional branches should be positioned above or below the target depending on its configuration.

Advanced designs are available from several manufacturers (Fig. 2) with off-the-shelf and patient-specific stent-grafts options. Most of these devices are

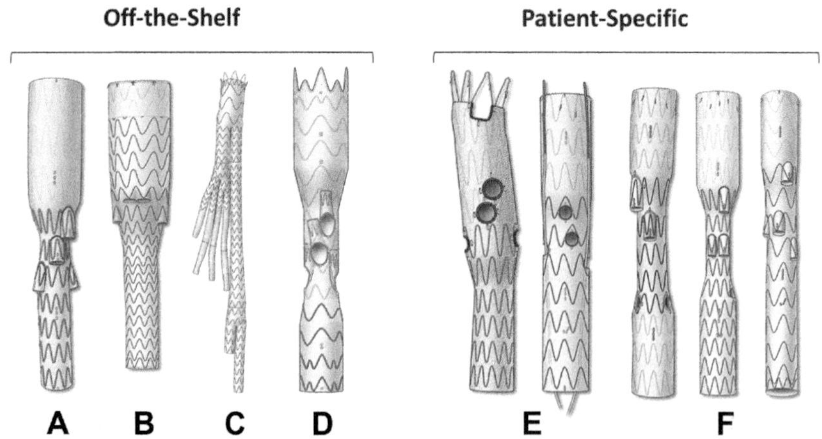

Fig. 2. Current off-the-shelf and patient-specific devices. Cook t-Branch (*A*), Gore TAMBE (*B*), Medtronic Valiant TAAA (*C*), E-nside TAAA Jotec (*D*), Zfen + Cook (*E*), and Patient-specific Cook platform (*F*). (Reproduced by permission of University of Texas Health Science at Houston for Medical Education and Research. All rights reserved.)

investigational in the United States and have access limited to a few centers. Cook Medical pioneered the manufacturing of fenestrated devices since the late 1990s. The Zenith Fenestrated AAA Endovascular Graft (ZFEN) system (William Cook Australia, Brisbane, AU) was the first to be approved for commercial use in the United States in 2012 but it is only applicable to treat short neck or juxtarenal aneurysms, which comprise one-third of all CAAAs [35]. Therefore, these devices are not ideally suited for aneurysms extending above the renal arteries, including TAAAs. To overcome the lack of device access in most centers, physicians often rely on the modification of manufactured devices (PMEGs).

The largest experience with FB-EVAR has been with cook-manufactured patient-specific fenestrated-branched stent-grafts with options of any combination of fenestrations or directional branches or off-the-shelf multibranched stent-grafts. Patient-specific devices have the option of lower profile fabric (18–20Fr sheath) and preloaded guidewire or catheter systems to facilitate access to fenestrations or directional branches. The Gore ThoracoAbdominal Multi-Branch Endoprosthesis (TAMBE, W.L. Gore & Associates Inc, Flagstaff, AZ) is currently undergoing clinical investigation on a Pivotal trial and will likely be the first commercially available 4-vessel device in the United States.

Arterial access

Total percutaneous femoral access is used whenever possible, except in patients with excessively calcified femoral arteries, high femoral artery bifurcation, or prosthetic grafts. The technique of preclosure using 2 percutaneous monofilament sutures has been widely applied. In patients with small or diseased iliac arteries, a permanent or temporary surgical conduit, or an endovascular conduit, is considered to avoid the risk of accidental arterial rupture, which is associated with increased risk of mortality and spinal cord injury (SCI) from sustained hypotension [36–39].

Upper extremity (UE) arterial access via the proximal brachial or distal axillary artery was widely used to facilitate catheterization of target vessels during FB-EVAR [40]. In these cases, we recommend open surgical exposure with primary repair using a small incision in the right axilla, although several centers also use a percutaneous approach for the axillary artery. The recent development of steerable sheaths has allowed the advancement of stents from femoral access and decreased the need to use UE approach. Currently, our preference is to use a total transfemoral approach with steerable sheaths whenever possible, reserving UE for difficult cases or when femoral approach is not possible.

Implantation technique

FB-EVAR procedures are performed in a hybrid operating room with fixed imaging and advanced applications, including onlay fusion and high definition cone beam computed tomography (CBCT). General endotracheal anesthesia is used in most cases with intraoperative motor evoked and somatosensory evoked neuromonitoring in patients with 5 cm or greater supraceliac coverage of the thoracic aorta. Preoperative placement of cerebrospinal fluid drainage (CSFD) is no longer used for TAAAs with few exceptions because of high rates of drain-related complications [41,42].

The patient is positioned supine with upper extremities overhead to optimize imaging on lateral projections and rotational CBCT [43]. Percutaneous femoral access is obtained using ultrasound guidance with a 0.018-inch micropuncture set, which is exchanged for a 0.035-inch Benson wire and a 6Fr sheath. The access sites are preclosed using 2 Perclose ProGlide closure devices (Abbott Vascular, Santa Clara, CA) oriented at 1:30 and 10:30 o'clock positions. Once the arterial access is completed, the patient is systemically heparinized with 80 to 100 units/kg to achieve a target activated clotting time greater than 250 seconds. The preoperative CTA fusion model is registered using bi-view fluoroscopy bony landmarks. Bilateral femoral access is established using catheters and guidewires, which are advanced to the ascending aorta and exchanged for a stiff 0.035-inch Lunderquist wire (Cook Medical, Bloomington, IN). Final calibration of the onlay fusion is performed using limited angiography at the level of the renal arteries or selective catheterization of one of the target vessels with a LIMA guide catheter. It can be optimized by precatheterization of one of the renal arteries. Specific technical steps vary according to device design and are summarized below.

Patient-specific 3 or 4-vessel fenestrated stent-graft with preloaded system

The main aortic device is usually introduced via the right femoral approach and has preloaded wires for immediate access to the renal fenestrations. The device is oriented extracorporeally, introduced via the femoral approach and deployed with adequate apposition between the fenestrations and the target vessels. Onlay fusion and the precatheterization assist with proper deployment. The device remains constrained by the diameter-reducing ties, which allow some movement in case of misalignment of fenestrations. Hydrophilic 6Fr sheaths are advanced via the preloaded systems into the renal fenestrations. Using a Van Schie 3 catheter and glidewire, both renal arteries are sequentially catheterized, and a 0.035-inch Rosen wire is positioned in the distal main renal artery. The 6Fr 90-cm Flexor Shuttle sheaths (Cook Medical, Bloomington, IN) are advanced into the renal arteries, followed by positioning of the balloon-expandable stents. Using the contralateral femoral approach, the precatheterization guide catheter is removed from the target vessel and used for selective catheterization of the fenestrated aortic component. An 18Fr Dryseal sheath (WL Gore, Flagstaff, AZ) is advanced into the fenestrated component. Using the 18Fr sheath, the SMA (3-vessel) or CA and SMA (4-vessel) are sequentially catheterized using guide catheter and glidewire, which are exchanged for 0.035-inch Rosen wires. A 7Fr 55-cm hydrophilic Ansel sheath (Cook Medical, Bloomington, IN) or 7Fr 55-cm Destino steerable sheath (Oscor, FL) is sequentially advanced, followed by positioned of balloon expandable stent-grafts. Once all vessels are catheterized, the fenestrated component is completely deployed by removing the diameter reducing ties. The top portion of the delivery system is partially withdrawn to the infrarenal aorta. The renal arteries, CA and SMA bridging stent-grafts, are sequentially deployed and flared using a 10-mm angioplasty balloon. Selective angiographies of each vessel are performed using diluted contrast. The sheaths and wires are removed from the target vessels. Balloon angioplasty of the proximal landing zone is optional but should be performed before deployment of the bridging stents if indicated. A bifurcated universal device is introduced via the femoral approach and deployed inside the fenestrated component with a minimum of 2 stent overlap. The contralateral gate of the bifurcated graft is catheterized, and the repair is extended to the contralateral common iliac artery using an iliac limb extension (Fig. 3). A completional rotational digital subtraction angiography (DSA) with high-definition CBCT with and without contrast is obtained for the technical assessment [44].

Mixed designs with fenestrations and directional branches

Devices are designed to tailor the patient's anatomy but the most common combinations are 2 or 3 fenestrations for the renal arteries and SMA and 1 or 2 directional branches for the CA and SMA. The initial steps of the procedure are identical to what has been described above. The fenestrated-branched component is oriented extracorporeally, introduced via the femoral approach, and deployed with apposition of the fenestrations to the target vessels. The directional branches are typically designed to be placed more than 2 cm proximal to the target vessel when caudally oriented. The preloaded system allows advancement of 6Fr 90-cm or 110-cm sheaths into the renal fenestrations. If the

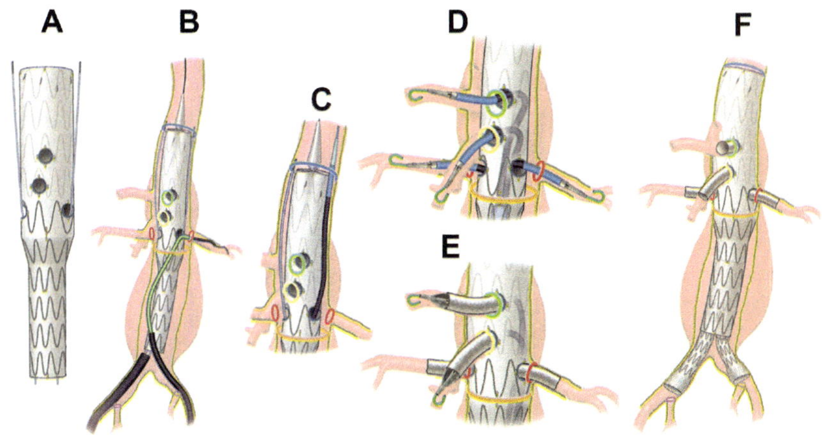

Fig. 3. A device with 4 fenestrations and 2 preloaded catheters for the renal arteries (*A*). A 7FR LIMA guide-catheter was used to precatheterize the left renal artery for onlay fusion calibration, followed by device deployment with adequate apposition between the fenestrations and the origin of the visceral arteries (*B*). The preloaded catheters were exchanged for 6Fr sheaths (*C*). A 0.018-inch wire is advanced to work as a "buddy wire" to secure the fenestration access, and a second catheter and guidewire are used to catheterize the renal arteries. The LIMA guide-catheter used for precatheterization of the renal artery is now used for selective catheterization of the celiac and superior mesenteric artery. After catheterization of all target vessels, the sheaths and bridging stents are advanced and deployed (*D, E*). Finally, a bifurcated stent-graft and iliac limbs are implanted, preserving the internal iliac artery (*F*). (Reproduced by permission of University of Texas Health Science at Houston for Medical Education and Research.)

SMA is targeted by a fenestration, the contralateral femoral access is used for catheterization of the SMA. Once hydrophilic sheaths and alignment stent grafts are positioned into each of the fenestrations over Rosen wires, the device is completely deployed by removing the diameter-reducing ties. Sequential stenting of the reinforced fenestrations is performed with balloon-expandable stent-grafts. Directional branches are usually stented with self-expandable stent-grafts or flexible balloon-expandable stent-grafts. The repair is extended into one of the iliac arteries using a bifurcated universal component. The proximal and distal landing zones and attachment sites are gently dilated with Coda balloon (Cook Medical Inc., Bloomington, IN).

The device sheath (18 or 20Fr) is downsized into a 12Fr 33-cm Dryseal sheath (WL Gore, Flagstaff AZ). Our preference for steerable sheath is the Destino Bidirectional 8.5Fr × 55 cm sheath (Oscor Inc., FL) coupled with a locking 0.014-inch wire, which are introduced into the 12Fr sheath via the Lunderquist using a coaxial 6Fr 90-cm sheath instead of the original dilator. The Lunderquist wire is removed and the 6Fr sheath is partially retracted, allowing the steerable sheath to form above the level of the CA. The locking wire is gently tacked with 2 hemostats to provide support for the steerable sheath during the advancement of catheters and stents. The most distal directional branch is catheterized using a 5Fr catheter and glidewire, which are exchanged for a 0.035-inch Amplatzer wire (Boston Scientific, Bloomington, IN). The 6Fr sheath is advanced over the catheter and used for selective angiography to confirm proper positioning of the wire and mark the first branch bifurcation. At this point, the 6Fr sheath and catheter are removed over the wire, and a balloon-expandable stent-graft is advanced bareback and deployed into the SMA or CA (Fig. 4). Once the stent is deployed, the balloon is removed and the 6Fr sheath is readvanced for selective angiography. The final steps consist of placement of the contralateral iliac limb extension into the common iliac artery, followed by rotational DSA and CBCT.

Multibranched stent-grafts

Multibranched stent-grafts can be off-the-shelf or patient-specific, with up to 5 directional branches positioned in different locations to fit the patient anatomy. Low-profile branched stent-grafts require an 18Fr sheath compared with 22Fr for the standard off-the-shelf device. The repair may require proximal thoracic stent-grafts depending on the location of the proximal landing zone, which may

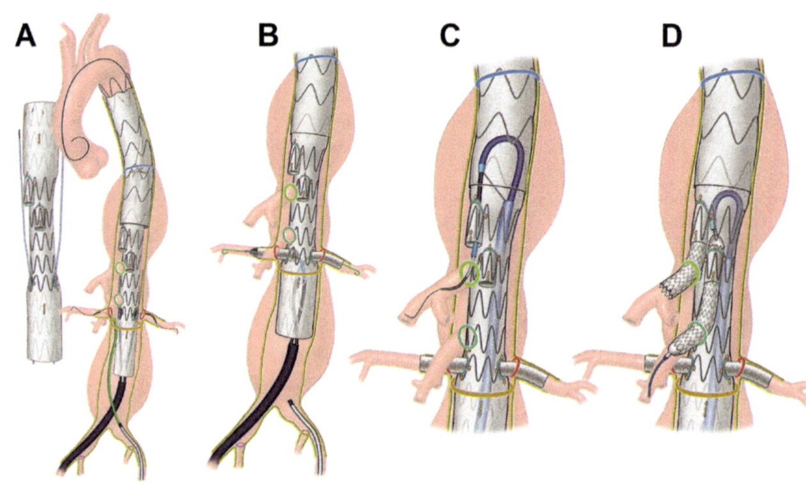

Fig. 4. A device with a combination of 2 fenestrations for the renal arteries, 2 directional branches for the CA and SMA, and preloaded catheters for the fenestrations (*A*). The device is deployed with apposition of the fenestrations to the target vessels using onlay fusion and the precatheterized renal artery (*A*). The preloaded system allows the advancement of 6Fr 90-cm or 110-cm sheaths into the renal fenestrations. Once hydrophilic sheaths and bridging stent-grafts are positioned into each of the fenestrations over Rosen wires, the device is completely deployed by removing the diameter-reducing ties followed by sequential stenting of the reinforced fenestrations (*B*). The CA is catheterized and stented from the femoral artery using a coaxial directional system (*C*). The same step from the groin is repeated for the SMA (*D*). The final stages consist of catheterization of the contralateral gate and placement of an iliac limb extension into the common iliac artery. (Reproduced by permission of University of Texas Health Science at Houston for Medical Education and Research.)

have been placed as part of a first-stage procedure. Once access is established in standard fashion and onlay fusion has been properly calibrated, the branched stent-graft is oriented extracorporeally, advanced, and deployed with each of the directional branches approximately 1 to 2 cm proximal to the intended target vessel. The distal bifurcated stent-graft and ipsilateral iliac stent-graft limbs are deployed but the contralateral gate is left open to allow access to the aneurysm sac. The proximal and distal landing zones and attachments are gently dilated, and the large delivery system is removed and exchanged over the wire for a 12Fr 33-cm Dryseal sheath. The steerable sheath system described above is introduced for sequential catheterization and stenting, starting with the renal arteries, followed by the SMA and CA. Our preference is to use 0.035-inch Rosen wires for the renal arteries and 0.035-inch Amplatzer wires for the mesenteric vessels. Stenting is performed using balloon-expandable stent-grafts, followed by selective angiographies (Fig. 5). The procedure is completed with the placement of the contralateral iliac limb extension, rotational DSA, and CBCT.

POSTOPERATIVE CARE

Patients are extubated in the operating room and admitted to an intensive care unit for 1 to 2 days. Permissive hypertension, normal coagulation profile, and

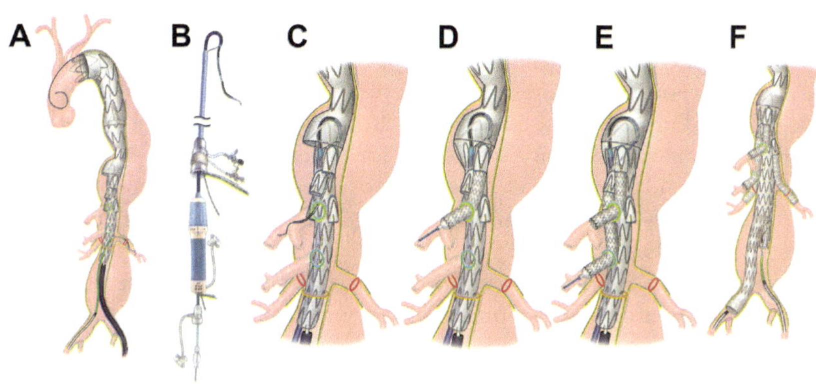

Fig. 5. A multibranched stent-graft is deployed using the onlay fusion, and the precatheterized renal artery as reference (*A*). Each of the directional branches are located approximately 1 to 2 cm proximal to the intended target vessel. The proximal and distal landing zones and attachments are gently dilated, and the large delivery system is removed and exchanged over the wire for a 12Fr 33-cm Dryseal sheath. Our preference for steerable sheath is the Destino Bidirectional 8.5Fr × 55 cm sheath (Oscor Inc., FL) coupled with a locking 0.014-inch wire, which are introduced into the 12Fr sheath via the Lunderquist using a coaxial 6Fr 90-cm sheath instead of the original dilator (*B*). With the coaxial system, the CA is catheterized (*C*) and stented (*D*), followed by the SMA (*E*), and both renal arteries. The procedure is completed with the catheterization of the contralateral gate of the bifurcated graft (*F*) and extension into the contralateral iliac limb. (Reproduced by permission of University of Texas Health Science at Houston for Medical Education and Research. All rights reserved.)

hemoglobin greater than 10 gm/dL are recommended in the first 48 hours. Patients remain in bed rest during the first 24 (Extent IV) or 48 hours (Extent I-III). A therapeutic CSFD placement and rescue maneuvers are needed in 10% of patients with Extent I-III TAAA and in 1% to 2% of those with Extent IV TAAAs to treat symptoms of SCI, with improvement in 75% of patients [41]. Vasodilator antihypertensive medications are held or titrated downward in the first weeks following repair but beta-blockers are administered to prevent supraventricular tachycardia. Perioperative antisalicylic acid is continued, and clopidogrel is added 2 weeks after the procedure to decrease the risk of renal stent thrombosis. We recommend not starting clopidogrel soon after the repair due to the potential risk of delayed SCI requiring placement of CSFD. Follow-up includes clinical examination, duplex renal and mesenteric ultrasound, and CTA at 6 to 8 weeks, 6 months, 1 year, and annually thereafter.

RESULTS

Several centers have shown significant improvements in mortality, morbidity, and early reinterventions of FB-EVAR after overcoming the initial learning curve, despite increase usage in patients with more complex anatomy [12–14,21]. Overall the technique has high technical success with 30-day mortality in the range of 0% to 6.7% for CAAAs and 1.3% to 10.6% for TAAAs [13,14,17,29,45–49]. The 5-year report of the US ZFEN Pivotal trial included a 1.5% 30-day mortality and a 97% freedom from aneurysm-related mortality at 5 years. Freedom from any secondary intervention was 64% at 5 years, with no aneurysm rupture or conversion to open surgical repair [50]. Oderich and colleagues reported the midterm results of 430 patients enrolled in a prospective, nonrandomized study. Mortality at 30 days was 0.9%, including a mortality of 0.6% among 165 patients treated for Extent I to III TAAAs. Freedom from any secondary intervention was 64% but freedom from major interventions (defined by any open surgical or large sheath endovascular procedure) was 87% at 5 years [13].

Results of FB-EVAR are also reproducible in multiple center experiences. The US Aortic Research Consortium (ARC) is an initiative from 10 centers with ongoing prospective, nonrandomized physician-sponsored investigational device exemption studies. The latest interim analysis of 1681 patients had a 30-day mortality of 3%, including 622 extent I-III TAAAs, 535 extent IV TAAAs, and 502 CAAAs, a remarkable improvement compared with the mortality of open surgical repair. A recent analysis of secondary interventions in the US ARC cohort showed freedom from secondary interventions of 59% at 5 years [51].

SUMMARY

FB-EVAR had evolved from an alternative to treat elderly and higher risk patients to the first line of treatment in most patients with suitable anatomy, independent of the clinical risk. Anatomic feasibility requires adequate landing zones, target vessels, and iliofemoral access. Open surgical repair is an alternative in good risk patients who are not well suited for endovascular approach and those with GenTADs. Limitations of FB-EVAR are limited availability due to prolonged regulatory process, the high cost of these devices, and the need for continued surveillance and secondary interventions. Nonetheless, the high technical success and low rate of late aortic related mortality is a testament to the effectiveness of the technique.

Disclosure

Dr G.S. Oderich has consulting fees and research grants from Cook Medical, WL Gore, and GE Healthcare and is part of the Scientific advisory board of Cook Medical and Centerline Biomedical.

References

[1] Kent KC, Zwolak RM, Egorova NN, et al. Analysis of risk factors for abdominal aortic aneurysm in a cohort of more than 3 million individuals. J Vasc Surg 2010;52(3):539–48.
[2] Schermerhorn ML, O'Malley AJ, Jhaveri A, et al. Endovascular vs. open repair of abdominal aortic aneurysms in the Medicare population. N Engl J Med 2008;358(5):464–74.
[3] Greenberg RK, Clair D, Srivastava S, et al. Should patients with challenging anatomy be offered endovascular aneurysm repair? J Vasc Surg 2003;38(5):990–6.
[4] Lobato AC. Sandwich technique for aortoiliac aneurysms extending to the internal iliac artery or isolated common/internal iliac artery aneurysms: a new endovascular approach to preserve pelvic circulation. J Endovasc Ther 2011;18(1):106–11.
[5] Silveira PG, Galego GN, Bortoluzzi CT, et al. RE: "Branched grafts for thoracoabdominal aneurysms: off-label use of FDA-approved devices. J Endovasc Ther 2012;19(1):130.
[6] Kasirajan K. Branched grafts for thoracoabdominal aneurysms: off-label use of FDA-approved devices. J Endovasc Ther 2011;18(4):471–6.
[7] Ohrlander T, Sonesson B, Ivancev K, et al. The chimney graft: a technique for preserving or rescuing aortic branch vessels in stent-graft sealing zones. J Endovasc Ther 2008;15(4): 427–32.
[8] Moulakakis KG, Mylonas SN, Dalainas I, et al. The chimney-graft technique for preserving supra-aortic branches: a review. Ann Cardiothorac Surg 2013;2(3):339–46.
[9] Lobato AC, Camacho-Lobato L. Endovascular treatment of complex aortic aneurysms using the sandwich technique. J Endovasc Ther 2012;19(6):691–706.
[10] Ahmad W, Mylonas S, Majd P, et al. A current systematic evaluation and meta-analysis of chimney graft technology in aortic arch diseases. J Vasc Surg 2017;66(5):1602–10.e2.
[11] Wanhainen A, Verzini F, Van Herzeele I, et al. Editor's Choice - European Society for Vascular Surgery (ESVS) 2019 Clinical Practice Guidelines on the Management of Abdominal Aorto-iliac Artery Aneurysms. Eur J Vasc Endovasc Surg 2019;57(1):8–93.
[12] Verhoeven EL, Katsargyris A, Oikonomou K, et al. Fenestrated Endovascular Aortic Aneurysm Repair as a First Line Treatment Option to Treat Short Necked, Juxtarenal, and Suprarenal Aneurysms. Eur J Vasc Endovasc Surg 2016;51(6):775–81.
[13] Oderich GS, Tenorio ER, Mendes BC, et al. Midterm Outcomes of a Prospective, Nonrandomized Study to Evaluate Endovascular Repair of Complex Aortic Aneurysms Using Fenestrated-Branched Endografts. Ann Surg 2021;274(3):491–9.
[14] Mastracci TM, Eagleton MJ, Kuramochi Y, et al. Twelve-year results of fenestrated endografts for juxtarenal and group IV thoracoabdominal aneurysms. J Vasc Surg 2015;61(2): 355–64.
[15] Park JH, Chung JW, Choo IW, et al. Fenestrated stent-grafts for preserving visceral arterial branches in the treatment of abdominal aortic aneurysms: preliminary experience. J Vasc Interv Radiol 1996;7(6):819–23.
[16] Antoniou GA, Antoniou SA, Torella F. Editor's Choice - Endovascular vs. Open Repair for Abdominal Aortic Aneurysm: Systematic Review and Meta-analysis of Updated Peri-

operative and Long Term Data of Randomised Controlled Trials. Eur J Vasc Endovasc Surg 2020;59(3):385–97.

[17] Geisbüsch S, Kuehnl A, Salvermoser M, et al. Editor's Choice - Hospital Incidence, Treatment, and In Hospital Mortality Following Open and Endovascular Surgery for Thoracoabdominal Aortic Aneurysms in Germany from 2005 to 2014: Secondary Data Analysis of the Nationwide German DRG Microdata. Eur J Vasc Endovasc Surg 2019;57(4): 488–98.

[18] Latz CA, Cambria RP, Patel VI, et al. Durability of open surgical repair of type I-III thoracoabdominal aortic aneurysm. J Vasc Surg 2019;70(2):413–23.

[19] Coselli JS, LeMaire SA, Preventza O, et al. Outcomes of 3309 thoracoabdominal aortic aneurysm repairs. J Thorac Cardiovasc Surg 2016;151(5):1323–37.

[20] Estrera AL, Sandhu HK, Charlton-Ouw KM, et al. A Quarter Century of Organ Protection in Open Thoracoabdominal Repair. Ann Surg 2015;262(4):660–8.

[21] Eagleton MJ, Follansbee M, Wolski K, et al. Fenestrated and branched endovascular aneurysm repair outcomes for type II and III thoracoabdominal aortic aneurysms. J Vasc Surg 2016;63(4):930–42.

[22] Chaikof EL, Dalman RL, Eskandari MK, et al. The Society for Vascular Surgery practice guidelines on the care of patients with an abdominal aortic aneurysm. J Vasc Surg 2018;67(1):2–77, e2.

[23] Brown PM, Zelt DT, Sobolev B. The risk of rupture in untreated aneurysms: the impact of size, gender, and expansion rate. J Vasc Surg 2003;37(2):280–4.

[24] Lederle FA, Johnson GR, Wilson SE, et al. Rupture rate of large abdominal aortic aneurysms in patients refusing or unfit for elective repair. Jama 2002;287(22):2968–72.

[25] Riambau V, Böckler D, Brunkwall J, et al. Editor's Choice - Management of Descending Thoracic Aorta Diseases: Clinical Practice Guidelines of the European Society for Vascular Surgery (ESVS). Eur J Vasc Endovasc Surg 2017;53(1):4–52.

[26] Lo RC, Lu B, Fokkema MT, et al. Relative importance of aneurysm diameter and body size for predicting abdominal aortic aneurysm rupture in men and women. J Vasc Surg 2014;59(5): 1209–16.

[27] Jones GT, Sandiford P, Hill GB, et al. Correcting for Body Surface Area Identifies the True Prevalence of Abdominal Aortic Aneurysm in Screened Women. Eur J Vasc Endovasc Surg 2019;57(2):221–8.

[28] Davenport MS, Perazella MA, Yee J, et al. Use of Intravenous Iodinated Contrast Media in Patients With Kidney Disease: Consensus Statements from the American College of Radiology and the National Kidney Foundation. Kidney Med 2020;2(1):85–93.

[29] Katsargyris A, Oikonomou K, Kouvelos G, et al. Comparison of outcomes for double fenestrated endovascular aneurysm repair versus triple or quadruple fenestrated endovascular aneurysm repair in the treatment of complex abdominal aortic aneurysms. J Vasc Surg 2017;66(1):29–36.

[30] Oderich GS, Ribeiro M, Hofer J, et al. Prospective, nonrandomized study to evaluate endovascular repair of pararenal and thoracoabdominal aortic aneurysms using fenestrated-branched endografts based on supraceliac sealing zones. J Vasc Surg 2017;65(5): 1249–59.e10.

[31] Banga P, Oderich GS, Farber M, et al. Impact of Number of Vessels Targeted on Outcomes of Fenestrated-Branched Endovascular Repair for Complex Abdominal Aortic Aneurysms. Ann Vasc Surg 2021;72:98–105.

[32] Kristmundsson T, Sonesson B, Dias N, et al. Outcomes of fenestrated endovascular repair of juxtarenal aortic aneurysm. J Vasc Surg 2014;59(1):115–20.

[33] Lima GB, Tenorio ER, Marcondes GB, et al. Differences in procedural metrics and clinical outcomes among patients treated by fenestrated-branched endovascular repair of thoracoabdominal aortic aneurysms using infrarenal aortic versus iliac sealing zones. J Vasc Surg 2021.

[34] Chait J, Tenorio ER, Mendes BC, et al. Effect of Gap Distance Between Fenestration and Aortic Wall on Target Artery Instability After Fenestrated-Branched Endovascular Aortic Repair. J Vasc Surg 2021;74(3):e87–8.

[35] Oderich GS, Greenberg RK, Farber M, et al. Results of the United States multicenter prospective study evaluating the Zenith fenestrated endovascular graft for treatment of juxtarenal abdominal aortic aneurysms. J Vasc Surg 2014;60(6):1420–8, e1-5.

[36] Hinchliffe RJ, Ivancev K, Sonesson B, et al. Paving and cracking": an endovascular technique to facilitate the introduction of aortic stent-grafts through stenosed iliac arteries. J Endovasc Ther 2007;14(5):630–3.

[37] Giannopoulos S, Malgor RD, Sobreira ML, et al. Iliac Conduits for Endovascular Treatment of Aortic Pathologies: A Systematic Review and Meta-analysis. J Endovasc Ther 2021;28(4):499–509.

[38] Criado FJ. Iliac arterial conduits for endovascular access: technical considerations. J Endovasc Ther 2007;14(3):347–51.

[39] Conrad MF, Crawford RS, Davison JK, et al. Thoracoabdominal Aneurysm Repair: A 20-Year Perspective. Ann Thorac Surg 2007;83(2):S856–61.

[40] Malgor RD, Marques de Marino P, Verhoeven E, et al. A systematic review of outcomes of upper extremity access for fenestrated and branched endovascular aortic repair. J Vasc Surg 2020;71(5):1763–70.e2.

[41] Kärkkäinen JM, Cirillo-Penn NC, Sen I, et al. Cerebrospinal fluid drainage complications during first stage and completion fenestrated-branched endovascular aortic repair. J Vasc Surg 2020;71(4):1109–18.e2.

[42] Kitpanit N, Ellozy SH, Connolly PH, et al. Risk factors for spinal cord injury and complications of cerebrospinal fluid drainage in patients undergoing fenestrated and branched endovascular aneurysm repair. J Vasc Surg 2021;73(2):399–409.e1.

[43] Marcondes GB, Tenorio ER, Baumgardt G, et al. Evaluation of Safety of Overhead Upper Extremity Positioning During Fenestrated-Branched Endovascular Repair of Thoracoabdominal Aortic Aneurysms. Cardiovasc Intervent Radiol 2021.

[44] Tenorio ER, Oderich GS, Sandri GA, et al. Prospective nonrandomized study to evaluate cone beam computed tomography for technical assessment of standard and complex endovascular aortic repair. J Vasc Surg 2020;71(6):1982–93.e5.

[45] Greenberg RK, Sternbergh WC 3rd, Makaroun M, et al. Intermediate results of a United States multicenter trial of fenestrated endograft repair for juxtarenal abdominal aortic aneurysms. J Vasc Surg 2009;50(4):730–7.e1.

[46] Early results of fenestrated endovascular repair of juxtarenal aortic aneurysms in the United Kingdom. Circulation 2012;125(22):2707–15.

[47] Marzelle J, Presles E, Becquemin JP. Results and factors affecting early outcome of fenestrated and/or branched stent grafts for aortic aneurysms: a multicenter prospective study. Ann Surg 2015;261(1):197–206.

[48] Van Calster K, Bianchini A, Elias F, et al. Risk factors for early and late mortality after fenestrated and branched endovascular repair of complex aneurysms. J Vasc Surg 2019;69(5): 1342–55.

[49] Spanos K, Kölbel T, Kubitz JC, et al. Risk of spinal cord ischemia after fenestrated or branched endovascular repair of complex aortic aneurysms. J Vasc Surg 2019;69(2): 357–66.

[50] Oderich GS, Farber MA, Schneider D, et al. Final 5-year results of the United States Zenith Fenestrated prospective multicenter study for juxtarenal abdominal aortic aneurysms. J Vasc Surg 2021;73(4):1128–38.e2.

[51] Zettervall SL, Tenorio ER, Schanzer A, et al. Secondary interventions after fenestrated/branched aneurysm repairs are common and nondetrimental to long-term survival. J Vasc Surg 2021.

Advances in Surgery 56 (2022) 321–335
ADVANCES IN SURGERY

Is There a Role for Rib Plating in Thoracic Trauma?

Chaitan K. Narsule, MD*, Anne C. Mosenthal, MD
Department of Surgery, Lahey Hospital and Medical Center, 41 Mall Road, Burlington, MA 01805, USA

Keywords
• Rib fractures • Rib plating • Surgical stabilization of rib fractures • Flail chest • Nonflail rib fractures

Key points

- Over the past decade, the surgical stabilization of rib fractures (SSRF) has become very common in the management of severe rib fractures at trauma centers throughout the United States.
- Though rib plating for the management of flail chest injury is associated with improved outcomes, more recent reports also support the role of rib plating for nonflail rib fractures, in elderly patients, and in patients with concomitant moderate to severe traumatic brain injuries (TBI).
- Cases of hardware infection or failure are notably rare occurrences, and can be managed both through a multimodal approach and often without the need for the restabilization of rib fractures.

INTRODUCTION

Rib fractures are a morbid consequence of blunt chest trauma. One prominent historical report has noted that rib fractures occur in up to 10% of all trauma patients, one-third of whom have a concomitant hemothorax or pneumothorax and one-quarter of whom have an associated pulmonary contusion. Moreover, more than half of such patients will require operative intervention or admission to the intensive care unit (ICU), 90% will have associated injuries, 35% will require discharge to an extended care facility, and 12% will die. [1] Subsequent reports have clarified the effect of pre-existing medical conditions [2,3]; age [4,5]; the number of fractured ribs [6,7]; complicated thoracic injuries including

*Corresponding author. *E-mail address:* chaitan.narsule@lahey.org
Twitter: @ChaitanNarsule (C.K.N.)

https://doi.org/10.1016/j.yasu.2022.02.009
0065-3411/22/

flail chest [8], the presence of bilateral rib fractures and pulmonary contusions [9]; and the development of pneumonia [2] on the morbidity and mortality of rib fractures.

In practice, patients afflicted with blunt chest trauma can have a highly variable presentation ranging from minor, nondisplaced rib fractures causing limited, manageable pain in highly compensated individuals to severely displaced rib fractures with concomitant pulmonary contusions and hemopneumothoraces leading to respiratory failure in badly injured healthy people or in frail, elderly populations. The mechanisms attributable to pulmonary insufficiency from rib fractures include: (1) fracture-related pain which causes impaired clearance of secretions and atelectasis due to splinting, (2) alteration of normal diaphragmatic and costovertebral muscular excursion, and (3) penetration of fractured ribs into the pleural space leading to pulmonary parenchymal injury, disruption of the endothoracic fascia and intercostal musculature, or both and causing pneumothorax, hemothorax, and/or pulmonary lacerations or contusions [10]. In extreme cases of severe blunt chest injury which leads to flail chest development, in which 3 or more consecutive ribs are fractured at 2 or more sites and paradoxical chest wall movement is present, mortality can approach 25% [11,12].

The open reduction and internal fixation of rib fractures, now more commonly referred to as the surgical stabilization of rib fractures (SSRF), was first conceived and reported in the 1950s [13,14]. Since then, due to an evolution of techniques [15,16], fixation technology, and general acceptance, the application of SSRF has substantially increased at trauma centers all throughout the United States and for multiple indications especially in the last decade [17]. This is particularly notable when observed as an increased prevalence of SSRF from 0.7% for patients with flail chest injury reported to the National Trauma Data Bank (NTDB) from 2007 to 2009 [18], to 5.8% for adults with 3 or more rib fractures reported to the NTDB from 2008 to 2014 [19], and to 7.1% for adults with flail and nonflail rib fractures reported to the Trauma Quality Improvement Program from 2010 to 2015 [20].

Clinical practice guidelines published both by the Eastern Association for the Surgery of Trauma and the Rib Fracture Colloquium in 2017 have conditionally recommended SSRF predominantly for the management of flail chest injury, owing to the limited data available at that time supporting the use of SSRF for other indications [21,22]. Even in the 4 years since then, numerous reports have emerged which have further clarified the role of SSRF–in particular, for subsets of patients who would benefit the most from the procedure–and cemented its place in the armamentarium of the trauma and acute care surgeon engaged in the management of patients with complex chest wall injuries.

The purpose of this summary is to review the most recent and current reports with respect to indications, preoperative evaluation and imaging, approaches, outcomes, and management of complications.

Table 1
Indications for the surgical stabilization of rib fractures [23]

1. Acute respiratory insufficiency despite optimal medical therapy	• Need for mechanical ventilation – OR – • Two or more of the following: o Tachypnea o Hypercarbia o Hypoxia o Uncontrolled secretions o Incentive spirometry < 75% predicted
2. Uncontrolled pain despite optimal medical therapy	• Two or more of the following: o Numeric pain score equal or >4 of 10 o Splinting o Lung hypoexpansion on imaging
3. Impaired pulmonary mechanics or anticipated chronic pain	• One or more of the following: o Flail chest o Hemithoracic volume loss equal to or >30% o 3 or more bicortically displaced rib fractures

INDICATIONS

General indications for the surgical stabilization of severe rib fractures have been well established in recent publications [23–25]. In particular, the Denver Health Medical Center criteria [23] for the SSRF are itemized in Table 1.

Additionally, SSRF is indicated for: (1) the impalement of ribs into the lung (Fig. 1), other solid organs, or the diaphragm and (2) the anticipated nonunion or malunion of rib fractures. In the scope of the authors' practice, flail chest injury, significant hemithoracic volume loss, bicortically displaced rib fractures, visceral impalement, and respiratory failure requiring mechanical ventilation specifically predominate among the major indications for SSRF.

Fig. 2 is an example of hemithoracic volume collapse. The patient is a 55-year-old woman with previous right shoulder reverse arthroplasty who crashed

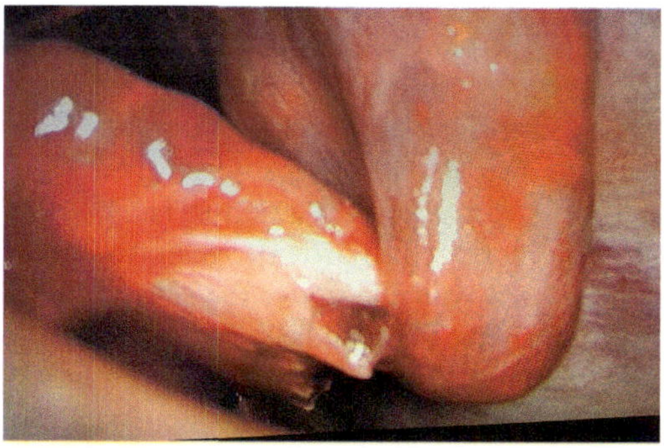

Fig. 1. Thoracoscopic image of a fractured rib impaling the left lower lobe of a patient who sustained blunt trauma to the lower chest.

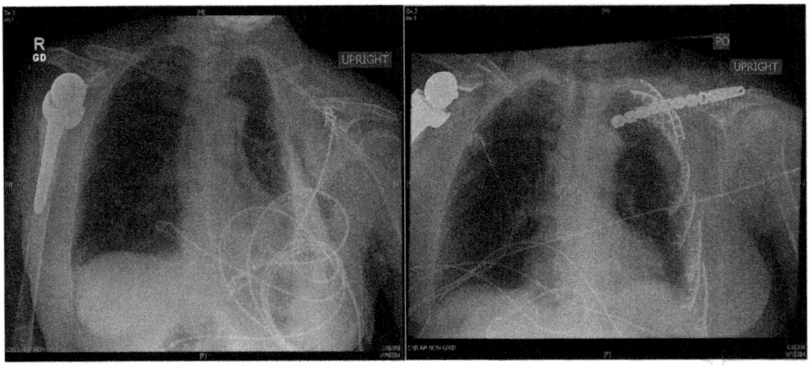

Fig. 2. Chest x-rays of a 55-year-old woman with left hemithoracic volume collapse following a moped collision. (The left x-ray was obtained preoperatively, and the right x-ray was obtained post-operatively.)

while riding a moped at high speed. Preoperatively, her left hemithorax caved in from multiple bicortically displaced rib fractures and she also had a concomitant left clavicle fracture. Following a period of management at an outside hospital with a left tube thoracostomy for a hemopneumothorax, she underwent surgical stabilization of her rib fractures with thoracoscopic evacuation of her retained hemothorax on transfer and subsequent fixation of her left clavicle fracture. Her preoperative and postoperative chest x-rays are seen in the figure. Note the restoration of the left hemithoracic volume. Her postoperative exercise capacity was at its baseline by her 8-week follow-up visit, and she required no pain medications after 3 weeks.

Fig. 3 illustrates the case of a 25-year-old woman who sustained blunt force trauma to the left torso during a motorcycle collision. Following intervention for other nonthoracic injuries, she persisted in having a "pseudo-flail" of paradoxical motion due to her substantially displaced left rib fractures and associated laceration of the endothoracic fascia and intercostal musculature (Fig. 3A demonstrates the 3-dimensional computed tomographic reconstruction of her rib cage). Fig. 3B demonstrates repair of the substantially displaced and adjacent rib fractures; the stabilized ribs were then re-approximated and covered by the latissimus dorsi, serratus anterior, and pectoralis major muscles which were generously mobilized to provide coverage over the hardware that would have otherwise been palpable under the skin of this thin patient.

Certainly, in cases of severe chest wall disruption, the role of plating can be self-evident. Making the case for plating minimally displaced fractures or pain-related reasons, however, can be challenging. In part, radiographic evaluation can underestimate the magnitude of rib fractures. In a study by Bauman and colleagues [26], radiologists and surgeons at the same institution compared rib fractures on CT scans in 410 patients who presented over a 1-year period,

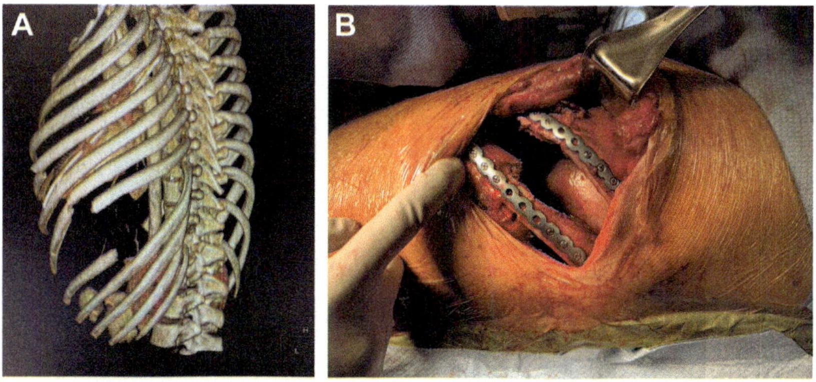

Fig. 3. (*A*). Three-dimensional computed tomography of the chest of a 25-year-old woman who sustained blunt chest trauma. Multiple left lateral rib fractures–with one severely displaced rib fracture creating a "pseudoflail" presentation from lacerated endothoracic fascia–is readily evident. (*B*). Intraoperative image following SSRF of 2 displaced left rib fractures.

and it was found that radiologists underreported both the number of existing rib fractures and their severity in terms of displacement when compared with interpretations by surgeons.

This discordance can have clinical implications. Fig. 4 is an intraoperative picture from the case of a 62-year-old woman who was in a motor vehicle collision and sustained left 7th through 10th rib fractures. On imaging, all fractures were deemed to be minimally displaced on CT imaging. Consequently, the patient elected initial nonoperative management with epidural catheter management for analgesia. During this period, however, she developed new subcutaneous emphysema associated with her fractures after postinjury day 3 and subsequently agreed to rib plating. In the figure, for which the latissimus dorsi muscle is reflected posteriorly and the serratus anterior muscle superiorly, the displaced nature of the rib fractures–including laceration of the intervening intercostal musculature–can be readily appreciated.

PREOPERATIVE EVALUATION AND IMAGING

In the work up of patients as candidates for rib fixation, high-resolution imaging is of utmost importance both to identify fracture patterns and for operative planning. In a study evaluating the value-added by the use of chest x-rays, 2-dimensional (2D) chest CT scans, and 3-dimensional (3D) reconstructed chest CT images for 35 patients by surgeons experienced at rib fracture fixation, it was found that while 2D CT scans were the most accurate modality for detecting rib fractures, 3D CT reconstructions were more helpful for local operative planning (in terms of length and position of incision) [27]. We similarly find that 2D CT scans are most helpful to identify candidate fractures for intervention, and 3D CTs for displaced fractures are also a great tool to help illustrate the burden of rib fractures to patients and their families.

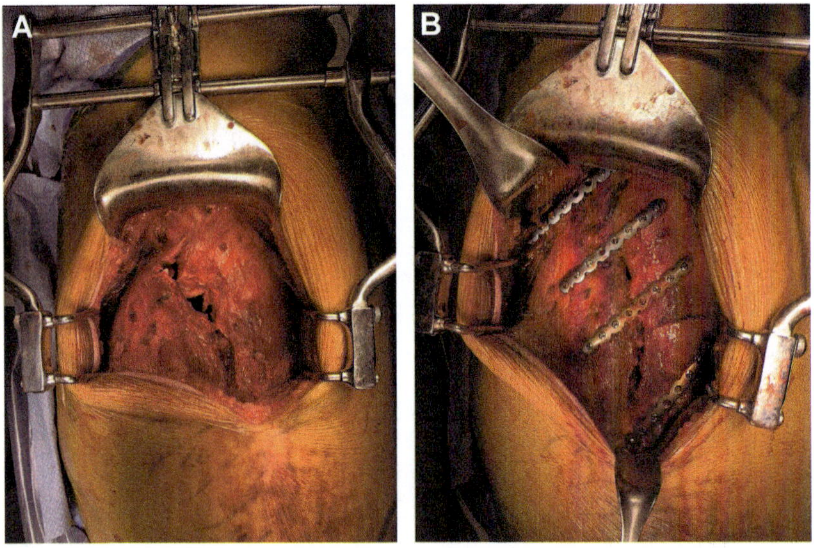

Fig. 4. (*A*). Intraoperative image of the lateral chest wall, following the mobilization of the latissimus dorsi and serratus anterior muscles, of a 62-year-old woman with fractures of the left 7th through 10th ribs. (The patient is in the right lateral decubitus position, the back is toward the right of the image, and the upper chest and neck are beyond the top of the image.) (*B*): Intraoperative picture after SSRF of the left 7th through 10th ribs.

Another method to stratify patients based on the radiographic pattern of rib fractures on chest CT imaging is the RibScore [10] developed by investigators from Denver Health Medical Center. Though other methods to catalog traumatic rib fractures exist, including the Rib Fracture Score [28,29], the organ injury scale (OIS) Chest Wall grade [30], and Chest Trauma Score [31,32], these methods account for laterality and number of fractures only. Conversely, the RibScore uses features of rib fractures that are associated with worse clinical outcomes. These include the presence of flail chest, 6 or more ribs fractured, bilateral rib fractures, 3 or more bicortically displaced rib fractures, first rib fracture, and fractures located each in the anterior, lateral, and posterior anatomic areas. Importantly, the association of the RibScore with pneumonia, acute respiratory failure, and tracheostomy has been validated. In our practice, though RibScore alone is not itself an absolute criterion in deciding on operative rib fixation, it is a valuable benchmark for cases of blunt chest wall injury and allows for a clinical prediction of outcomes that rib fixation may hopefully prevent.

Furthermore, the assessment of forced vital capacity (FVC) can also be useful in the preoperative assessment of rib fractured patients. The utility of FVC in predicting pulmonary complications has been reported in several recent studies [33–35]. A recent report by Billings and colleagues [36] also used the percentage of predicted FVC among patients with rib fractures and demonstrated better resource allocation–in terms of fewer transfers to the ICU, and both shorter ICU and hospital length of stay. Preoperative assessments of FVC might be especially helpful in guiding decisions about rib fixation in non-flail injury patients.

ASPECTS OF TECHNIQUE AND OTHER KEY POINTS

The modern and recent American and international experience with the SSRF largely conforms to muscle-sparing techniques, approaches, and opinions recently published by Pieracci and colleagues [15], Ali-Osman and colleagues [16], and the Rib Fracture Colloquium [22]. Accordingly, additional aspects of technique reported here are those that are worthy of emphasis from the authors' perspective.

Timing of rib plating is an important logistical concern as patients who sustain severe blunt chest trauma may also have multi-system injuries and are also at risk of pulmonary contusions, traumatic pneumatoceles, and hemopneumothoraces that can lead to the interval development of early-onset acute respiratory distress syndrome. This, in turn, can dramatically affect a patient's stability for operative intervention, especially in cases in which concomitant thoracoscopy for the evacuation of a retained hemothorax–thus, requiring lung isolation–is planned. Also, the interval development of septic complications–bacteremia, pneumonia, and urinary tract infections–might complicate decisions favoring rib plating and hardware placement. Pieracci and colleagues [37] evaluated the outcomes of 551 patients who underwent SSRF from 2006 to 2016 at 4 trauma centers to determine the effect of early (<1 day), mid (1–2 days), and late (3–10 days) timing of SSRF on clinical outcomes. They found that early SSRF was optimal as each additional hospital day before SSRF was associated with a 31% increased likelihood of pneumonia, a 27% increased likelihood of prolonged mechanical ventilation, and a 26% increased likelihood of tracheostomy. Additionally, Prins and colleagues [38] looked further into the question of timing by reviewing all available literature in which early and late cohorts of patients undergoing SSRF were described. Nine retrospective studies were identified and reviewed. Though in these studies specific reasons for early versus late SSRF were not enumerated, early SSRF (defined as within 48–72 hours following admission) had benefits over late SSRF that included shorter ICU and hospital length of stay, shorter duration of mechanical ventilation, and lower rates of pneumonia and tracheostomy placement. Currently, no prospective studies have yet examined the issue of timing further, and future prospective studies would be helpful to overcome aspects of selection bias that affect retrospective reports.

Generally, we advocate strongly for concomitant ipsilateral thoracoscopy during rib plating procedures. The reasons are 3-fold: (1) a hemothorax is a frequently associated complication of rib fractures, and performing pneumolysis (Fig. 5) and combining all loculated hemothoraces for evacuation proactively avoids having to manage a retained hemothorax later on, (2) a properly positioned posterior and apical chest tube can be placed (Fig. 6),

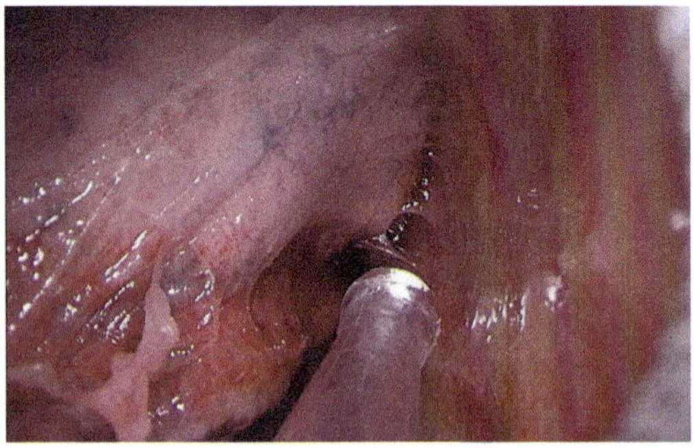

Fig. 5. Thoracoscopic view of pneumolysis and evacuation of retained hemothorax.

and (3) the surgeon is provided with the opportunity to perform an intercostal nerve block with bupivacaine for better perioperative analgesia (Fig. 7). To perform thoracoscopy, we anticipate the need for selective lung isolation by having our patients intubated with left-sided dual-lumen endotracheal intubation tubes.

Specific hardware for use with rib fixation operations has had a historic evolution from primitive stabilization devices such as Krischner wires and Judet staples to absorbable plates and, more recently, external nonabsorbable plates and intramedullary nails. More recently, intrathoracic fixation systems adaptable to a thoracoscopic approach for rib fracture stabilization have also been introduced, though reports on experiences with these systems are limited [39]. While the authors do not endorse one product over the other, generally hardware systems supporting open external plating through strategically placed incisions that both are muscle-sparing and positioned over the fracture line facilitate the rib fixation process. Also, the development of self-tapping screws

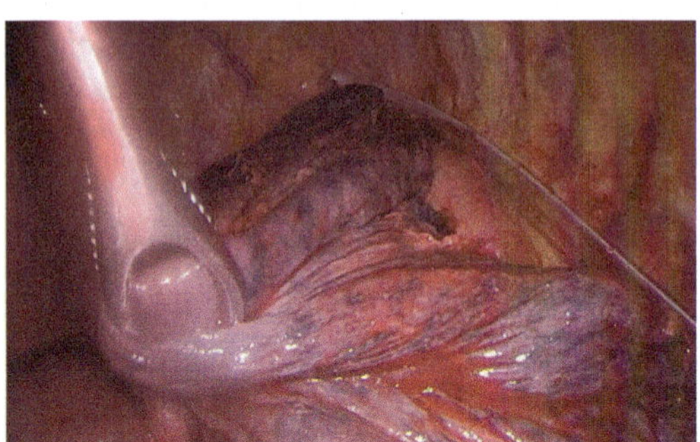

Fig. 6. Thoracoscopic view of the left chest demonstrating apical and posterior chest tube placement. The apex is at the top of the image, the left lower lobe is retracted anteriorly with ring forceps, and the back is along the right side of the image.

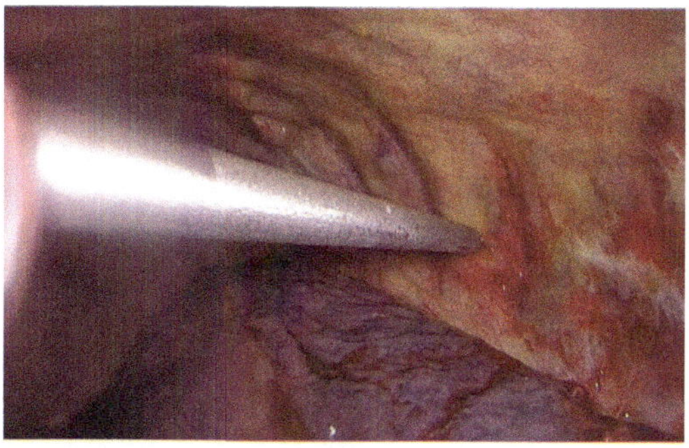

Fig. 7. Thoracoscopic view of posterior intercostal nerve blocks.

for fixation is an advance over an earlier generation of plating systems that required predrilling and saves a step that is especially useful for hard-to-reach locations. Moreover, the authors find the use of intramedullary nails to be not-so-straightforward and, consequently, do not advocate for their use. Further, while most reports describe experiences using external rib plating systems, the use of an intrathoracic fixation system has key advantages–including minimizing periosteal disruption and wound morbidity–that may lead to its more widespread adoption as providers gain more experience with these systems.

As most fractures are anterolateral in location, we recommend longitudinal incisions along the lateral thorax in the space between the latissimus dorsi and pectoralis major muscles for these fractures. The actual incision itself should be oriented to be over the key fracture line as much as possible. From this vantage point, it is often straightforward to locate and mobilize the latissimus dorsi muscle posteriorly and the pectoralis muscle anteriorly as needed. Generally, the serratus anterior musculature can also be mobilized or split, depending on the fracture line location, providing exposure to the rib cage. Authors have described avoiding the first, second, and third ribs because of the minimal participation of the rib cage with respect to respiratory mechanics. Akin to the surgical management of superior sulcus (Pancoast) tumors whereby the apex of the rib cage is not reconstructed following resection [41], the morbidity of treating fractures of the first, second, and third ribs likely outweighs the benefits. Similarly, because morbidity outweighs the benefit for exposure of the fractures involving the tenth rib or below, it is recommended to avoid treating these fractures unless the displacement of the rib fracture makes visceral injury likely. Finally, it is best to avoid interventions on posterior rib fractures that are within 5 cm of the costovertebral joint as there is not enough room for external prosthetic placement. Despite this limitation, whenever possible, the stabilization of both fracture lines of a flail chest injury is recommended as the stabilization of only one of the 2 fractures lines of a flail chest injury has been shown to be inferior [40]. Typically, for this reason, anterolateral flail chest injuries are easier to repair than posterolateral injuries.

SUMMARY OF SELECT OUTCOMES OF SURGICAL STABILIZATION OF RIB FRACTURES

Over the past decade, and especially over the past 5 years, many reports have surfaced reinforcing the role of SSRF. Key reports pertaining to specific patient populations will be emphasized here.

With respect to the management of flail chest injuries, a practice management guideline from the Eastern Association for the Surgery of Trauma reviewed 22 studies–only 3 of which were prospective studies–that included 986 patients with flail chest injury [21]. On meta-analysis, SSRF for flail chest injury was clearly associated with improved mortality, duration of mechanical ventilation, ICU and hospital length of stay, incidence of pneumonia, and need for tracheostomy. A subsequent study evaluating outcomes of SSRF for flail chest injury reported similar findings and also demonstrated cost-effectiveness (32.6 quality-adjusted life years, vs 30.84 for nonoperatively managed flail chest injuries) [42]. Most recently, a retrospective analysis of the Agency of Healthcare Research and Quality's 2012 to 2014 National Inpatient Sample revealed that SSRF was cost-effective for patients with flail chest (~$150,000/QALY gained), but not for patients without flail chest [43]. However, the effect of cost-effectiveness on the surgical management of nonflail chest injuries might inherently be limited by the timeframe of the study.

In the ongoing effort to refine indications for SSRF in nonflail fracture patterns, in elderly patients, and in other special groups, a number of publications have been recently published. Notably, the Chest Wall Injury Society recently reported outcomes from a multicenter, prospective clinical trial of patients who underwent SSRF within 72 hours at 12 centers who had 3 or more ipsilateral, severely displaced rib fractures without flail chest [44]. One hundred and ten patients met the criteria for enrollment and, of these, 51 underwent SSRF. The numeric pain score was significantly lower at 2-week follow-up compared with the nonoperative cohort (2.9 vs 4.5, $P < .01$). Also, the respiratory disability-related quality of life score was significantly improved in the operative cohort (21 vs 25, $P = .03$), which also had a significantly lower rate of pleural space complications (0% vs 10.2%, $P = .02$). Notably, for the SSRF cohort, evacuation of a concomitant hemothorax and pleural lavage was performed in 37 and 39 patients, respectively, which is an advantage of the operative approach to mitigate pleural space problems. This study reinforces the role of SSRF in nonflail rib fractures in the improvement of postoperative pain and also highlights the role for pleural space management at the time of surgery to minimize potential future pleural space complications.

The matter of cost-effectiveness of SSRF in cases involving 3 or more displaced rib fractures was evaluated in a recent single-center review [45]. Two hundred and seventy-nine patients admitted from 2010 to 2019 were analyzed and, of these, 182 patients underwent SSRF. In comparison with those who were nonoperatively managed, patients who underwent SSRF had decreased hospital charges most strongly associated with hospital length of stay.

Moreover, outcomes on the SSRF of patients 80 years of age and older have recently been reported [46]. In a multicenter, retrospective cohort study involving eight centers experienced with SSRF, octogenarians and older patients who underwent SSRF from 2015 to 2020 were enrolled and matched to controls. In total, 360 patients were enrolled, 133 of whom underwent SSRF. Though the operative cohort was more badly injured than the nonoperative cohort, SSRF was associated with a decreased risk of mortality compared with patients who were treated nonoperatively. However, the patients who underwent SSRF were more likely to develop pneumonia and had an increased duration both on mechanical ventilation and with ICU length of stay. Notably, the operative group was significantly less likely to be discharged on narcotic pain medications.

In addition, as patients who sustain severe blunt chest trauma often have additional traumatic injuries, determining the role–let alone the timing–of SSRF in managing these patients with concomitant injuries becomes increasingly important. In one of the first multicenter reports to address the role of SSRF in patients with specific traumatic injuries that typically portend poor clinical outcomes, the Chest Wall Injury Society retrospectively analyzed the effect of SSRF (vs nonoperative management) in patients with concomitant moderate to severe traumatic brain injuries (TBI) through a multicenter trial [47]. The study population included 456 patients treated between January 2012 and July 2019, of which 111 underwent SSRF. For both moderate and severe TBI patients, the odds of 30-day mortality in the SSRF cohort were significantly lower, and for moderate TBI patients, the odds of developing pneumonia were also significantly lower.

MANAGING HARDWARE INFECTIONS AND FAILURES

With SSRF, both infections and hardware failures are infrequent and rare events, respectively. Hardware infection risk after SSRF had been construed to be in the range of 0% to 10%, with variability owing to the derivation of these data from individual case series [48–50]. In 2016, investigators from the Mayo Clinic reported on their experience pertaining to hardware infections [25]. In approximately 4.5 years, 122 patients underwent SSRF, and 5 patients (4.1%) were found to have a hardware infection on average by the 12th postoperative day. This cohort underwent wound debridement, and variably underwent partial removal of hardware (1 patient), negative-pressure wound therapy, local antibiotic bead placement, and suppressive antibiotic therapy. Thereafter, 3 of the 5 patients underwent hardware removal between 140 and 192 days following SSRF. At the latest follow-up of these patients (which occurred at a minimum of at least 6 months), no patient required reintervention for fracture nonunion, no patients were on narcotic pain medications or suppressive antibiotics, no mortalities had occurred, and all patients objectively had evidence of bone healing by CT imaging. Notably, in all cases, gram-positive bacteria were cultured from microbiology specimens. This limited evidence suggests that though the management of hardware infections can be morbid, by using a multi-modal approach it is possible to still achieve bony union and control of sepsis without the need for repeat surgical stabilization of fracture mal-/nonunions.

The Chest Wall Injury Society has recently reported on characteristics of hardware failure in patients undergoing SSRF [51]. In a multicenter, retrospective analysis from 2010 to 2017, 1224 patients had undergone SSRF and, of these, only 38 patients (3%) had hardware failure. The operative surgeons were experienced, with a median of 100 SSRF cases. Hardware failures were most common for lateral (45.5%) and posterolateral rib fractures (40%). With respect to the mechanism of hardware failures, screw migration occurred in 44.7%, plate fracture occurred in 47.4%, and plate migration occurred in 26.3% of all patients. Notably, 40% of patients with hardware failure were asymptomatic, with the finding detected on routine chest x-ray. Pain occurred in 42%, and persistent clicking while breathing occurred in 13% of patients. Infection developed in 8% of patients. Hardware was explanted in 55% of cases and, of these, reimplantation was necessary for 10% of patients as most fractures had shown evidence of healing at the time of hardware removal. The data from this study suggest that–because almost half of all hardware failures are asymptomatic and, for those who present with symptomatic hardware failure, redo SSRF is infrequently needed–working patients up for hardware failure based on symptomatology alone, as opposed to routine surveillance imaging, may be a reasonable approach.

SUMMARY AND FUTURE DIRECTIONS

The SSRF has a firm place in the management of thoracic trauma. Based on the evidence described herein, trauma surgeons across the United States are performing these procedures in increasing numbers each year. Contemporary data suggest that rib plating is safe and has a favorable complication profile and, in most cases in which there is a hardware infection or occurrences of hardware failure, patients can be managed through a multi-modal approach with the explantation of hardware often happening after bony union has occurred, thus limiting the need for restabilization in most cases. Recent reports reinforce the use of SSRF for nonflail rib fractures, and in the elderly and other select populations. Ongoing clinical focus on the outcomes of SSRF, both in patients with multisystem traumatic injuries as well as the timing of SSRF for patients with severely compromised respiratory physiology as a complication of the traumatic injuries, will further entrench SSRF in the management of blunt chest trauma.

CLINICS CARE POINTS

- Though SSRF has been historically considered in patients with severe flail chest injury, it should also be considered in cases of non-flail rib fractures, elderly patients, and patients with concomitant brain injuries as recent evidence demonstrates favorable outcomes in these populations.

- In working up candidates for SSRF, 2D and 3D chest CT scans are helpful in identifying candidate fractures and for operative planning, respectively.
- During SSRF, ipsilateral thoracoscopy is recommended to manage the pleural space and drain any retained hemothoraces, optimally place a posterior and apical chest tube for pleural drainage, and perform a multi-level intercostal nerve block for enhanced post-operative analgesia.
- Both hardware infections and failure are infrequent post-operative events. Typically, a multimodal approach can enable a patient to still achieve bony union even if hardware explantation is necessary, thus limiting the need for repeat rib fixation.

DISCLOSURE

The authors have nothing to disclose.

References

[1] Ziegler DW, Agarwal NN. The morbidity and mortality of rib fractures. J Trauma 1994;37(6):975–9.
[2] Battle CE, Hutchings H, Evans PA. Risk factors that predict mortality in patients with blunt chest wall trauma: a systematic review and meta-analysis. Injury 2012;43(1):8–17.
[3] Brasel KJ, Guse CE, Layde P, et al. Rib fractures: relationship with pneumonia and mortality. Crit Care Med 2006;34(6):1642–6.
[4] Bulger EM, Arneson MA, Mock CN, et al. Rib fractures in the elderly. J Trauma 2000;48(6): 1040–6.
[5] Battle CE, Hutchings H, Evans PA. Risk factors that predict mortality in patients with blunt chest trauma: a systematic review and meta-analysis. Injury 2012;43(1):8–17.
[6] Lien YC, Chen CH, Lin HC. Risk factors for 24-hour mortality after traumatic rib fractures owing to motor vehicle accidents: a nationwide population-based study. Ann Thorac Surg 2009;88:1124–30.
[7] Lee RB, Bass SM, Morris JA, et al. Three or more rib fractures as an indicator for transfer to a Level I trauma center: a population-based study. J Trauma 1990;30(6):689–94.
[8] Liman ST, Kuzucu A, Tastepe AI, et al. Chest injury due to blunt trauma. Eur J Cardiothorac Surg 2003;23:374–8.
[9] Pape HC, Remmers D, Rice J, et al. Appraisal of early evaluation of blunt chest trauma: development of a standardized scoring system for initial clinical decision making. J Trauma 2000;49(3):496–504.
[10] Chapman BC, Herbert B, Rodil M, et al. RibScore: a novel radiographic score based on fracture pattern that predicts pneumonia, respiratory failure, and tracheostomy. J Trauma Acute Care Surg 2016;80(1):95–101.
[11] Cannon RM, Smith JW, Franklin GA, et al. Flail chest injury: are we making any progress? Am Surg 2012;78:398–402.
[12] Leinicke JA, Elmore L, Freeman DB, et al. Operative management of rib fractures in the setting of flail chest: a systematic review and meta-analysis. Ann Surg 2013;258:914–21.
[13] Coleman FP, Coleman CL. Fracture of ribs; a logical treatment. Surg Gynecol Obstet 1950;90:129–34.
[14] Proctor H, London PS. The stove-in chest with paradoxical respiration. Br J Surg 1955;42: 622–33.
[15] Pieracci FM, Rodil M, Stovall RT, et al. Surgical stabilization of severe rib fractures. J Trauma Acute Care Surg 2015;78(4):883–7.

[16] Ali-Osman F, Mangram A, Sucher J, et al. Geriatric (G60) trauma patients with severe rib fractures: is muscle sparing minimally invasive thoracotomy rib fixation safe and does it improve post-operative pulmonary function? Am J Surg 2018;216(1):46–51.

[17] Kane ED, Jeremitsky E, Pieracci F, et al. Quantifying and exploring the recent national increase in surgical stabilization of rib fractures. J Trauma Acute Care Surg 2017;83: 1047–52.

[18] Dehghan N, de Mestral C, McKee MD, et al. Flail chest injuries: a review of outcomes and treatment practices from the National Trauma Data Bank. J Trauma Acute Care Surg 2014;76(2):462–8.

[19] Cheema FA, Chao E, Buchsbaum J, et al. State of rib fracture care: a NTDB review of analgesic management and surgical stabilization. Am Surg 2019;85(5):474–8.

[20] Rockne WY, Girgorian A, Christian A, et al. No difference in mortality between level I and level II trauma centers performing surgical stabilization of rib fracture. Am J Surg 2021;221(5):1076–81.

[21] Kasotakis G, Hasenboehler EA, Streib EW, et al. Operative fixation of rib fractures after blunt trauma: a practice management guideline from the Eastern association for the surgery of Trauma. J Trauma Acute Care Surg 2017;82:618–26.

[22] Pieracci FM, Majercik S, Ali-Osman F, et al. Consensus statement: surgical stabilization of rib fractures rib fracture colloquium clinical practice guidelines. Injury 2017;48:307–21.

[23] Pieracci FM, Rodil M, Stovall RT, et al. Surgical stabilization of rib fractures. J Trauma Acute Care Surg 2015;78(4):883–8.

[24] Pierraci FM, Lin Y, Rodil M, et al. A prospective, controlled clinical evaluation of surgical stabilization of severe rib fractrues. J Trauma Acute Care Surg 2016;80(2):187–94.

[25] Thiels CA, Aho JM, Naik ND, et al. Infected hardware after surgical stabilization of rib fractures: Outcomes and management experience. J Trauma Acute Care Surg 2016;80(5): 819–23.

[26] Bauman ZM, Binkley HJ, Pieper CJ, et al. Discrepancies in rib fracture severity between radiologist and surgeon: a retrospective review. J Trauma Acute Care Surg 2021;91(6): 956–60, ePub ahead of Print.

[27] Pulley BR, Taylor BC, Fowler TT, et al. Utility of three-dimensional computed tomography for the surgical management of rib fractures. J Trauma Acute Care Surg 2015;78:530–4.

[28] Easter A. Management of patients with multiple rib fractures. Am J Crit Care 2001;10(5): 320–7.

[29] Maxwell CA, Mion LC, Dietrich MS. Hospitalized injured older adults: clinical utility of a rib fracture scoring system. J Trauma Nurs 2012;19:168–74.

[30] Moore EE, Cogbill TH, Jurkovich GJ, et al. Organ Injury Scaling III: chest wall, abdominal vascular, ureter, bladder, and urethra. J Trauma 1992;33(3):337–9.

[31] Pressley CM, Fry WR, Philp AS, et al. Predicting outcome of patients with chest wall injury. Am J Surg 2012;204(6):910–3.

[32] Chen J, Jeremitsky E, Philp F, et al. A chest trauma scoring system to predict outcomes. Surgery 2014;156(4):988–93.

[33] Carver TW, Milia DJ, Somberg C, et al. Vital capacity helps predict pulmonary complications after rib fractures. J Trauma Acute Care Surg 2015;79(3):413–6.

[34] Carrie C, Stecken L, Scotto M, et al. Forced vital capacity assessment for risk stratification of blunt chest trauma patients in emergency settings: a preliminary study. Anaesth Crit Care Pain Med 2018;37(1):67–71.

[35] Warner R, Knollinger P, Hobbs G, et al. Forced vital capacity less than 1: a mark for high-risk patients. J Trauma Acute Care Surg 2018;85(2):271–4.

[36] Billings JD, Khan AD, Clement LP, et al. A clinical practice guideline using percentage of predicted forced vital capacity improves resource allocation for rib fracture patients. J Trauma Acute Care Surg 2021;90(5):769–75.

[37] Pieracci FM, Coleman J, Ali-Osman F, et al. A multicenter evaluation of the optimal timing of surgical stabilization of rib fractures. J Trauma Acute Care Surg 2018;84(1):1–10.

[38] Prins JTH, Wijffels MME, Pieracci FM. What is the optimal timing to perform surgical stabilization of rib fractures? J Thorac Dis 2021;13(Suppl 1):S13–5.
[39] Pieracci FM. Completely thoracoscopic surgical stabilization of rib fractures: can it be done and is it worth it? J Thorac Dis 2019;11(Suppl 8):S1061–9.
[40] Dartevelle P, Macchiarini P. Surgical management of superior sulcus tumors. Oncologist 1999;4:398–407.
[41] Marasco S, Liew S, Edwards E, et al. Analysis of bone healing in flail chest injury: do we need to fix both fractures per rib? J Trauma Acute Care Surg 2014;77(3):452–8.
[42] Swart E, Laratta J, Slobogean G, et al. Operative Treatment of Rib Fractures in Flail Chest Injuries: A Meta-analysis and Cost-Effectiveness Analysis. J Orthop Trauma 2017;31(2): 64–70.
[43] Choi J, Mulaney B, Laohavinij W, et al. Nationwide cost-effectiveness analysis of surgical stabilization of rib fractures by flail chest status and age groups. J Trauma Acute Care Surg 2021;90(3):451–8.
[44] Pieracci FM, Leasia K, Bauman Z, et al. A multicenter, prospective, controlled clinical trial of surgical stabilization of rib fractures in patients with severe, nonflail fracture patterns (Chest Wall Injury Society NONFLAIL). J Trauma Acute Care Surg 2020;88(2):249–57.
[45] Coleman JR, Leasia K, Douglas IS, et al. Quantifying the expense of deferring surgical stabilization of rib fractures: Operative management of rib fractures is associated with significantly lower charges. J Trauma Acute Care Surg 2020;89(6):1032–8.
[46] Pieracci FM, Leasia K, Hernandez MC, et al. Surgical stabilization of rib fractures in octogenarians and beyond—what are the outcomes? J Trauma Acute Care Surg 2021;90(6): 1014–21.
[47] Prins JTH, Van Leishout EMM, Ali-Osman F, et al. Outcome after surgical stabilization of rib fractures versus nonoperative treatment in patients with multiple rib fractures and moderate to severe traumatic brain injury (CWIS-TBI). J Trauma Acute Care Surg 2021;90(3): 492–500.
[48] Wiese MN, Kawel-Boehm N, Moreno de la Santa P, et al. Functional results after chest wall stabilization with a new screwless fixation device. Eur J Cardiothorac Surg 2015;47(5): 868–75.
[49] Nirula R, Allen B, Layman R, et al. Rib fracture stabilization in patients sustaining blunt chest injury. Am Surg 2006;72(4):307–9.
[50] Mayberry JC, Kroeker AD, Ham LB, et al. Long-term morbidity, pain, and disability after repair of severe chest wall injuries. Am Surg 2009;75(5):389–94.
[51] Sarani B, Allen R, Pieracci FM, et al. Characteristics of hardware failure in patients undergoing surgical stabilization of rib fractures: A Chest Wall Injury Society multicenter study. J Trauma Acute Care Surg 2019;87(6):1277–81.